A PRACTICAL ENGLISH—CHINESE LIBRARY OF TRADITIONAL CHINESE MEDICINE

PUBLISHING HOUSE OF SHANGHAI COLLEGE OF TRADITIONAL CHINESE MEDICINE

EDITOR—IN—CHIEF   ZHANG ENQIN

CHINESE MASSAGE

Written by Wang Guocai, Fan Yali, Guan Zheng

Revised by Zhang Enqin, Shi Lanhua, Zhang Wengao

Translated by Yu Wenping, Wang Ruiying, Mu Junzhen
Xia Yunbin, He Zhijiang, Cong Laitin

Revised by Wang Zhikui, Dang Yi, Zhang Enqin
Zhang Qingling, Bao Xianmin

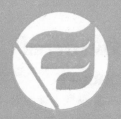

英汉对照
实用中医文库

主　编　张恩勤

中国推拿

编著	王国才	范亚莉	管　政
审校	张恩勤	史兰华	张文高
翻译	于文平	王瑞英	牟俊贞
	夏运斌	何之江	从莱庭
审校	王治奎	党　毅	张恩勤
	张庆龄	包献民	

上海中医学院出版社

Preface

The books in series, entitled "*A Practical English-Chinese Library of Traditional Chinese Medicine*", are edited with a view to disseminating the theory and knowledge of traditional Chinese medicine (TCM) across the world, promoting academic exchanges on medical science between China and other countries, and meeting with the ever-increasing international interest in TCM, so as to make it serve the interests of all nations and benefit entire mankind. This library is the first of its kind in China.

The library is composed of 12 books: *Basic Theory of TCM* (in two volumes), *Diagnostics of TCM, The Chinese Materia Medica, Prescriptions of TCM, Clinic of TCM* (in two volumes), *Health Preservation and Rehabilitation, Chinese Acupuncture and Moxibustion, Chinese Medicated Diet* and *Chinese Qigong.* The two other English-Chinese books —— *Rare Chinese Materia Medica* and *Highly Efficacious Chinese Patent Medicine* —— chiefly edited by me are also published simultaneously along with this library.

The authors and editors of the series strive to abide by the following principles: maintaining the systematism, integrity, practicability and adaptability in terms of TCM theory; paying full attention to the organic connection between basic theory and clinical treatment, taking in the available results of scientific researches carried out at home and abroad in the

1

field of TCM; and being concise, precise, and easy to understand in the Chinese version, and correct and fluent in the English one. Some of the books mentioned above contain figures and coloured photos. It is our sincere hope that the books will turn out to be good teachers and reliable friends of those abroad who have begun to learn and practise TCM and Chinese, and provide help for those at home who wish to study TCM documents in English.

The component books of this library are written, translated, and edited through joint efforts of professors, associate professors, lecturers and medical research workers from Shandong TCM College and its affiliated hospital, Shandong Medical University and its affiliated hospital, Shandong University, Shandong Teachers Training University, Shandong Medical Academy, Shandong Provincial Anti-epidemic Station, China Academy of TCM, Nanjing TCM College, Shanghai TCM College, Beijing TCM College, etc.

In order to ensure that the present library is of good quality, we have sent its Chinese version for revision to Professor Zhou Fengwu, Professor Li Keshao who was once my tutor when I was a postgraduate student, Professor Xu Guoqian and Professor Zhang Zhenyu at Shandong TCM College, Professor Qiu Maoliang at Nanjing TCM College, and Professor Lu Tongjie, director of the Affiliated Hospital of Shandong TCM College; and the English version for proofreading to Professor Huang Xiaokai of Beijing Medical University, Professor Lu Chengzhi, head of the Foreign Languages Department of Shandong Medical University, Professor Huang Jiade of Shandong University, Mr. Huang Wenxing, professor of pharmacology, Mme. Zou Ling, professor of gynecology and obstetrics, both working in Shandong Medical University, and our foreign friends, Ms. Beth Hocks, Australian teacher of English, Mr. Howard G. Adams, American teacher of English, and some others working in Jinan.

I am deeply indebted to Mr. Li Dichen, Editor-in-Chief of Publishing House of Shanghai TCM College, and his colleagues, Mme. Xu Ping, director of the Editorial Depatmrent, and Mr. Yao Yong, responsible editor, for their advice about drawing up an outline for compiling the library to ensure a success of it; to Mr. Chen Keji, professor of China Academy of TCM and advisor on traditional medicine to WHO, Professor Zhang Zhiyuan and Associate Professor Shao Guanyong of Shandong TCM College, Mr. Liu Chonggang, deputy head of the Yellow River Publishing House, for their valuable, instructive suggestions; and to responsible members at various levels, such as Mr. Hu Ximing, Chairman of the World Acupuncture and Moxibustion Association, vice-minister of the Ministry of public Health and chief of the Administrative Bureau of TCM and Pharmacy of the People's Republic of China, Mr. Zou Jilong, president of Shandong TCM College, Mr. Yan Shiyun, vice-president of Shanghai TCM College, Mr. Gao Heting, president of Beijing TCM College, Mr. Xiang Ping, vice president of Nanjing TCM College, and Mr. Shang Zhichang, president of Henan TCM College for their warm encouragement and indispensable [support as well as their personal participation in compiling and checking the books.

TCM, which dates back to ancient times, has a unique

and profound theoretical system. The greater part of its terminology has particular denotations, and is matter-of-factly difficult to understand and translate. Inaccuracies in the library, therefore, are unavoidable. I hope that my friends in the TCM circle will oblige me with timely corrections.

May TCM spread all over the world and everyone under the heaven enjoy a long happy life.

May 20th, 1988 Dr. Zhang Enqin

Editor-in-Chief of *A Practical English-Chinese Library of Traditional Chinese Medicine,* Director of the Advanced Studies Department of Shandong TCM College

前　言

　　为扩大中医学在国际上的影响，促进中外医学学术交流，适应国外日趋发展的"中医热"形势，使传统的中医学走向世界，造福人类，我们编写了这套《英汉对照实用中医文库》。在国内，这尚属首部。

　　该文库包括《中医基础理论》(上、下册)、《中医诊断学》、《中药学》、《方剂学》、《中医临床各科》(上、下册)、《中医养生康复学》、《中国针灸》、《中国推拿》、《中国药膳》和《中国气功》，共十二个分册。与《文库》同时出版的还有其配套书——英汉对照《中国名贵药材》和《中国名优中成药》。

　　《英汉对照实用中医文库》的编译宗旨是：在理论上，努力保持中医学体系的系统性、完整性，突出实用性和针对性；在内容上，充分注意基础理论与临床治疗的有机联系，汲取国内外已公布的科研成果，以反映当代中医学术水平；在文字上，力求中文简明扼要，通俗易懂，译文准确流畅，并配有图表、彩照。我们竭诚希望《英汉对照实用中医文库》能成为国外读者学习中医、汉语的良师益友，同时也为国内读者学习中医专业英语提供帮助。

　　负责文库编写、翻译和审校的主要是山东中医学院及其附属医院、山东医科大学及其附属医院、山东大学、山东师范大学、山东省医学科学院、山东省卫生防疫站、中国中医研究院、南京中医学院，上海中医学院和北京中医学院等单位的部分教授、副教授、讲师和科研人员。

　　为确保文库质量，各分册中文稿还先后承蒙山东中医学院周凤梧教授、李克绍教授、徐国仟教授、张珍玉教授，南京中医学院邱茂良教授，山东中医学院附属医院院长吕同杰教授等审阅；英文稿先后承蒙北京医科大学英语教研室黄孝楷教授，山东医科大学英语教研室主任卢承志教授，山东大学外文系黄嘉德教授，山东医科大学药理教研室黄文兴教授、妇产科教研室邹玲教授以及澳大利亚籍教师 Beth Hocks 女士和美籍教师 Howard G. Adams 先生等审阅。

上海中医学院出版社总编辑李迪臣、编辑部主任徐平和责任编辑姚勇，亲自帮助我们修订编写大纲，指导编译工作；世界卫生组织传统医学顾问、中国中医研究院陈可冀教授，山东中医学院张志远教授、邵冠勇副教授，黄河出版社副社长刘崇刚，也为本文库的编译工作提出了许多宝贵的指导性意见；编译工作还得到了各级领导的支持和帮助，世界针灸学会联合会主席、中华人民共和国卫生部副部长兼国家中医药管理局局长胡熙明先生，山东中医学院院长邹积隆先生，上海中医学院副院长严世芸先生，北京中医学院院长高鹤亭先生，南京中医学院副院长项平先生和河南中医学院院长尚炽昌先生等，亲自参加编审并给予指导，在此一并表示衷心感谢！

由于中医学源远流长，其理论体系独特，不少名词术语深奥难解，译成英文，难度较大。故书中错误、欠妥之处在所难免，敬希国内外同道指正。

愿中医流传世界，求普天下人健康长寿。

主编　张恩勤
1988年5月20日

CONTENTS
目　　录

Chinese Massage

中国推拿

Chapter One

General Introduction

Section 1

An Outline

1. A Brief Account of Chinese Massage

Chinese massage has a long history and dates back to the ancient times. Archaeological studies in recent years have shown that as early as the late period of the New Stone Age around 2700 B.C., the Chinese ancestors in the Yellow River valley primarily summed up the primitive experiences in massage which had been gradually accumulated by their forefathers in their struggle for life and fight against nature. This turned the spontaneous medical behavior that originated from self-defence instinct into a medical mode for the early human race. It was recorded in *Statesman, Patriot and General in Ancient China* that a famous doctor in the reign of Emperor Huang (equating the period of Longshan Culture) Yu Fu had applied the antient massage technique *"anwu"* to his clinical practice.

At the time of the Shang Dynasty, primitive witch doctors ran rampant. They were socially very prestigious, dominant in administering incantation, praying, 'fortune telling and the medicine, and they often used folk methods including massage to show their "miraculous power" for the religious and superstitious purposes. That is why the witch officials were also called "miraculous doctors" or "witch doctors". It was recorded in the unearthed oracle inscriptions on bones or tortois shells of the Shang Dynasty

第 一 章

总 论

第一节 概 说

1. 中国推拿简介

中国推拿源远流长。据近年考古发现证实，早在新石器时代晚期（约公元前 2700 年），生息在黄河流域的中华祖先，就初步总结了洪荒时期先辈们为求生存在与大自然搏斗中逐渐积累起来的原始推拿经验，使推拿这一起源于人类自卫防御本能的自发医疗行为，逐步发展成为人类早期的医学模式。据《史书》记载，黄帝时代（相当龙山文化时期）的名医俞跗，已将"案扤"这一古代推拿术应用于临床。

殷商时期，原始巫医盛行。巫吏有很高的社会地位，掌握着禁咒、祈祷、占卜和医药，并常利用包括按摩在内的一些民间治疗方法的效验来印证其神力，以此为宗教迷信服务。故巫吏又被称为"神医"或"巫医"。在出土的殷商甲骨文卜辞中，就有女巫姁为

that the female witch doctor Bi could treat the patients with massage. This testifies to the fact that massage technique of that time had reached quite a high level.

In the time of the Spring and Autumn and Warring States, owing to the collapse of slavery system, the idealistic conception of religious authority began to shake while the simple materialistic theory of *yin* and *yang* were developed. Those witch doctors of the old days came among the people and gradually became doctors with practical medical skills. This social change promoted the development of antient medicine, with no exception of massage. Take medical terminology for example, the treatment with hand pressing, kneading and stroking was then called "massage"; the treatment of making the patients flex and extend their hands and feet and breath in prone or supine position was called "leading" (pressing) or "stepping" while the combination of the two manipulations was called "pressing and stepping" or "stepping and rubbing". In practice, the forms of manipulation gradually become perfect, with its application range obviously enlarged and its therapeutic effect enhanced. Massage had become a mature, widely used method for medical treatment. Bian Que, a famous doctor at the time, was an example in using massage and acupuncture as a comprehensive treatment. He got crown prince Guo's syncope cured with a miraculous effect of bringing the dead back to life. In addition, record of the folk use of massage therapy can be found in many unauthoritative medical writings of the time: *Lao Zi*, *Meng Zi*, *Xun Zi* and *Mo Zi*.

Up to the dynasties of Qin, Han and the Three Kingdoms, people come to enrich and sum up the experience that had been accumulated and improvement in the methods that had been invented in the earlier times, contributing greatly to the publication of the first medical book on massage, not only in the history of China and but also in the history of the world, ten volumes of *Classics on Massage of Yellow Emperor and Qi Bo*,

人按摩治病的记录。可见当时按摩术已达到一定水平。

春秋战国时期，随着奴隶制的崩溃，神权唯心思想开始动摇，朴素唯物的阴阳学说得到发展。昔日的巫医流入民间，逐渐变成操有实际医疗技术的医者。这一社会变革促进了包括推拿术在内的古代医学的发展。如在命名上，当时已将用手抑压和揉抚的疗法称为"按摩"；将使患者屈伸手足、呼吸俯仰的疗法，称为"导引"、"蹻引"；两法合用，则称为"按蹻"或"挢摩"。在实践上，手法的形式亦日臻完善，其适用范围明显扩大，治疗效果得到了进一步的提高。按摩基本成为一种比较成熟的医疗手段而被广泛应用。如当时的名医扁鹊，就曾用按摩、针灸等综合疗法，治愈虢太子的"尸厥"证，获得了起死回生的奇效。此外，在当时成书的《老子》、《孟子》、《荀子》、《墨子》等许多非医学名著中，都可看到按摩疗法在民间应用的记载。

至秦、汉、三国时期，人们开始对在早期医疗实践中获得的经验与创造的方法初步地进行充实、提高和总结，因而诞生了我国，也是世界医学史上的第一部按摩专著——《黄帝岐伯按摩经》十卷，可惜此书已佚。然值得庆幸的是，在与上书同时成书的中医

Unfortunately this book was lost. Yet, it is quite lucky that another great medical book *The Yellow Emperor's Internal Classic* published in the same period devoted many chapters and sections to massage. This book is almost all inclusive, covering extensively such fields as the sources, manipulating methods, clinical application, indications, therapeutic principles and teaching of massage. For example, in terms of massage manipulations, a dozen manipulating methods such as pushing, pressing, rubbing, stepping and pulling are mentioned in this book and in talking of indications, acute and chronic diseases of various specialities such as fear, syncope with flacidity, cold and heat, spleen-wind, blockage of channels, abdominal pain due to cold, and many others are listed. Incisive expositions were made in the book especially on mechanism of manipulation therapy and some of them are still guiding today's clinical practice. Later, Zhang Zhongjing, a medical saint of the Eastern Han Dynasty, put forward for the first time the *"gaomo"* treatment in his book *Treatise on Febrile and Miscellaneous Diseases*. This method prescribes that some prepared ointment should be smeared on a certain part of the patient's skin. Then manipulations of stroking-transversely, rubbing, scrubbing and kneading should be administered on this part to achieve a combined double effect of manipulation and medicine. This can not only raise the therapeutic effect, but also enlarge the application range of massage. For instance, a famous doctor of the Three Kingdoms Hua Tuo was especially good at treating febrile diseases and removing superficial pathogen from the skin with *gaomo* therapy.

The period of Eastern and Western Jins and Northern and Southern Dynasties saw great development in *gaomo* therapy. A doctor of Western Jin, Wang Shuhe introduced a "wind-ointment" method to treat numbness and pain in his book *The Pulse Classic*. Ge Hong, a Taoist of Eastern Jin, systematically summarized for the first time in his *Handbook of Prescrip-*

经典著作《黄帝内经》中，还可看到不少论述按摩的章节。该书对按摩的起源、手法、临床应用、适应病症、治疗原理以及按摩教学等各方面内容，已无所不涉。如书中提到的按摩手法，就有推、按、摩、跻、掣等十几种；列举的适应症，有惊恐、痿厥、寒热、脾风、经络不通、寒腹痛等各科急、慢性病症；特别是对手法治疗的机理，书中已阐述得相当精辟，有的至今仍指导着临床。嗣后，东汉医圣张仲景在《伤寒杂病论》中，首倡"膏摩"疗法。该法是先将配制好的中药膏剂涂抹在患者体表的治疗部位，然后再用手法在其上抚摩擦揉，具有手法与药物的双重治疗作用。这不仅提高了疗效，而且扩大了按摩的应用范围。如三国名医华佗，即擅用膏摩治疗伤寒与驱除肌肤的浮淫。

两晋南北朝时期，膏摩术有了进一步的发展。如西晋医家王叔和，在《脉经》中提出用"风膏"治疗痹痛。东晋道家葛洪，在《肘后备急方》中首次系统总结了膏摩的方、药、证、法和摩膏的制作

tions for Emergencies the prescriptions, drugs, indications and therapeutic principles of *gaomo* massage and the method of making the ointment, introducing eight medical formula and including diseases of various departments in the indications such as internal and external diseases, diseases of gynecology and diseases of the eye, ear, nose and the throat. He also mentioned in *Bao Puzi's, Inner Treatise* the publication of *Ten Volumes of Classics on Massage and Physical and Breathing Exercise* (lost). Tao Hongjing, a famous medical scientist, Taoist and alchemist of the Northern and Southern Dynasties also wrote a special volume "Physical and Breathing Exercises and Massage" included in the book *Record on Preserving Health and Prolonging Life*, which is very rich in content, with many pages elaborating on a series of actions of physical and breathing exercise and massage, such as teeth-pecking, eye hot-compressing, eye pressing, ear guiding, hair raising, face massaging, dry bathing, etc. That helped to originate the "self-massage" technique for the purpose of health-preservation and self-treatment of diseases.

Sui and Tang Dynasties were a flourishing age for Chinese massage. In the Office of the Imperial Physicians of the Sui Dynasty, a massage doctor was authorized to be in charge of daily medical treatment and teaching affairs. A massage speciality was set up in the Office of the Imperial Physicians of the Tang Dynasty and the massagists were classified as massage doctors (massagists with doctorate), massagists and massage workers. Helped by the massagists and massage workers, the massage doctors taught the massage students "to master the physical and breathing exercise to treat diseases and rectify injuries." Massage treatment and teaching became unprecedentedly prosperous. At that time, self-massage and *gaomo* therapy were more extensively used and raised to a high level. *General Treatise on the Causes and Symptoms of Diseases* written by Chao Yuanfang of Sui Dynasty included physical

方法，共介绍膏摩方8首，其适应症遍及内、外、妇、五官各科；

葛洪还在《抱朴子·内篇·遐览》中提到撰有《按摩导引十卷》，但已佚。南北朝时期著名医药学家、道家、炼丹家陶弘景，也在《养性延命录》一书中设有"导引按摩"专卷，并以相当多的篇幅详细介绍了啄齿、熨眼、按目、引耳、发举、摩面、干浴等成套导引、按摩动作，内容十分丰富。这就为后世以养生保健、疾病自疗为目的的"自我推拿"术的形成，开示了源头。

隋唐时期是中国推拿的盛世。如隋太医署内设有按摩博士职位，负责日常医疗与教学工作。唐太医署内增设按摩科，把按摩医生分为按摩博士、按摩师和按摩工的等级。按摩博士在按摩师和按摩工的辅助下，教授按摩生"掌导引之法以除疾，损伤折跌者正之。"其按摩医疗与教学盛况空前。此期的自我按摩与膏摩疗

and breathing exercise and massage in the last part of each volume of the book. In his *Prescriptions Worth a Thousand Gold*, Sun Simiao of the Tang Dynasty further developed the prescriptions and drugs of *gaomo* therapy and broadened its application scope. This book had a systematic description of the treatment of infantile diseases with *gaomo* therapy. It listed a dozen applicable infantile diseases which could be treated with this therapy such as "convulsion seizure due to fright" and "dying due to stiffness of nape", "nose blocked with discharge", "night crying", "abdominal distension and fullness" and "being unable to suck". It was also recorded in the book that "ointment can often be applied to the top of the head, on the palms and soles of the infants in the early morning to protect them from cold wind, even though they are not sick." This is the first report of the application of ointment massage to infantile health-preservation. Sun also introduced some other methods of massage and physical and breathing exercise, e.g., over ten manipulations described in *The Massage Therapy of Lao Zi*: pressing, rubbing, scrubbing, holding and twisting, embracing, pushing, dabbing, hitting, turning, and right falling stroke. *Six Classics in the Tang Dynasty*, one of the other medical classics written in this period, reported that massage could treat the diseases caused by eight factors: wind, cold, heat, dampness, hunger, overeating, fatigue and leisure, which greatly broadened the application range of massage. Another example is Wang Tao's *Medical Secrets of an Official* that presented a lot of experience in massage treatment and recorded a number of ointment prescriptions with their sources indicated. These historical facts bear a strong evidence that, by the time of Sui and Tang Dynasties, massage as a TCM branch for clinical practice had reached quite a high level in its basic theory, diagnostic technique and treatment. It is believed that the embryonic form of modern massage took shape in that very period. Thanks to the rapid development of China's politics, economy, culture

法亦得到更广泛地应用和进一步地提高。如隋巢元方的《诸病源候论》，在每卷之末都附有导引、按摩之法。唐孙思邈的《千金方》更是发展了膏摩的方药，扩大了其应用范围，尤其是对膏摩治疗小儿疾病，进行了系统论述。该书例举了"中客忤强项欲死"、"鼻塞不通有涕出"、"夜啼"、"腹胀满"、"不能乳食"等十几种小儿病证的膏摩治疗。书中还载有"小儿虽无病，早起常以膏摩囟上及手足心，甚辟寒风"，这是首次将膏摩用于小儿保健的最早文献。孙氏还介绍了《老子按摩法》等按摩、导引方法，单手法就有按、摩、擦、捻、抱、推、搌、打、捩、捺等十余种之多。这个时期的其他医学名著，如《唐六典》介绍了按摩可以治疗"风、寒、暑、湿、饥、饱、劳、逸"八疾，大大拓展了按摩的应用范围；王焘的《外台秘要》介绍了许多按摩治病的经验，辑录了大量膏摩方剂，并注明其出处。以上史料说明，至隋唐时期，按摩作为一门中医临床学科，在基础理论、诊断技术与治疗方法诸方面，都已达到了相当高的水平。可以认为，近代推拿学的雏形，在此期已

and transportation and the excellent situation of cultural exchange with foreign countries during that period, massage was also introduced into Korea, Japan, Arabian countries, etc., together with the traditional Chinese medicine as a whole, and promoted the development of this branch of medical science in those countries. "Laws and Decrees of Tai Bao" issued during the Tai Bao years (701—703) of Japan's Civil and Military Dynasty, stipulated that massage was one of the compulsory courses for medical students. This laid a solid foundation for "the three manipulating skills" that remain current now in Japan.

Though there is no massage department in the medical organizations of the government in the Song, Jin and Yuan Dynasties, the title of massage doctor remained unchanged. The massage treatment affairs came under the supervision of carbuncle department and war wound department of the Bureau of the Imperial Physicians in the Song Dynasty, but under the administration of the bone-setting department of the Institute of the Imperial Physicians in the Yuan Dynasty. Meanwhile, the department of pediatrics was opened in this period, with doctors in charge of the massage for infants. Owing to the fact that the massotherapy of this period was used mainly for the treatment of bone injuries and infantile illnesses, massage afterwards was divided into bone-setting massage and massage for treating infantile diseases. This period placed much importance on the analysis of massage manipulations. For instance, *General Collection for Holy Relief* written in the Song Dynasty pointed out: "Pressing and rubbing are used and sometimes combined, so this is generally called pressing-rubbing. Pressing is not rubbing while rubbing is not pressing; pressing is done only by hand while rubbing done in combination with the use of ointment. As to which of the two manipulations is to be used, it just depends on the situation. ... Generally speaking, every type of massage aims at either eleminating something or restraining something; the former makes obstruction disperse while the latter brings hy-

经形成。由于这一时期，中国的政治、经济、文化与交通均有了较大发展，对外文化交流出现了欣欣向荣的局面，推拿也随中医学传到朝鲜、日本、阿拉伯等地，促进了这些国家推拿医学的发展。如在日本文武朝太宝年间(公元701～703年)颁布的"太宝律令"中规定，推拿作为医学生的必修课程之一。这为日本现代盛行的"手技三法"的形成，奠定了基础。

宋、金、元时期，政府的医疗机构中虽未设按摩科，但仍设按摩博士职位。按摩医疗工作，在宋代，归属于太医局的疡科及金镞科；在元朝，归属于太医院的正骨科。此外，此期又增设小方脉科，小儿按摩则由小方脉科的医师掌管。由于此期的按摩疗法主要用于骨伤科和小儿病证的治疗，这就孕育了后世推拿学中正骨推拿与小儿推拿的学科分化。这一时期比较重视推拿手法的分析，如宋《圣济总录》指出："可按可摩，时兼而用，通谓之按摩。按之弗摩，摩之弗按，按止以手，摩或兼以药，曰按曰摩，适所用也。……大抵按摩之法，每以开达抑遏为义，开达则壅蔽者以

peraction under control." This was a great contribution to the development of massage theory.

The Ming Dynasty was the second age for Chinese massage to flourish in its long history of development. Massage was again included in the thirteen departments of TCM in the official Institute of the Imperial Physicians. Rich clinical experience and theoretical knowledge were gradually accumulated in the treatment of infantile diseases with massage during this time. In 1601, China's first treatise on massage therapy of infantile diseases *The Canon of Massage for Children* came into being. Soon after, *Complete Classic of the Secret Principles of Massage to Bring Infants Back to Life*, and *Secret Pithy Formula of Massage for Children* among other works on child massage were published in succession. By that time, as an academic branch, child massage had taken shape and an independent system of massage diagnosis, manipulation, application points and treatment had been established. Furthermore, "massage", the term we use today to refer to this academic branch, was put forward right in this period.

There was no massage department in Institute of Imperial Physicians in the Qing Dynasty, but owing to its marked therapeutic effect, it was practiced and spread as extensively as before, both in the government and among the people. Child massage was further developted in this period, especially in the early and middle Qing Dynasty. There emerged a number of famous doctors of child massage and such professional classics which greatly influenced the later generations as Xiong Yingxiong's *Elucidations of Massage for Children*, Luo Rulong's *Secrets of Massage of Pediatric Speciality*, Xia Yunji's *The Massage for the Care of Infants* and Zhang Zhenjun's *Revised Synopsis of Massage*. In addition, the massagists of Qing Dynasty made striking achievements in treating injuries with massage. Take the book *The Golden Mirror of Medicine* for example which regarded the following manipulations as the

之发散，抑遏则慓悍者有所归宿。"这是对推拿理论的一大贡献。

明代是中国推拿发展史上的第二个盛世。在政府太医院所设的十三科中，又重新设置了按摩科。在按摩治疗小儿疾病方面，初步积累了丰富的临床经验和理论知识。至1601年，中国第一部小儿推拿专著——《小儿按摩经》问世；尔后，《小儿推拿方脉活婴秘旨全书》、《小儿推拿秘诀》等小儿推拿著作相继刊行。至此，小儿推拿作为推拿学科的一个分支已经形成，并在辨证、手法、穴位、治疗等方面形成了独特的体系。此外，我们今天采用的"推拿"这一学科名称，正是这一时期首先提出来的。

清朝政府的太医院虽未设推拿科，但由于其疗效卓著，无论是在官方还是民间，其应用、流传，仍相当广泛。特别是在清朝的初、中叶，小儿推拿又得到了进一步的发展，出现了一批著名的小儿推拿医师和对后世影响较大的小儿推拿专著，如熊应雄的《小儿推拿广意》，骆如龙的《幼科推拿秘书》，夏云集的《保赤推拿法》，张振鋆的《厘正按摩要术》等。此外，清代推拿医师在运用推拿治疗伤科疾病方面，取得了令人瞩目的成就。如《医

eight methods for treating injuries: touching, reuniting, holding, lifting, pressing, rubbing, pushing and grasping. Judging from the above, the branch of injury massage had basically taken shape in this period.

In the past century, thanks to the joint effort of the massagists both at home and abroad, Chinese massage has undergone great development. In 1956, China organized her first massage training class in Shanghai. In 1958 in Shanghai, a massage clinic opened and the same year saw the establishment of a special school of massage to which many distinguished experts from all over the country were invited to teach and in which quite a number of students were trained to become specialists. Massage departments were established in hospitals of different places and many folk massage doctors with rich practical experience were sent to work in those hospitals. In the year 1974, Shanghai TCM College initiated a department of accupuncture, massage and traumalogy, followed then by a department of massage. Subsequently, the TCM colleges in Beijing, Anhui, Nanjing, Zhejiang and Shandong set up massage specialities one after another and created favourable conditions for training professional massagists. After the national massage association was organized in 1987, academical activities of massage, nation-wide and world-wide, were carried out and gradually increased. In the last ten years, treatises and theses on massage have reached the highest level in history both in number and in quality. Massage treatment of cervical spondylopathy, prolapse of lumbar intervertebral disc, infantile diarrhea, coronary heart disease and cholecystitis has achieved excellent therapeutic effect Researches in massage documents and foundamental study on massage are being progressively carried out. Since 1981, the scientific researchers in Shandong and Shanghai have begun one after another their study in massage mechanics and massage information from the point of view of kinetic biomechanics and have made great progress.

宗金鉴》一书，将摸、接、端、提、按、摩、推、拿列为伤科八法。由上不难看出，伤科推拿这一推拿分支，此期已基本形成。

近百年来，通过海内外推拿医师的共同努力，中国推拿得到了很大发展。1956年，中国上海开办了第一届推拿训练班；1958年又成立了上海推拿门诊部；同年，又开设了推拿专科学校，邀请当时全国著名专家任教，培养了一批推拿专业人材；各地医院相继成立推拿科，把有实践经验的民间推拿医生请进医院工作。1974年，上海中医学院首先成立针（灸）推（拿）骨伤系，后又专设推拿系；嗣后，北京、安徽、南京、福建、浙江、山东等地的中医学院相继设立了推拿专业，为培养高层次推拿人材创造了条件。1987年，全国推拿学会成立，国内外推拿学术活动得以逐步开展。近十年来，有关推拿方面的专著与论文，无论是数量上还是在质量上，都已达到历史最高水平。推拿治疗颈椎病、腰椎间盘突出症、小儿腹泻、冠心病、胆囊炎等，取得了良好疗效。推拿的文献与基础研究，正在逐步展开。自1981年以来，山东、上海等地的科研人员相继从运动生物学角度开展对推拿力学信息的研究，并取得了可喜的成绩。

At present, massage in China is playing an important role in the fields of medical service, rehabilitation and health preservation. Along with the nation-wide and world-wide academic exchange in massage, this branch of Chinese medicine will undoubtedly be accepted as a safe, effective, comfortable, harmless and free-of-side-effect therapy by the people of the world and contribute greatly to their health and life-prolonging.

2. The Main Schools of Chinese Massage

Influenced by its different academic sources, lineages, indications and complicated backgrounds of society, provincialism and mores, Chinese massage grew gradually into many academic schools and branches in its long and tortuous history of development.

A comprehensive survey shows that all the massage schools have roughly three common characteristics: ① They all have quite long histories and have been popularized within specified regions; ② They have respective theoretical guidances, substantial practical experiences, expert indication circles, special training exercises and methods. ③ Each school has its own special manipulations, also called "chief manipulations" or "school manipulations", and several or dozens of auxiliary manipulations as well. In terms of technical forms and treatment styles, each has its own provincialities and touch of mores. For example, most of the manipulations of different massage schools in North China are lucid and vigorous while those in South China are exquisite and gentle. The present chief schools and academic branches of massage in China are: one finger meditation massage, rolling massage, internal exercise massage, digital acupoint pressure massage, bone-setting massage, traumatic pressing-rubbing therapy, massotherapy, child massage, viscera and channels massage, keep-fit massage, health-preserving massage, gastropathy massage, tendon-pinching and patting-beating therapy, finger-pressing massage, finger-pressure

目前，中国推拿正在医疗、康复、保健等多方面发挥着重要作用。随着国内外推拿学术交流的广泛开展，中国推拿必将以安全、有效、舒适、无害、无副作用等优点为世界人民所接受，并为世界人民的健康与长寿做出贡献。

2. 中国推拿的主要流派

中国推拿在其漫长而曲折的发展过程中，由于学术渊源、师承关系、主治对象以及社会、地域、人情等复杂原因，逐渐形成了许多各具特色的学术流派与分支。

综观各推拿流派，大多具有以下三个特点：①有较长的发展史，并在一定地域内流传、盛行；②有一定的学术理论指导和丰富的实践经验，并有其擅长的主治范围和独特的练功及专业训练的方法；③每一推拿流派各有一特长手法，称之为"主治手法"或"流派手法"，并有几种或几十种辅助手法。此外，在手法的术式与治疗风格上，往往带有明显的地域、人情色彩。如中国北方各推拿流派，其手法多明快刚健；而南方各推拿流派，其手法则多细腻柔和。当今中国推拿的主要流派与学术分支有一指禅推拿、滚法推拿、内功推拿、点穴推拿、整骨推拿、外伤按摩疗法、按摩疗法、小儿推拿、脏腑经络推拿、保健推拿、养生按摩、胃病推拿、捏筋拍打法、指压推拿、指针疗法、指拨疗法、捏脊疗

therapy, finger-plucking therapy, chiropractic therapy, self-massage, massage with ointment, physical exercise massage, sports massage, beauty massage, extra-ordinary points massage, midnight-noon ebb-flow massage, channel points massage, *Qiao*-point massage, etc. Now here is a brief introduction to some of the schools with greater influence.

1) One-finger Meditation Massage

One-finger meditation massage has ever been spreading in the region south of Changjiang River, particularly in Jiangsu, Zhejiang and Shanghai, since the period of Xianfeng in the Qing Dynasty. Guided by the basic theory of TCM such as *yin-yang*, five elements, viscera, channels and collaterals, *ying-wei-qi-xue*(blood), etc. and taking the four diagnostic methods and eight principal syndromes as its means of diagnosis, it lays stress on both examining the syndrome and searching for causes and holds that diagnosis and treatment should be based on the overall analysis of symptoms and signs, the cause, nature and location of the illness and the patients' physical conditions. One-finger meditation massage serves as its chief treatment manipulation accompanied by other eleven methods: grasping, pressing, rubbing, rolling, holding and twisting, sweeping, foulage, quick pushing, kneading, rotating and shaking. It requires that manipulations be soft and penetrating, soft but powerful, with softness being coordinated with strength; it emphasizes that softness is the most valuable. Just because its chief manipulations are extremely difficult, great attention is always paid to its basic training while a series of scientific methods are used for special function training. Its students are required to practise, first, external strong exercise *"yijinjing"*, and then based on this, the primary manipulating actions on the bags of rice. In treatment, one-finger meditation massage mainly selects fourteen channels, points on regular channels, channel tendons, extra-channel points and non-fixed points and in manipulation it pursues the principle of "massaging the points

法、自我推拿、膏摩疗法、动功按摩、运动按摩、美容按摩、经外奇穴推拿、子午流注推拿、经穴推拿、窍穴奇术推拿等。这里仅将影响较大的几种推拿流派简介如下：

1）一指禅推拿

自清朝咸丰年间以来，一指禅推拿一直流传于江南，特别是在江苏、浙江、上海一带盛行。它以中医的阴阳五行、脏腑经络和营卫气血等基本理论为指导，以四诊八纲为诊察手段，强调审症求因与辨证论治。其手法是以一指禅推法为主治手法，还有拿、按、摩、捻、抄、搓、缠、揉、摇、抖等常用手法，共12种。手法要求柔和深透，柔中寓刚，刚柔相济，强调以柔和为贵。由于一指禅推拿的几种主要手法技术难度较大，故非常重视其基本功训练，并有一整套科学的训练方法。训练时，要求学员先练外壮功"易筋经"，并在此基础上再在米袋上练习手法的基本动作。在治疗时，主要选用十四经脉、经穴、经筋、经外奇穴和阿是

along the channels". It covers quite extensive indications, being able to treat diseases of channels and collaterals, physical and internal organs due to both internal and external causes. In particular it can be applied to the treatment of such cases as headache, vertigo, insomnia, internal injuries due to overwork, hypertension, irregular menstruation, stomachache, long-lasting diarrhea, constipation and other miscellaneous diseases. It also produces remarkable results in curing diseases of motor system such as omalgia, servical spondylopathy and lumbar pain, infantile diarrhea, and infantile bed-wetting.

2) Rolling Massage

Rolling massage developed on the basis of single-finger massage in the 40's of the current century. Its chief manipulation is rolling, and the other commonly used manipulations are kneading, pressing, grasping, holding and twisting and foulage. In the process of massage, it often coordinates with the passive movement of the limbs and guides the patients in their initiative movement after massage so as to enhance and consolidate the curative effect. In clinical practice, TCM is often combined with Western medicine, examining the symptoms to search for causes, making clear diagnosis and giving treatment on the overall analysis of the cases. Simultaneously, Western physical diagnosis is adopted so as to make sure what kind of disease it is and how to treat it. Massage should be done at the points along the channels, to move the joints, rectify deformity, restore and treat injured soft tissues, press and stroke nerves on the basis of the channel and collateral doctrine of TCM and the Western medical theory in anatomy, physiology and pathology, etc. Its special training method is the same as that of one-finger meditation, which emphasizes exercises and training of the basic manipulation on rice bags. Rolling manipulation has not only the same strong points as those of one-finger meditation massage such as soft and rhythmic stimulation to the body, but also its own characteristics—big manipulation area and

穴。操作时，要求遵循"循经络、推穴位"的原则。其适用范围比较广，无论是外感、内伤所致的经络、形体或内脏疾病，一般皆可用之。尤擅长于治疗头痛、眩晕、不寐、劳倦内伤、高血压、月经不调、胃脘痛、久泻、便秘等疾病。对漏肩风、颈椎病、腰痛等运动系统病症以及小儿泄泻、小儿遗尿等病症，亦有卓效。

2）滚法推拿

滚法推拿是在一指禅推拿的基础上，于本世纪四十年代发展起来的一推拿学派。其主治手法是滚法，其他常用手法有揉、按、拿、捻、搓5种。在施术过程中，常须配合肢体的被动运动。术后还指导病人进行自主性运动，以加强、巩固疗效。临诊时，常运用中西医结合的诊断方法，明确诊断，审症求因，辨证论治。施术时，则循经走穴，运动关节，矫正畸形，理顺筋肉，按抚神经。一招一式均以中医的经络学说与西医的解剖、生理、病理等基础理论为指导。其专业训练方法与一指禅推拿相同，强调练功和米袋上的手法基本功锻炼。滚法既保持了一指禅推法对人体具

strong power. Therefore, the clinical curative effect is manifested more distinctively in treating some diseases in the motor system and nerve system. Rolling massage is, in the main, applied to hemiparalysis, infantile paralysis, peripheral paralysis, deviation of mouth and eyes, various kinds of chronic joint diseases, sprain of the joints of waist and the four limbs, tenontothecitis, scapulohumeral periarthritis, cervical spondylopathy, prolapse of lumbar intervertebral disc, headache and sternocostal pain, etc.

3) Internal Exercise Massage

Internal exercise massage is chiefly based on palm-pushing (including flat-pushing, thenar-eminence-pushing and side-pushing). It requires that massagers should be well-trained in *Shaolin* internal exercise. In the course, the operator, should direct *qi* inside, but produce power outside. The manipulation should be vigorous and powerful but soft, with *yin-yang* in good order and gentleness and strength running parallel. Academically, guided by the TCM theory, it emphasizes the concept of wholism and follows the principle of strengthening the body's resistance to diseases and eliminating pathogenics without neglect of either. Clinically, it emphasizes "outside treatment with internal exercise", that is, the patients should, while being manipulated, practise *Shaolin* internal exercise so as to strengthen the body resistance and keep fit. The manipulations of internal exercise massage are: flat-pushing, thenar-eminence-pushing, side-pushing, five-finger grasping, tri-finger grasping, lifting-grasping, digital-pressing, pressing, adhesion separating, joining, sweeping, arching-pushing, motioning, crossing, restoring, shaking, foulage, traction and counter-traction, palm-striking (shaking), fist-striking (shaking), stick-striking, etc. This whole set of manipulations are vigorous, sprightly and smooth, penetrating, and imbued with typical Northern China style. Its clinical manipulations follow these procedures: pushing Qiao-gong (the left side first and right side next for males, and

有柔和的节律性刺激这一特点，又有施力面积大和力量强等优点。故临床上用于治疗运动、神经系统病症，效果尤著。㨰法推拿的主要适应症有半身不遂、小儿麻痹后遗症、周围神经麻痹、口眼歪斜、各种慢性关节病、腰及四肢关节扭伤、腱鞘炎、肩周炎、颈椎病、腰椎间盘突出症、头痛、胸胁痛等。

3）内功推拿

内功推拿是以掌推法（包括平推法、鱼际推法、侧推法）为主要治疗手法的一种推拿疗法。施术者须有坚实的少林内功基础。施术时要运功于内，发力于外。手法要刚劲有力，刚中含柔，阴阳有序，温力并行。在学术思想方面，内功推拿以传统中医理论为指导，强调整体观念，遵循扶正祛邪、正邪兼顾的原则。在临床治疗时，注重"外治内练"，即要求患者在接受手法治疗的同时，结合锻炼少林内功，以扶正强身。内功推拿的手法有平推法、鱼际推法、侧推法、五指拿、三指拿、提拿、点、压、分、合、扫、散、运、盘、理、抖、搓、拔伸、掌击（震）、拳击（震）、棒击（震）等。全套手法刚健雄劲，明快流畅，力透肌骨，具有典型的中国北方推拿流派风格。其临床操作有一套常规顺序，即推桥弓（男先左后右，女反之），分印堂，分眉棱，扫散太阳穴，

for females just the other way round), separating Yintang (Extra 1) and supra-orbital (bone), sweeping across Taiyang (Extra 2), five-finger grasping the top of the head, tri-finger grasping the big tendons at the neck, flat-pushing or thenar-eminence pushing against the chest and back, flat-pushing against the hypochondriac regions (but no pushing in the liver region), pushing-scrubbing and lifting-grasping at the upper limbs (from wrist to shoulder), foulaging the upper limbs (from shoulder to wrist), arc-pushing the shoulder joints, pressing-gripping the five fingers, splitting the finger seam, palm-striking on the fist (from the forefinger to the medial of the little finger), foulaging and shaking the upper limbs, patting on Jianjing (GB 21) points of both shoulders (patients in standing position, and the same for the following), patting on the two legs (from the base of the thigh to the shank), then again five-finger grasping the top of the head, and finally tri-part striking, i.e., fist-striking Dazhui (Du 14) (promoting *yang-qi* of the whole body), fist-striking Mingmen (Du 4) and the Ba-liao (UB 31—34) to invigorate the kidney-*yang* and premordial *qi* and conduct the fire back to its origin, palm-striking Fengan point on top of the head (like striking water with stone) for tranquilization. The entire regular practice covers the head, face, waist, chest, abdomen and the lower limbs, involving twelve channels and eight extra-channels. It is effective in dredging the channels and collaterals, regulating *qi* and blood, strengthening the body resistance and nourishing the viscera. Based on this regular practice, massagers take different diseases and consequences into full consideration, increase or reduce their manipulations to form prescriptions. Internal exercise massage is good for the treatment of internal diseases due to deficiency and overwork and diseases of the departments of surgery and gynecology.

4) Finger-pressing Massage

Finger-pressing massage is also called "digital point

五指拿头顶，三指拿项后大筋，平推或鱼际推前胸及后背，平推两胁(肝区禁推)，推擦与提拿上肢(自腕至肩)，搓上肢(自肩至腕)，运肩关节，理(拭)五指，劈指缝，掌击拳面(握拳时，食～小指近侧指骨处)，搓、抖上肢，拍双侧肩井(患者站势，下同)，拍二腿(从大腿根拍至小腿)，再五指拿头顶，最后以三处击法结束，即拳击大椎，以通调一身阳气，拳击命门、八髎，以壮肾阳，补元气，引火归元；掌击头顶风安穴(顽石击水法)，以安神定魄。整个常规操作从头面至腰骶、胸腹及下肢，涉及十二经脉和奇经八脉，具有疏通经络、调和气血、强健身体、荣灌脏腑等作用。临床应用时，可在此操作常规的基础上，根据其具体病情与辨证分型，随证加减，组合成一治疗处方。本法擅治内科虚劳杂病、外科病症以及妇人经带诸疾。

4) 指压推拿

指压推拿又称"点穴推拿"或"指针疗法"，系指用按点法、按

pressing massage" or "finger-pressure therapy" — a massage therapy used in clinical practice to prevent and treat diseases chiefly with digital pressing, pressure massage or nipping on the channel and collateral points. Its basic manipulation is "finger-pressing" which mainly uses the finger tip to press the points. While pressing, the finger either remains unmoved, or presses side-wise, or kneads lightly, vibrates slightly, moves along or press-and-lifts heavily. Besides, there are also manipulations like fingernail-nipping, elbow-pressing and tapping, etc. Because the above manipulations offer the patients a point-like pressing stimulation in the treatment, they should be performed on their selected points on the channels and collaterals, Ashi points or tenderness points and other point-like parts. Finger-pressing manipulation has combined the therapeutic functions of acupuncture and massage, so its treatment induction is powerful and it is safe and comfortable with quick effect but little damage. In the clinical practice, under the guidance of the Chinese medical theory concerning viscera, channels and collaterals, and *ying*, *wei*, *qi* and *xue*, massagers should select effective points on the channels to form a prescription based on the differentiation of syndromes. And then, they should follow the prescription and perform finger-pressing massage in proper order. Mainly based on pressing and on-the-point pressing, finger-pressing is an ancient massotherapy. Many, many years ago, *The Yellow Emperor's Internal Classic* discribed the curative effect of pressing as "pressing can resolve blood stasis, dispel *qi* and relieve pain", "pressing produces heat and the heat can relieve pain". Therefore, this therapy is effective in regulating *qi* and blood, dredging the channel, adjusting the viscera function and dispersing cold and relieving pain. It can cure all the commonly encountered diseases in the departments of internal medicine, surgery, gynecology, pediatrics and eyes, ear, nose and throat.

5) Digital Point Pressure Therapy

Digital point pressure therapy, which is popular in

压法或掐法,在人体经络穴位上操作以防治疾病的一种推拿疗法。指压推拿的基本手法是"指按法",主要用手指指端按压穴位。可按而静止不动,亦可按而左右拨动,按而轻轻揉动,按而微微颤动,按而滑行移动,按而起伏用力。此外,还有爪掐、肘压、叩点等治疗手法。由于上述手法在施术时给受术者是一点状的按压刺激,故施术主要选择经络俞穴、阿是穴或压痛点等点状部位。指压推拿具有针刺与推拿两法的治疗作用,故治疗时感应强、作用快、安全舒适,且损伤小。运用时,先以中医的脏腑、经络、营卫气血理论为指导,根据辨证分型,选择有效经穴组成推拿治疗处方;然后再按处方规定的顺序,依次点穴施治。以按点为主治手法的指压疗法是一种古老的推拿术,早在《黄帝内经》中就有"按之则血气散,故按之痛止","按之则热气至,热气至则痛止矣"的论述。这说明本法具有调和气血、疏通经络、调理脏腑和散寒止痛等作用,能治内、外、妇、儿、五官等各科常见病症。

5) 点穴疗法

点穴疗法是由中国传统武术中的点穴、打穴、拿穴、踢穴和

Qingdao, Laoshan and the whole Jiaodong peninsula in Shandong China, evoluted from digital acupoint pressing, point-hitting, point-capturing, point-kicking, point-opening and other actions of the traditional Chinese martial arts. All the digital point pressing methods mentioned above are taken both as means for attack in striking and as therapy for injury treatment. Taking for reference the technical actions of striking and point-hitting, and based on the summarized practical experiences of its own in treatment, digital point therapy has become a well-known school of massage in preventing and treating diseases under the guidance of the theoretical principles of channels and collaterals, *qi* and blood of traditional Chinese medicine. Its chief manipulation is digital-hitting therapy (see "digital-hitting therapy" in the section of "manipulation"). The other important manipulations are patting, tapping, pressing, nipping, clutching-grasping, thumping and orthotherapy. The whole set of manipulations take the various ways of digital pressing, hitting, patting and thumping as its basic forms which are vigorous, swift and energetic. During the performance, massagers are required to have quite strong fingers and arms as well as the supporting power of the whole body. That is why beginners should first practise digital point pressing, of which the chief exercises are: squating-standing-up, strength directing and patting, contra-pulling, lying-on-the-back, back-bumping, sentipede-jumping, eagle's claw-power, paper-thumping, hill-pushing, waist-picking and so on. It is theoretically believed that any flaccidity and arthralgia could mean the imbalance of *yin* and *yang* as a result of the struggle between the pathogenic factor and vital *qi*, the disorder of channel *qi* and blockage of *ying*, *wei*, *qi* and *xue's* circulation. Therefore, in treatment, stronger digital hitting manipulations are "to be used on the relative or opposite in order to make the closed ones feel shaking and open gradually so as to let the blocked *qi* and blood slowly restore their circulation." It

解穴等动作演化而来的一种推拿疗法，在中国的青岛、崂山及胶东一带盛行。武术中的上述点穴法，既是一种击技的进攻手段，又是一种治疗损伤的方法。而点穴疗法则是借鉴了武术击技点穴的技术动作，总结了其医疗点穴的实践经验，并在中医经络、气血学说指导下用以防治疾病的一种推拿流派。其主治手法为击点法（详见手法节"击点法"），其他主要手法有拍打法、叩打法、按压法、掐法、扣压法、抓拿法、捶打法和矫形法等。整套手法以各种点、打、拍、捶为基本形式。施术风格峻猛刚健，捷速强劲。由于施术时要求术者有较强的指力、臂力与全身的支持力，故初学者首先要进行点穴练功。主要功法有蹲起功、运气拍打功、对拉功、仰卧功、撞背功、蜈蚣跳、鹰爪力、捶纸功、推山功及扎腰功等。在病理上，认为当人体发生痿、痹等病症时，由于邪正相搏，阴阳失调，经络之气随之逆乱，营卫气血运行因而受阻。故在治疗上，要运用较强的点打手法，"从其穴之前导 之，或 在对位之穴启之，使其所闭之穴感受震激，渐渐开放，则所阻滞之

is also pointed out that "when the channels get unobstructed, their diseases will relieve themselves." This shows digital point pressing therapy plays a curative role in dredging the channel, promoting the flow of *qi* and blood circulation, regulating *ying* and *wei* and strengthening the vital *qi* to expel external pathogenic factors. Digital acupoint pressing therapy has obtained remarkable curative effect in its clinical treatment for various types of paralysis, numbness and obstinate rheumatalgia.

From the brief introduction above, it can be seen that each massage school has formed its own system on the basis of its own origin, history, theory, chief manipulations, training method, therapeutic style and adaptable sphere. This contributes to a great variety of schools and branches of modern Chinese massage.

3. How to Learn Chinese Massage

Chinese massage is, in theory and practice, a powerful clinical subject of TCM. Professional doctors of massage should have not only the elementary knowledge of Chinese and Western medicine, a good command of the professional theory and TCM's method of diagnosis and treatment based on overall analysis of symptoms and signs, but also a good physical consstitution and proficient manipulation technique for clinical massage. So, the students in the massage speciality of TCM colleges in China must systematically study *Classics on Massage*, *Theory on Massage Exercise*, *Manipulation of Massage*, *Basis of Massage*, *Massage Therapeutics*, *Children Massotherapy* and other specialized courses in addition to all that required. Moreover, they have to carry on strict constitutional exercise and technical training in manipulations.

In the aspect of basic medical courses, special emphasis is laid on the study of TCM's *yin-yang*, the five elements, *ying-wei-qi-xue*, channels and collaterals, viscera, causes of the illnesses, four diagnostic methods and eight-principal-syndrome diagnosis

气血亦缓缓通过其穴，以复其流行矣。"认为"经脉既行，其病自除"。这说明点穴疗法具有疏通经络、行气活血、调和营卫、鼓舞正气、驱除邪气等治疗作用。本法用以治疗各种瘫痪、麻痹及风湿顽痹，效果显著。

综上所述，各种推拿流派均以其各自的历史源流、学术理论、主治手法、训练方法、医疗风格及适用范围而自成体系，从而构成了当代中国推拿界丰富多彩的流派与分支。

3. 怎样学习中国推拿

中国推拿是一门理论性和实践性都比较强的中医临床学科。推拿专科医生不仅要通晓中、西医基础知识，掌握专业理论和中医辨证论治的方法，而且还要具备能适应推拿临床工作的身体素质和熟练的手法操作技能。所以，中国各中医院校推拿专业的学生，除了学习中医医疗专业学生规定的中、西医必修课程外，还需系统学习《推拿文献学》、《推拿练功学》、《推拿手法学》、《推拿基础学》、《推拿治疗学》和《小儿推拿学》等专业课程。此外，还要进行严格的身体素质锻炼与手法操作技能训练。

在医学基础课程方面，要特别强调中医的阴阳五行、脏腑经络、营卫气血、病因病机、四诊八纲、辨证论治等内容的学习，

and treatment based on overall analysis of symptoms and signs and on the study of anatomy, physiology, pathophysiology, patho-anatomy and physical diagnosis in Western medicine. Special stress is laid on the intimate knowledge of the courses of the four-teen regular channels and their relationship to the internal organs, the commonly used points on the fourteen regular chan-nels, the location of extra-ordinary points and the special points for massage, point selection, indications, human histology, motion function, etc. This knowledge is of high practical value and of great importance in guiding clinical massage.

So far as professional technical training is concerned, the first thing is to carry on conscientious training step by step according to the commonly used exercises and their training methods introduced in the section of "exercise] training". During the training, attention should be paid not only to cons-titutional qualities such as strength, endurance, pliability and toughness but also to the culture of psycology, i. e., the indo-mitable will power and quality to bear hardships and strenuous work so as to get physically and psycologically prepared for the long-term professional massage. Furthermore, stress should also be laid on the serious study of "the movement struc-ture" and "technical essentials" of various manipulations intro-duced in the section of "commonly used manipulations" in this book, strict following-up of the training methods and steps, and assiduous and persevering practice of manipulating tech-nique in its proper sequence so as to accomplish the trainings at three elementary stages such as rice-bag training, human-body training and manipulating training for combating com-mon diseases.

In a word, for those with some knowledge of medical scien-ce, it is easy to practise massage on trial basis within a short time as a result of conscientious training, but difficult to come up to professional standards, particularly to gain a perfect and serviceable command of the technically difficult manipulations

以及西医的解剖、生理、病理生理、病理解剖、物理诊断等课程的学习。尤其是要熟知十四经脉的循行路线及其内脏的络属关系、常用十四经穴、经外奇穴及推拿特定穴的位置、取穴方法、功能主治，以及人体结构、运动生理等。这些对将来从事推拿工作具有较高的指导意义和实用价值。

在专业技能训练方面，首先要根据本书"练功"一节所介绍的常用功法及其练习方法，按步骤地进行认真练功。在练功过程中，不仅要注意力量、耐力、柔韧性等身体素质的锻炼，而且还要加强心理素质的培养。即在提高身体素质的同时，培养自己吃苦耐劳、坚韧不拔的精神，以便为将来长期从事推拿专业工作打下良好的基础。此外，还要注意认真学习本书"常用手法"一节所介绍的各种手法"动作结构"与"技术要领"，严格遵循所规定的训练方法与步骤，循序渐进、持自以恒地进行锻炼，保质保量地、按步骤地完成米袋练习、人体练习与常见病操作练习三个基本阶段的训练。

总而言之，对具有一定医学基础的人来说，经过一段时间的认真训练，推拿是不难在短期入门的。但要想达到推拿专业医师的水平，特别是要熟练掌握一指禅推法、滚法等技术难度较高的手法，

of single-finger massage, and rolling therapy without going through long-term special training or accumulating "special skills."

Section 2
Acting Principle of Massage

Massage is a Chinese medical therapy with various manipulations applied to certain locations of the human body (including specified passive movement of the limbs) to prevent diseases. One of its chief curative factors is the "quality" of the manipulation and the other factor is the exceptional effect of the manipulated locations, channels and collaterals, and points. Therefore, generally speaking, on the one hand, when the curative effect of massage is working on one specified location of the body through manipulations, the direct effect of its stress can act locally to promote blood circulation and remove blood stasis, restore and treat injured soft tissues, correct deformity and abnormal location of bones and soft tissues in anatomic site. On the other hand, dynamic wave signals of the manipulation can reflexively influence the physiological function and pathological state of the body fluid, *qi* and blood, *ying*, *wei*, cerebrospine, viscera, mind and emotion, etc. through the conducting channel of points $\rightleftharpoons$ channels and collaterals $\rightleftharpoons$ viscera so as to effect a recuperative medical function all over the body. The chief acting principles are as follows:

1. Regulating *Yin* and *Yang*

Yin and *yang* are a pair of concepts in the ancient Chinese philosophy, representing respectively "exposure to the sun" and "facing the opposite direction of the sun", the former situation being *yang* and the latter *yin*. Later, this meaning was extended to explain any two opposite things or phenomena that nourish

并能得心应手地运用于临床，则必须经过长时间的专业训练，积累一定的"功夫"。否则是难以实现的。

第二节　推拿作用原理

推拿是在人体的一定部位上，运用各种手法（包括特定的肢体被动运动）来防治疾病的一种中医疗法。其产生疗效的主要因素，一是手法的"质量"，二是施术的部位、经络与穴位的特异作用。因此，从整体上说，推拿的治疗作用，一方面是通过手法作用于人体体表的特定部位后，其应力的直接作用发挥了活血化瘀、理筋整复、矫正畸形、纠正人体骨与软组织解剖部位的异常等局部作用；另一方面，手法动态力的波动信号，可通过穴位⇌经络⇌脏腑的传导途径，反射性地影响津液、气血、营卫、脑髓、脏腑以及精神、情志等生理活动和病理状态，从而起到全身性的调治作用。其主要作用原理包括以下几方面：

1. 调整阴阳

阴阳，是中国古代的一个哲学概念。最初，阴阳是指日光的向背，即向日光的地方为阳，背日光的地方为阴。后来，这个概

each other, supplement each other or wane and wax mutually (one wanes, the other waxes or vice versa) and transform to each other, which gradually developed into *yin-yang* theory. As early as more than two thousand years ago, *yin-yang* theory was introduced into TCM and became an important part of its basic theory, being able to explain the organic structure, the physiological function and the pathologic change of the human body and guide clinical diagnosis and treatment.

According to *yin-yang* theory, every part of the human body is constituted of two opposite but unified materials or functions, i.e. *yin* and *yang*. So far as the structure of the human body is concerned, the exterior is *yang* whereas the interior is *yin*; the upper part is *yang* and the lower part is *yin*; the back is *yang* and the abdomen *yin*. So far as the *zang* and *fu* organs are concerned, the six *fu*-organs are *yang* and the five *zang*-organs *yin*. So far as *qi* and blood are concerned, *qi* is *yang* and blood *yin*. In terms of function and material, function is *yang* and material *yin*. In terms of functioning status, excitement is *yang* and restrain *yin*; activity is *yang* and stasis *yin*; growth is *yang* and decline *yin*. As for the functional activity of *qi*, upward is *yang* and downward *yin*; outward is *yang* while inward *yin*, etc. If *yin* and *yang* are in dynamic equilibrium, life activity of the body will remain in a healthy state of "*yin* and *yang* in equilibrium". But if the relative balance of *yin* and *yang* is destroyed due to the six pathogenic factors, seven emotions or traumatic injuries and so on, there can be such pathogenic changes as an excess of *yang* causing heat syndrome and an excess of *yin* cold one; an excess of *yin* leading to disorder of *yang*, excess of *yang* disorder of *yin*; insufficiency of *yang* causing exterior cold syndrome, deficiency of *yin* interior heat one, etc. Clinically syndromes of different degrees and properties such as *yin*, *yang*, exterior, interior, cold, heat, deficiency, excess may be present.

Massage treatment follows the principle described in *The Yellow Emperor's Internal Classic*: "examining carefully

念被进一步引伸，用以解释自然界中一切相互对应、相互资生、相互消长、相互转化的事物现象，从而逐渐形成了阴阳学说。早在两千多年前，阴阳学说就被引用到中医学中，成为中医基本理论的一个重要组成部分。中医用阴阳来解释人体的组织结构、生理功能、病理变化等，并指导着临床诊断与治疗。

阴阳学说认为，人体是由两种既对立、又统一的物质与功能，即阴和阳构成的。就人体部位而言，体表为阳，体内为阴；上部为阳，下部为阴；背部为阳，腹部为阴。就人体脏腑而言，六腑为阳，五脏为阴。就人体气血而言，气为阳，血为阴。就功能与物质而言，功能为阳，物质为阴。就功能活动的状态而言，兴奋为阳，抑制为阴；活动为阳，静止为阴；增长为阳，减退为阴。就气机运行而言，上升为阳，下降为阴；向外为阳，向内为阴等。当阴阳双方处于相对动态平衡状态时，人体的生命活动便处于"阴平阳秘"的健康状态。如因六淫、七情或跌仆损伤等因素的作用使阴阳的相对平衡状态遭到破坏时，就会导致一系列"阴阳失调"的病理变化，如阳盛则热，阴盛则寒；阴盛则阳病，阳盛则阴病；阳虚生外寒，阴虚生内热等。临床可表现为阴、阳、表、里、寒、热、虚、实等多种不同层次、不同性质的病证。

推拿治病遵循《黄帝内经》"谨察阴阳所在而调之，以平为期"

the conditions of *yin* and *yang* so as to get them in relative balance". That is to say, massagists should, according to differential diagnosis, use different manipulations with stimulations of different degrees which may be mild, powerful, slow, quick, vigorous or soft in order to treat the illness of deficiency type by tonifying methods, excess syndromes with the purgative and reductive manipulation, heat syndromes with methods of cold or cool nature, cold syndromes with hot-natured methods, stasis by dissipation, stagnation and accumulation of pathogen by diffusion, exopathogens in the superficies of the body by dispersion and half exterior and half interior syndromes by mediation so as to change the relative excessiveness of *yin* and *yang*, regulate their relationship and restore their relative balance, eliminate pathogen and recover the vital-*qi*. The deficiency of *yin*, deficiency of *yang* or deficiency of both *yin* and *yang* of the corresponding viscera can be reinforced if the light, soft and slow pushing with one-finger meditation, kneading and rubbing therapies are used to stimulate the specified Front-*Mu* points, *Shu* points and other adjunct points while the relatively strong or powerful manipulations of rubbing, scrubbing or squeezing and pressing therapies can expel pathogen and reduce excessiveness. For the diseases of such as cold and deficiency and *yin* types, relatively slow and soft rhythmical manipulations should be performed at the treatment location for comparatively a longer time to make the patients feel deep warmth and heat so as to promote *qi* by warming *yang*. Furthermore, scrubbing mildly at the waist can nourish *yin* and remove fire so as to clear away deficiency heat from the blood. Pushing mildly of *Du* channel from Dazhui (Du 14) to sacrum and coccyx can clear away excessive heat from *qi* system while pushing forcefully along the same route can cool the blood and clear away excessive heat from the blood system.

的原则，根据辨证分型，术者采用或轻、或重、或缓、或急、或刚、或柔等不同刺激量的手法，使虚者补之，实者泻之，热者寒之，寒者热之，壅滞者通之，结聚者散之，邪在皮毛者汗而发之，病在半表半里者和而解之，以改变人体内部阴阳失调的病理状态，从而达到恢复阴阳的相对平衡、邪去正复之目的。如应用轻柔缓和的一指禅推法、揉法与摩法，刺激特定的募穴、俞穴及其他配穴，能补益相应脏腑的阴虚、阳虚或阴阳两虚；而使用力量较强的摩擦或挤压类手法，则能祛邪泻实；对阴寒虚冷的病证，要用较慢而柔和的节律手法在治疗部位上做较长时间的操作，使患者产生深沉的温热感，有温阳益气的作用。此外，轻擦腰部，能养阴泻火，以清血中虚热；自大椎至尾椎轻推督脉，可清气分实热；在同一路线上重推督脉，则能清热凉血，以泻血分实热。

2. Regulating the Function of Channels and Collaterals, *Qi* and Blood, and Viscera

The function of the channels and collaterals is to propel the circulation of *qi* and blood in order to nourish *yin* and *yang*, and facilitate the bones, tendons and joints. The channels and collaterals connect with visceral organs and the extremities and all the internal and external parts of the body. The five *zang*-organs and six *fu*-organs, four limbs and entire skeleton, five sense organs and nine orificies, muscles and bones of the body must rely on the nourishment of *qi* and blood and the connection by the channels and collaterals so that they can give full play to their own physiological function and become an organic entirety by mutual coordination. Any blockage in the channels and collaterals will cause stagnant circulation of channel *qi* and blood and many other diseases such as atrophy and non-effective function of the skin, muslces, tendons, channels and vessels, and joints due to the loss of nutrients, and malnutrition of the five *zang*-organs, dysfunction of the six *fu*-organs, etc. may occur.

Qi refers to two aspects: one, the refined nutritive substance that builds up the human body and maintains its life activities, the other, the physiological function or motility of *zang* and *fu*, channels and collaterals. *Qi* has the function of promoting metabolism and transformation, consolidating the liquid substances and the organs in the abdominal cavity and warming the body. Among all the *qis* in human body, the most essential ones are *yuanqi* (primordial *qi*), *yingqi* and *weiqi* (defensive *qi*.) Primordial *qi*, also called vital *qi* or genuine *qi*, is the primary substance and a concentrated expression of the life activity. Defensive *qi* which is located and circulates outside the blood vessels, can nourish the viscera and muscles, protect the exterior part of the body, regulate and control the pore of sweat duct and resist external pathogen. *Yingqi* circulates inside the blood vessels, shares the function of interpro-

2. 调整经络、气血与脏腑的功能

经络有"行气血、营阴阳、濡筋骨、利关节"的生理功能，且内属脏腑，外联肢节，沟通表里，联络全身。人体的五脏六腑、四肢百骸、五官九窍、皮肉筋骨等，只有通过气血的濡养与经络的联络作用，才能充分发挥各自的生理功能，并相互协调，形成一个有机的整体。如经络不通，则经气不畅，经血滞行，可出现皮、肉、筋、脉及关节失养而萎缩、不用，或五脏不荣、六腑不运等。

气的含义有二：一是指构成人体和维持人体生命活动的精微物质，二是指脏腑、经络的生理功能或动力。气有化生、推动、固摄、温煦等作用。人体诸气之中，最基本的气有元气、营气、卫气等。其中，元气又称正气或真气，是人体生命活动的集中体现；卫气分布于脉外，依旁着脉道运行，有温养脏腑和肌肤、保护体表、调节和控制汗孔与抵御外邪等作用；营气运行于脉内，

moting blood and nourishing the whole body. Diseases in the
qi system are chiefly manifested in the three forms: stagnation
deficiency, and reversed flow of *qi*.

Blood is a red nutritious liquid which flows in the blood
vessels. It comes from food which is processed by the spleen and
stomach. Circulating throughout the whole body along the
blood vessels, it provides the viscera, tissues and organs with
nutrition to maintain their normal physiological function. If the
blood circulation is blocked due to a certain cause, all the component organs of *zang fu*, tissues and organs won't get nutrients
of blood, which will result in the imbalance, blockage and
even loss of their normal physical function and subsequently
various kinds of diseases of blood such as blood stasis and
deficiency of blood or bleeding, etc.

The modulation of channels and collaterals, *qi*, blood and
viscera function is accomplished by massage on the channel
and collateral system through manipulations. Because, in the
massage treatment, all manipulations are used firstly on the
superficial portion of the body to "push the points along channels and collaterals"; secondly, massage is directed to the
projected superficial portion of the body corresponding to a certain organ of viscera, thus, on the one hand, the local effect
of manipulation can produce a direct curative effect on the diseases of channels and collaterals, *qi*, blood and viscera at the
manipulated location. For instance, it can cure local swelling and
pain due to blood stasis after trauma, limb pain and numbness
due to cold attack on the channels and collaterals, gastrointestinal spasm caused by cold, stomach distension caused by improper diet, etc. On the other hand, the stimulating effect of
manipulations arouses the special function of the points on
regular channels and the whole channel and collateral system
and conducts wave action of the dynamic force of manipulation along the channels and collaterals to their corresponding
viscera and all the tissue organs such as brain, marrow, uterus

能化生血液，营养全身。气的主要病证有气虚、气滞和气逆三类。

血是循行于脉管内富有营养作用的赤色液体，主要由脾胃化生的水谷精微通过心肺的作用变化而成。它随血脉循行全身，为各脏腑、组织、器官提供营养，以维持它们的正常生理功能。如因某种原因导致血液运行障碍，脏腑、组织、器官等就得不到血液的濡养，其生理功能便会失调、障碍，甚至丧失，从而产生血瘀、血虚或出血等多种血分病证。

推拿调整经络、气血、脏腑的功能是通过手法作用于经络系统来完成的。因为推拿施治时，一是运用各种手法在人体体表"推穴道，走经络"；二是在脏腑投影的相应体表部位施以手法能起到对其"直接"按摩的作用。这样，一方面可由手法的局部作用，对受术部位的经络、气血、脏腑病证起到直接的治疗作用。如外伤所致的局部瘀血肿痛、麻木不仁，以及受寒所致的胃肠痉挛，饮食不节引起的胃脘闷胀等，均可通过手法的局部作用而得到调治。另一方面，由于手法的刺激激发了经穴乃至整个经络系统的特异作用，使手法动态力的波动作用沿着经络传至所属的脏腑及其所过之处的组织、器官，如脑、髓、胞宫等，从而改善、

and so on, where they passed by, thus improving and restoring the physiological function of these viscera, tissues and organs. For instance, massage at the concerned channel points of the spleen and stomach channels can promote the generation of *qi* and blood of the body. Meanwhile, massage at the points of the liver channel can improve the dredging function of the liver and promote the functional activities of *qi*. Massage with powerful pressing-digging and pressing-intervally or light pressing-kneading therapies can cure bradycardia or tachycardia by stimulating Neiguan (P 6) to influence the heart function through the special conducting function of the pericardium. Pressing-digging and pressing-intervally at Hegu (LI4) can cure toothache and facial paralysis. Pushing-pressing at Sanyinjiao (Sp 6) can regulate women's menses, etc. All the above mentioned can show the function of integrated modulation of massage treatment.

3. Recovery of the Function of Tendons, Bones and Joints

In TCM, soft tissues and joints include fascia, muscle, muscle tendon, tendon sheath, ligament, joint capsule, synovium, fibrous ring of verterbral disc, articular cartilage disc and other soft tissues of the body. Any direct trauma, indirect trauma and long-term strain can cause them a series of pathogenic changes. Their injuries can be local bruise, muscle sprain, fibrous rupture, tendon avulsion, slipped tendon, ligament rupture, laceration of joint capsule, semi-dislocation of bones, joint dislocation, chondroclasis and joint or soft tissue strain, etc. Massage has quite a good curative effect on all the above mentioned illnesses, and its chief principles are as follows:

1) Relaxing Muscles and Tendons and Dredging the Channels and Collaterals

After trauma, signals of spasm and pain can be sent off by the attaching points of muscles, fasciae, tenden, joint capsules,

恢复这些脏腑、组织器官的生理功能。如通过推拿脾经与胃经的有关经穴，可促进人体气、血的生成；同时通过推拿肝经的经穴，可改善肝的疏泄功能，以促进气机的调畅；再如运用较强的拿按法或轻柔的按揉法刺激内关穴，可通过心包经的传导作用，影响心脏的功能，以治疗心动过缓或心动过速；拿按合谷穴，可治疗牙痛、面瘫；推按三阴交穴，可调理妇女的经血等。这都是推拿整体性调治作用的体现。

3. 恢复筋骨、关节的功能

中医所说的筋骨、关节，包括筋膜、肌肉、肌腱、腱鞘、韧带、关节囊、滑膜、椎间盘、关节软骨盘等人体软组织。这些组织可因直接或间接外伤或长期劳损而产生一系列的病理变化。其损伤包括局部挫伤、肌肉拉伤、纤维破裂、肌腱撕脱、肌腱滑脱、韧带破裂、关节囊撕破、骨缝开错(半脱位)、关节脱位、软骨破裂以及关节或软组织劳损等。推拿对治疗上述诸病证，有良好的疗效。其作用原理主要有以下几方面：

1) 舒筋通络，解痉止痛

损伤后，肌肉附着点和筋膜、韧带、关节囊等受损害的软组

etc. to alert the concerned tissues through the reflexion of the nerve. Muscular contraction, tension and even spasm are the very reflexion of this alertful status. This is a protective reaction of human body which aims at reducing the activities of the limbs and avoiding the tracting stimulation to the injured part so as to relieve pain. But if no timely treatment is given or the treatment is not thorough-going, adhesion, fibrosis or cicatrization of different degrees of the injured tissues will occur and even damaging impulsion will be produced to increase the pain, tenderness and muscular contraction and tension, and subsequently secondary pain foci and malignant pain rings will appear in the surrounding tissues. Both the primary and secondary foci can stimulate and compress the terminals of nerves and the small nutrient blood vessels, resulting in partial obstruction in blood circulation and metabolism. Massage is a very effective way to remove muscular tension and spasm, in which it can not only relax the muscles but also get rid of the cause that leads to the muscular tension. The function and mechanism of massage consist of three parts: firstly, it can locally promote blood circulation and raise body temperature; secondly, it can increase the threshold value of pain of tissues with appropriate stimulation; thirdly, it can extend the tense and spasmodic muscles so that the illness can be eliminated.

2) Restoring and Treating Injured Soft Tissues and Reducing Dislocated Joints

Massage manipulations of tracting, traction and counter-traction, rotating and pulling or flicking-poking can reduce joint dislocation, join semiluxation, return the sprained soft tissue to normal position, restore slipped tendon, resituate herniation of pulpiform nucleus, take out the embedded synovium and eliminate the pathogenic state of muscle spasm and local pain to promote the recovery and reconstruction of the injured soft tissues.

3) Tripping Adhesion, Dredging Stenosis

织，可发出疼痛信号，通过神经的反射作用，使有关组织处于警觉状态。肌肉的收缩、紧张乃至痉挛，就是这一警觉状态的反映。这是人体的一种保护性反应，其目的在于减少肢体活动，避免对损伤部位的牵拉刺激，从而减轻疼痛。但对此如不及时处理，或治疗不彻底，损伤组织可形成不同程度的粘连、纤维化或疤痕化，以至不断地发出有害冲动，加重疼痛、压痛和肌肉收缩、紧张，继而又可在周围组织引起继发性疼痛病灶，形成恶性疼痛环。不管是原发病灶还是继发病灶，均可刺激和压迫神经末梢及小的营养血管，造成局部血运及新陈代谢障碍。推拿是解除肌肉紧张、痉挛的有效方法。这是因为它不但能放松肌肉，并能解除引起肌肉紧张的原因。其作用机理有三：一是能加强局部的血液循环，使局部温度升高；二是通过适当的刺激，提高了局部组织的痛阈；三是将紧张或痉挛的肌肉充分拉长，从而解除其紧张、痉挛，以消除疼痛。

2）理筋整复

运用推拿的牵引、拔伸、摇扳或弹拨手法，可使关节脱位者整复，骨缝错开者合拢，软组织撕裂者对位，肌腱滑脱者理正，髓核脱出者还纳，滑膜嵌顿者退出，从而消除引起肌肉痉挛和局部疼痛的病理状态，有利于损伤组织的修复和功能重建。

3）剥离粘连，疏通狭窄

When the soft tissues are injured, adhesion of the muscle, tendon, ligament, joint capsule, and others. due to local bleeding and organization of hematoma may cause a long-term pain and hinder the joint activities. Treatment, such as flicking-poking, joint lift-dragging, traction and counter-traction, rotating and pulling, can remove adhesion and smooth joints.

In the parts with such fiber-sheathed vessels of bones as the tendon vessel of the long head of biceps, tendon vessle and tendon sheath of lexor hallucis longus and flexor digitorum at the processus styloideus of radius, there may, due to hyperosteogeny, chronic strain or attack of wind, cold and dampness, occur tumefaction and hyperemia of the tendon and tendon sheath or exudation inside the sheath and then in time fibrosis, which will thicken the wall of the sheath, fetter the tendon inside the sheath and affect the extention-flexion movement of the joints. If it is a light case, the sheath will become constrictive and it makes snapping sounds while moving. If the case is a serious one, the local adhesion will become indurative, making the joint lose its extension-flexion function. For tendons and sheaths with pathologic changes, local massage by plucking and continuous rhythmic finger-kneading or rolling in coordination with rolling-pulling, traction and counter-traction and other manipulations of passive movement of the joint can subdue swelling and stop pain, strip adhesion, enlarge constriction and relieve the snapping sound to restore the tendon to its normal sliding function in the sheath.

4. The Tonifying and Purging Function of Massage Manipulation

Massage treatment takes manipulation as the most important means. In the course of diagnosis and treatment, according to the deficiency and excess of the patient's condition of constitution and illness, the massagist can make choice among such manipulations as tonifying, purging, mediating, exciting

肌肉、肌腱、腱鞘、韧带、关节囊等软组织的损伤，均可因局部出血、血肿机化而产生粘连，从而引起长期疼痛和关节活动受限。运用局部的弹拨手法和关节提拉、拔伸、摇扳等手法，能起到松解粘连、滑利关节的作用。

在人体具有骨纤维性鞘管的部位，如二头肌腱长头腱管，桡骨茎突部腱管和屈拇、屈指肌腱鞘，由于骨质增生，慢性劳损或遭受风、寒、湿三者的侵袭，该处的肌腱、腱鞘肿胀、充血，鞘内渗液，久之纤维化，鞘壁增厚，使肌腱束缚于腱鞘内，影响关节的屈伸活动。轻者腱鞘狭窄，活动时弹拨作响，重者局部粘连硬结，关节丧失屈伸功能。对病变肌腱、腱鞘，局部运用弹拨手法与持续的节律性指揉或揉法并配合摇扳、拔伸等关节被动运动类手法，有消肿止痛、剥离粘连、扩大狭窄、解除弹响等作用，从而恢复肌腱在腱鞘内的正常滑动。

4. 推拿手法的补泻作用

手法是推拿治病的主要手段。临床诊治时，推拿医师根据患者的体质强弱和病情的虚实，或补，或泻，或调和，或兴奋，或抑制。而这一切，全赖手法的巧妙应用。纵观古今推拿大师们的

or restraining, all depending on whether the manipulations can be skillfully applied. A comprehensive survey of the clinical experience of the masters of both ancient and modern Chinese massage shows that the tonifying and purging effect of the manipulation is directly related with factors such as whether using a mild or powerful manipulation, whether with vigorous or soft performance, and whether with a quick or slow frequency, what direction the force takes and how much time it lasts. Generally speaking, the tonifying manipulation refers to the manual stimulation with less strength, soft performance and slow frequency along the route of channels and collaterals (anti-clockwise manipulation at the abdominal region), which excites, stimulates and strengthens the human body. On the contrary, more powerful, vigorous but soft manual stimulations with quick frequency moving in the opposite direction of the channels and collaterals (clockwise manipulation at the abdominal region) for a short time are known as purging manipulation which has the function of restraining, tranquilizing the body and directly expelling pathogen. Besides, to-and-fro stimulations performed with moderate strength, frequency and time along the channels and collaterals are known as uniform reinforcing-reducing method, which is also called mediation method, with the function of regulating *yin* and *yang* and increasing the function of the related internal organs. But, all those manipulations mentioned above concerning tonifying and purging are relative and changeable in their clinical practice, so flexible application and differentiation should be made in accordance with the specific conditions. Take the tonifying method for example. It may be divided into two kinds, namely, slow tonifying and quick tonifying. For quick tonifying, strong manipulation is used to stimulate the points along the regular channels while slow tonifying performed gently and slowly for a longer time along the related channels. The purging method consists of quick purging and slow purging. For quick purging, deep

临床经验，其手法的补泻作用与手法用力的轻、重，操作的刚、柔，频率的快、慢，加力的方向与持续的时间等各方面的因素有关。一般来说，凡用力轻浅，操作柔和，频率缓慢，顺着经络行走的方向加力（在腹部则为逆时针方向施术），并持续时间较长的刺激手法为补法，对人体有兴奋、激发与强壮作用；反之，用力深重，操作刚中有柔，频率稍快，逆着经络行走方向加力（在腹部则为顺时针方向施术），并持续时间稍短的刺激手法为泻法，对人体有抑制、镇静和直接驱邪作用；此外，强度、频率与操作时间适中，在经络线上做来回往复操作的刺激手法为平补平泻法，又称和法，有调和人体阴阳、改善内脏生理功能的作用。必须明确，上述有关补泻手法的作用是相对的，在临床应用时并非一成不变的，临床应用时应根据具体情况，辨证地灵活应用。如补法又可分缓补与急补两种。急补时，手法较重，顺经刺激经穴；缓补时，手法要轻柔而缓慢，时间较长，循经操作。泻法也

finger-nail pressing is applied with more strength in the anti-channel direction while slow purging is performed with less strength in the anti-channel direction.

5. The Studies on the Mechanical Principles of Massage Manipulation

"Manipulation" is taken as the chief means of massage to prevent and treat diseases. Both ancient and modern massage masters have obtained desirable curative effect and accumulated rich experience in their long-time medical practice of how to apply proper manipulation. Their experience can be summed up as follows: Firstly, manipulations with different actions have different specified curative indications. For example, one-finger pushing therapy is good at treating internal and gynaecological diseases; quick pushing manipulation is curative for carbuncles and boils and other surgical diseases while digital hitting manipulation for paralysis. Secondly, due to their different technical levels, different massagists may, with the same manipulation, produce different effect — "highly skilled massagists produce a high curative effect while poorly skilled poor effect". That is why traditional Chinese massage emphasizes the standardization of the manipulation technology and "the more effort, the more effect" principle. In essence, the therapeutic effect is closely related with the output form of action force and the due dosage —"mechanical forms" which represent the mechanical characteristics of manipulation. That is to say, the former is caused by different manipulations with different mechanical forms while the latter is related with the quality of action force produced by manipulations of different technological standards. It can be seen that the mechanical features of manipulation are important factors to determine the adaptable sphere and curative effect of massage. Therefore, to establish a set of efficient research methods is by all means important for the systematic study on the action laws of various

有急泻与缓泻之分。急泻时，逆经深掐，力量较重；缓泻时，逆经施法，用力较轻。

5. 推拿手法的力学原理研究

"手法"是推拿防治疾病的主要手段。古今的推拿大师通过长期的医疗实践，在如何正确运用手法获取理想的疗效方面，积累了丰富的经验。在这些经验中，我们可以看到以下两种情况：一是动作方式不同的手法，其特效的主治范围不同。如一指禅推法擅长于治疗内、妇科杂病，缠法可治疗痈疖等外科病证，而点击法则对各种瘫痪有特效等。二是由于技术水平的差异，不同的操作者，尽管施用的是同一手法，但可出现"技高者效高，技差者效差"的结果。所以中国传统的推拿学十分重视手法动作技术的规范化，强调"一分功夫，一分疗效"。究其实质，疗效与推拿手法作用力的输出形式及应用剂量(即表示手法力学特征的"动力形式")有密切关系。也就是说，前者是由于不同手法的动力形式不一所造成；而后者则是与不同技术水平的手法所产生的作用力的"质量"有关。由此可见，手法的力学特征是决定推拿适应范围与疗效的重要因素。所以，建立一套有效的研究方法，对各种经典

classic manipulations, the step-by-step clearing-up of the characteristics of its kinetic biomechanics and finally to bring to light the action principles and treatment mechanism of massage manipulations. For this reason, ever since 1980, scholars of various disciplines have made joint efforts in researches on the mechanic laws of traditional manipulation. Now a brief account of it is made as follows:

1) Professional Facilities Manufactured for the Kinetic Biomechanism of Manipulation

In 1982, Shandong TCM College in cooperation with other institutions manufactured the first dynamic ergograph Model TDL-I for massage manipulation. And later, Shanghai and other places succeeded in succession in manufacturing manipulation ergograph of various models, which provide due means for the study in kinetic biomechanism of massage manipulations. The dynamic ergograph Model TDL-I (**Fig.** 1—1) is a special sensor designed and manufactured in accordance with the theory and technique of modern mechanical electric-test to determine the characteristics of manipulation mechanism. It mainly consists of an ergodisc and three groups of straining sensing elements that are coupled with the ergodisc in a floating way. While being used, it makes up the mechanical information test system aided by its corresponding secondary meter (Fig. 1-2, 1-3). While the ergodisc being operated, the ergograph can decompose the manipulation force into three directions, vertical, longitudinal and horizontal. This decomposed force is transformed into corresponding electro-signals, through the test of the secondary meter, to indicate and record such mechanical parameters as intensity, acceleration, frequency and dynamic curve of the three-dimensional force.

Based on the above mentioned progress, in 1985, Shandong TCM College produced "the system of computer-handled mechanical information of massage manipulation" (Fig. 1—4). The hardware of the handling system consists of the massage manipula-

手法的动作规律进行系统研究，逐步弄清其运动生物力学特征，以揭示推拿手法的动作原理与治疗机制，无疑是十分重要的。中国自1980年以来，通过多学科合作攻关，在研究传统手法的力学规律方面做了大量的工作，现简介如下：

1）研制出手法运动生物力学实验研究的专用设备。

1982年，山东中医学院等单位，首先研制出"TDL—I型推拿手法动态力测定器"。后来，上海等地也相继制成各种类型的手法测定器。这就为手法的运动生物力学研究提供了必要的手段。TDL—I型推拿手法动态力测定器（图1—1），是利用现代力学电测原理与技术设计而成的一种能测定手法力学特征的专用传感器，主要由测力盘及与之成浮动式组合的三组应变式传感元件组成。应用时，与相应二次仪表组成"推拿手法力学信息测录系统"（图1—2，图1—3），当在测力盘上进行操作时，测定器即可将手法作用力分解为垂、纵、横三个方向，并转换为相应的电信号，经由二次仪表测定、显示和记录其三维力的大小、加速度、频率及动态曲线等力学参数。

在此基础上，1985年山东中医学院又推出"推拿手法力学信息计算机处理系统"（图1—4），"处理系统"的硬件由推拿手法测定

tion ergograph, resistance straining meter, digital-analog control converter, analog-digital control converter and microcomputer. This is a mixed system for processing analog-digital signals, with the microcomputer as the center, and designed on the basis of electric test technology of modern medicine. It can convert the analogue information gained by the manipulation ergograph, through sampling and modulus, into a group of discrete digit value — digitized information which can be and is to be processed by computers. It can also restore the digital signal, through digital analogue, to analogue signals and display the analogue curve for further recognization and analysis by computers. Therefore, it is primarily sufficient for the practical functions needed in the characteristic research of manipulation mechanism in the aspects of combined-machinery test and recording, storage, analysis and processing, figure display and recognition, data management, duplication and manipulation teaching, etc.

Recently, the Massage Teaching and Research Section of Shandong TCM College again manufactured the "massage mechanical information detector", which consists of two parts: a mechanical information detector, Model TDL — II, and a strainometer for this special purpose. In addition to sharing all the functions of manipulation Model I, Model II makes the manipulation conditions of the detected person basically the same as that of the practical manipulation training of traditional massage so that the reliability of the measurement result is guaranteed because it adopted the the combining structure for the ergodisc board with additional pinching facility and the ergodisc working-plane which is made of rice bags on the ergodisc board. It also measures the mechanical functions of lifting, pressing-digging, pinching and other manipulations of the kind, further perfecting the function of the ergograph. And that is beyond the ability of detector Model I. A series of new designs have been adopted for the special strainometer,

器、电阻应变仪、模/数、数/模转换控制器及微型计算机联机组成。这是一种以现代力学电测技术为基础、以微机为中心的模拟与数字信号的混合型处理系统。它通过相应的管理程序、处理分析程序、数据计算程序及数据库等应用软件,可将由手法测定器获得的模拟信号,经过采样和量化即进行模数转换为一组离散的数字值——计算机所能进行处理的数字化信息,然后,由计算机来处理;也可以将数字信号经数模转换,还原成模拟信号并显示出模拟曲线,再由计算机来识别分析。因此,在实际工作中可基本满足手法力学特征研究所需要的联机测录、储存、分析处理、图形显示识别、资料管理、复制再现及手法教学等方面的应用功能。

最近,山东中医学院推拿教研室又研制成"推拿力学信息测定仪"。该仪器包括TDL—II型推拿力学信息测定器与专用应变仪两部分。II型手法测定器除保持有I型手法测定器的全部功能外,又因其测力盘面板上采用了组合式的结构方式,增加了捏力器与用米袋做成的测力盘工作面,故在实用时,不但使被测者的手法操作条件与传统推拿学在实际进行手法训练时所用的工作条件基本相同,从而保证了测量结果的可靠性;而且还可测量使用I型测定器不能测量的提、拿、捏一类手法的力学性能,使手法测力器的功能更臻完备。专用应变仪则在缩小体积、方便使用、

for instance, in volume reduction, handy operation, increase of precision and some special functions, thus distinctively increasing the functional value of the entire machine.

2) Experiment and Research on Kinetic Biomechanism of Manipulation

Since 1981, with the above mentioned instruments, extensive researches have been made on the various manipulations practised by different academic schools — one-finger massage, rolling massage, internal exercise massage and digital-acupoint massage, etc; on-the-spot detection has been done with regard to the "kinetic style" of various manipulations. Systematic analysis has also been made of the great amount of data of the wave-form curve of the three dimensional mechanism at different levels. Having got the methematical model, they have also made more precise and deep-going analysis of the manipulation action and its mechanical type with computer technology. In addition, they have set up a mechanical information data bank of traditional Chinese massage, in which are stored lots of valuable manipulation data, including those of the nine famous modern specialists in Chinese massage, such as Zhu Chunting, Ding Jifeng, Wang Jisong and Li Xijiu. The aforesaid work has primarily established a series of effective methods for the kinetic biomechanical research of manipulations, summarized the mechanical features of some manipulations and provided objective quantitative indexes and scientific expressions for the manipulation experience which could once only be sensed but beyond words. With the help of these achievements, we can pry out the microdynamic type and technological secrets of the motion of the manipulations through its macroappearance. Through the diagram of the three-dimensional dynamic wave curve, especially the three-dimensional co-axial curve diagram (Fig. 1—5) provided by computers, we can easily see the stereoscopic images of the three-dimensional space of the manipulation motion in any time phase. There-

提高仪器精度与增加专用功能方面，进行了一系列的新设计，使整机的实用价值得到了明显的提高。

2) 开展手法运动生物力学实验研究

自1981年以来，我们应用上述仪器，先后对一指禅推拿、㨰法推拿、内功推拿、点穴推拿等推拿学术流派传人的手法，做了广泛的研究，对各种手法的"动力形式"进行了现场测定，并对所采集的大量数据与手法三维力学波形曲线图，进行了各个层次的系统分析。在获得"数学模型"的基础上，又利用计算机技术对手法动作及其动力形式，做了更精确、深入的剖析，并建立了"中医推拿力学信息数据库"。把包括当代中国著名推拿专家朱春霆、丁季峰、王纪松、李锡九等的手法数据在内的一批有价值的手法资料，整理入库。上述工作，为手法运动生物力学研究，初步建立了一套有效的实验研究方法；总结了部分手法的力学特征，从而使这些以前只能"心授"不可"言传"的手法经验，有了客观的定量指标与科学的表达语言。借助这些成果，可使我们透过宏观的手法动作外形，窥探到微观的手法动力形式与手法动作的技术奥秘。因为从手法三维动态力波形曲线图，特别是通过由计算机提供的"三维同轴曲线图"（图1—5），能比较容易地观察到手法动作在任何时相内的三维力空间立体形象。因此，从图形提供的手法

fore, objective index can be found for such quantitative descriptions of manipulation motions of traditional massage as strong, lasting, even, soft and deep-going, so on and so forth through the manipulation cycle, frequency, external shaking period, internal shaking period, direction selection, ratio of the mechanics and other important data indicating the kinetic features of manipulations and all the kinetic parameters, such as the initial term angle, basic intensity, main wave intensity, echo wave intensity, power spectrum and frequency spectrum of the manipulation wave. Another significance lies in its direct relationship with the research on the cause of the manipulation motion and with the exposition of the quantity and form of its stimulation to the human body. The specified effect and quality nature of various manipulations all depend on the forms of the dynamic force generated during manipulation — "kinetic forms" of the manipulation which are composed of the fixed quantity, frequency, speed and direction. Massage is curative just because its manipulation effect, and in a fixed dynamic form, is absorbed as a kind of mechanical shaking-wave by various microstructures in the body, which can be explained by the theory of resonance absorption, and then some specific biological effect is caused accordingly. Therefore, it is of far-reaching academic significance to bring to light the dynamic form of the manipulation with the testing method for explaining the relationship between the quantity of manipulation stimulation and clinical curative effect and for exponding the treatment mechanism of massage. In order to provide further knowledge of the curative effect, a chapter on manipulation in this book will give a brief account of the dynamic form of some chief manipulations in the light of the manipulation motion structure.

周期、频率、外摆时、内摆时以及三向力的取向与比值等提示手法运动学特征的重要数据和手法波的初项角、基强度、主峰强度以及功率谱、频率谱等各项运动学参数，可为传统推拿学中对手法动作的定性描述，如有力、持久、均匀、柔和、深透等，找到客观指标。其意义还在于：对研究产生手法动作的原因以及阐明手法对人体作用的刺激量大小与作用形式有直接关系。由于各种手法的特异作用与"质量"的优劣取决于手法动作时所产生的由一定大小、频率、速度、方向组合成的动态力的形式，即手法的"动力形式"，推拿之所以有效，正是由于具有一定动力形式的手法作用力，以一种机械振荡波的形式，被人体内各种微观结构基于共振吸收的原理而吸收其能量，继而引起某些特异性生物效应的结果。所以，应用实验方法来揭示手法的动力形式，对解释手法刺激量与临床疗效的关系，以最终阐明推拿的治病机制，具有重要的学术价值。为了进一步了解手法的治疗作用，本书在手法章内，将结合手法的动作结构，对部分主要手法的动力形式，做简要介绍。

Section 3

Exercise as the Basic Training of Massage

The basic training of massage can be professional or thera-peutic. The former refers to a series of exercises designed for a massagist—a professional doctor to build up his own constitution, while the latter means the exercises done systematically by the patients themselves to facilitate rehabilitation in cooperation with the massagist. The traditional subject of massage attaches great importance to the basic training of massage, emphasizing "the more effort, the more effect", and considers it to be the key link in guaranteeing the quality of medical service. To a massagist, basic training of massage is not only a kind of medical technology that he must grasp, but also a compulsory measure to train his technique.

1. The Functions of the Basic Training (*Lian Gong*)

Literally, "*lian*" means practice, training or exercise, and "*gong*" refers to two things, one is the function or ability, the other the skill or specific training method. So the basic training of massage can be explained as a process for the learner to acquire the function of the organism and its loading ability to practise massage through long-term repeated and arduous practice and training of the specific skills. The functions of the basic training can be summarized as follows:

1) To improve the health status and an overall develop-ment of the constitution of the practitioners, including the development of strength, endurance, sensibility and flexibility; and on this basis, to raise the quality of endurance which a professional must have, including general endurance and en-durance of the muscles, the heart and blood vessels and of the respiratory system which may render the massagist the loading

第三节 推拿练功

推拿练功系指培养推拿专业医生的身体素质而进行的一系列专门训练。此外，为增强患者自身的康复能力，配合手法治疗，令患者进行的系统自我锻炼亦属推拿练功的范围。前者又称为专业性推拿练功，后者则称为医疗性推拿练功。中国传统的推拿学十分重视推拿练功，强调"一分功夫，一分疗效"，认为这是保证医疗质量的重要环节。故对推拿医生来说，推拿练功不仅是一种必须掌握的医疗技术，而且也是一项对自身进行专业技能训练的必要措施。

1. 练功的作用

"练"，即练习、训练、锻炼之意。"功"，其含义有二：一是指功能与能力；二是指功法，即特定的锻炼方法。故推拿练功也可以说是指通过对特定功法的长期反复的刻苦锻炼，使学习者逐渐获得从事推拿专业工作的机体功能与负荷能力的过程。其作用主要表现在以下几方面：

1) 通过推拿练功，提高练功者的健康水平，使力量、耐力、灵敏性、柔韧性等各项机体素质得到全面发展；并在此基础上，定向培养推拿专业工作者所必须具备的耐力素质，包括全身耐力、心血管耐力及呼吸系统耐力等，从而使其获得长时间进行手法操

ability in persistent, continuous hand manipulation of massage.

2) To improve the structural and functional status of the local manipulating parts of organs. For example, the muscle fibers may be increased, the area of the cross section of the muscles augmented, the fiber constitutent of the red muscles which are needed in endurance motion increased, the capability of the muscles in storing oxygen and energy raised, the muscular elasiticity improved and the initial length of the muscles prolonged, the ligaments, connective tissues and tendons thickened and strengthened, their extensibility and ability against tension (pulling force) raised, the capillary network enlarged with vesiculation present, the joints and bones thickened and reinforced and the function of nerve readjustment improved. These are the basic requirements for learning and improving hand manipulations, which may heighten the effect and ensure the quality of hand manipulation.

3) To gradually improve and finally unify the adjusting functions of the nerve and endocrine system, the coordination and mutual support between the internal organs, especially that between the cardiovascular system and the respiratory system, and that between hand manipulation and the internal organs.

4) To cultivate the "vital-qi" of the patients, in particular, through therapeutic basic training of massage which, combined with treatment by hand manipulation, can achieve the result of "strengthening the body resistance to eliminate pathogenic factors by combining external massage treatment and internal health cultivation" and raise the efficiency of massage.

In a word, basic training can make the massagist full of vigour and high in working efficiency and can upgrade his professional skill to ensure the quality of manipulation and the effect of treatment. It is also quite effective in the prevention of professional injury.

The Chinese massage is composed of a variety of schools.

作的持久负荷能力。

2）通过推拿练功，能改造与提高手法动作器官局部组织的结构与功能状态，如使肌纤维增多，肌肉横截面积增大，完成耐力性运动的红肌纤维成份增加，肌肉贮氧能力提高，弹性增强，初长度增加，韧带、结缔组织、肌腱厚实、粗壮，伸展性及抗拉伸力增强。毛细血管网增大并出现囊泡状，关节、骨骼增粗而坚固，神经调节机能改善等。这样就具备了学习与发展手法技术的基本条件，满足了手法技能训练的基本要求。因此，可提高与保证手法练习的效果与质量。

3）通过推拿练功，人体的神经、内分泌系统的调节机能，内脏器官特别是心血管系统与呼吸系统的配合、支持作用，以及与手法动作器官之间的协调功能可逐渐增强，进而达到高度统一。

4）医疗性推拿练功，能培养患者的"正气"，再配合手法治疗，可达到"外治内练、扶正祛邪"的目的，能明显提高推拿的疗效。

总之，通过推拿练功，可使推拿工作者保持旺盛的精力与高度的工作效率，在培养专业技能，保证手法质量，增强医疗效果以及防止职业性损伤等方面有着明显的效益。

The basic training methods they select vary obviously with the structures of the manipulations used in treatment, the ways they exert strength, and the indications. Introduced here are the main training skills of *"Yi Jin Jing"* (Sinew-transforming Exercise), and *"Shaolin Neigong"* (*Shaolin* Internal Cultivation Exercise) which are largely required in "massage with one-finger meditation", "rolling massage" and "internal skill massage".

2. Main Exercises for the Basic Training

1) Sinew-transforming Exercise (*Yi Jin Jing*)

Sinew-transforming Exercise is composed of twelve forms. Introduced hereof are the five commonly practised.

(1) Weituo's posture of Presenting the Pestle (Fig. 1—6)

Pithy Formula:

Keep erect when standing,

Hold the hands before the chest as if praying,

Set the breath even and the mind calm,

With a heart pure, soft and warm.

Movements:

① Preparatory posture: Stand erect. Step out with the left foot to set the feet apart at shoulder-width, with the feet on the ground steadily, the head picturing supporting an object on it, the eyes looking straight ahead, the chest tucked in and the back straightened, the tongue rested against the palate and the mouth slightly open; at the same time, raise the arms laterally to shoulder level to form a straight line, with palms facing the ground and fingers closed together.

② Move the two arms forward slowly to get the palms closed with fingertips pointing to the front.

③ Bend the elbows slowly to form an angle of 90 degrees, and keep the wrists, elbows and shoulders at the same level with the fingertips pointing upward.

④ Turn the arms and hands slowly inwards to point the fingertips toward the chest at the level of Tiantu (Ren 22),

中国推拿有许多流派，各流派因其治疗手法的动作结构、发力方式及主治范围不同，其选练的功法也有明显区别。现将本书介绍的"一指禅推拿"、"滚法推拿"与"内功推拿"所主练的"易筋经"、"少林内功"的主要功式介绍如下。

2．主要功法

1）易筋经

本功法全套共有十二个势式组成，推拿练功时最常用的有以下五势。

（1）韦驮献杵势（图1-6）

原文：立身期正直，环拱手当胸，气定神皆敛,心澄貌亦恭。

动作：①预备姿势：立正，左足向左平跨一步与肩等宽，双足平行，掌趾踏实，两腿站直，腘部微松，头如顶物,双目平视，含胸拔背，舌抵上腭，口唇稍开，同时两臂侧平举,掌心向下,五指并拢。

②两掌心向前慢慢合拢，指尖朝前。

③徐徐将肘关节屈曲至90°，使腕、肘、肩相平,五指朝上。

④两臂与手慢慢向内旋转，使指尖对胸与天突穴平。

Essentials: The practitioner should do the exercise with rapt attention. The muscles of all parts should be relaxed. Respiration should be orthodromic-abdominal, characterized by quick inhaling and slow exhaling and nasal inhaling and mouth exhaling. The mind is concentrated on *Dantian* and *qi* gathered in the lower abdomen. Beginners of the exercise may do it for three minutes each time and, one or two weeks later, increase the time by one or two minutes each week till they can do it for 20 minutes each session.

Note: Persistent training can increase the strength and the endurence of the muscles of the shoulder girdle and the circumflex muscles of the forearm and improve the flexibility of the wrist joint. It can raise the ability of the massagist's shoulders to support suspension during operation.

Another training can be adopted after step ① is practiced: turn hands slowly until they are before the chest to form a ball-holding posture, with the shoulders abducted at an angle of 45 degrees, the five fingers slightly bent and apart from each other, the centre of the palm dent, and the fingertips and the point Laogong of the two hands pointing at each other (Fig. 1—7).

(2) The Posture of Plucking and Resetting the Stars (Fig. 1—8)

Pithy Formula:

Over the head hold the sky with one palm,

Stare at the palm centre in calm,

With nasal inhaling frequently regulating the breath,

And shift the eyesight to another palm with strength.

Movements:

① Preparatory posture: Stand erect. Step forward with the right foot to form a T-shaped stance, the right heel pointing at the middle of the left foot with a space of about one fist. Make simultaneous movements of the two hands; the left, in "hollow" fist, is raised backwards to rest against the lumbosacral portion, and the right dropped to the internal side of the

要领：练习本势时，应全神贯注，各部肌肉放松，采用腹式顺呼吸，紧吸慢呼，鼻吸口呼，意守丹田，藏气于少腹。初练每次 3 分钟，1—2 周后，每周酌量增 1—2 分钟，一般增至 每次 20 分钟即可。

按语：本势久练能增强肩带肌肉与前臂旋肌的力量与耐 力，并能锻炼腕关节的柔韧性。提高术者手法操作时肩部的悬吊支持能力与前臂旋摆的持久力与灵活性。

另外，本势在动作①之后，也可改成以下练法：双手徐徐向前在胸前成抱球势，肩外展 45°左右，五指微屈自然分开，掌 心内凹，双手指端及劳宫穴相对（图 1-7）。

（2）摘星换斗势（图 1-8）

原文：只手擎天掌复头，更从掌内注双眸，鼻端吸气频调息，用力收回左右侔。

动作：①预备姿势：立正。右足向前外方跨出，成丁字步，右足跟与左足内缘中点相对，间距约为一拳。两手同时动作，左

right leg.

② Bend the left leg and squat down slowly till the angle at the knee is about 120—160 degrees. Simultaneously raise the right heel to get the right foot on tiptoe. The upper body should be kept straight without leaning foreward or backward.

③ Raise the right hand, with the palm facing downward and the five fingers close to each other like a hook, from the medial side of the leg slowly up along the midline of the abdomen and the chest till it reaches the head. Then tuck the upper arm in, turn the forearm sidewise and make the five fingers into "a hook" and the wrist bent, with the angle between the shoulder and the trunk being 90 degrees, the angle at the elbow 90 degrees and the angle at the wrist 90—100 degrees. Keep the upper part of the right arm static at the right side of the body.

④ Turn the fingertips sidewise as far as possible, meanwhile raise the head to stare at the centre of the palm.

When the left hand is trained, carry out the procedures in the same way.

Essentials: When squatting, the knee should not exceed the foot. The body weight should be shifted mainly to the leg at the back, the leg in the front only bears about 30% of the whole body weight. The raised hand should not be too high and it is desirable to have one-fist distance between the fingertips and the head. During practice, the five fingers should be in a pinch, the forearm should be abducted as far as possible to get the fingers pointing laterally, and the wrist should be flexed as much as possible. Keep the abducted forearm and the flexed wrist unmoved to sense the soreness, distention and pain for 10 seconds or so and then relax them for 10 seconds, and abduct them again. Do the exercise once and again within the time span required for the exercise. The practitioner should be attentive. The respiration method needed for it is as the same as that for the exercise "Weituo Presenting the Pestle", which should be as natural as possible. Do not hold breath

手握空拳，屈肘向后靠于腰骶部；右手向前垂于右大腿内侧。

②左腿屈膝徐徐下蹲（屈至约120°—160°左右），同时，右足跟提起，足尖点地，上身保持正直，不可前倾后仰。

③右手掌心朝下，五指握拢如钩状，自两腿间沿腹、胸中线缓缓举起，至头面部时，上臂内收，前臂外旋，钩手屈腕，呈肩前伸90°、屈肘90°、屈腕90°～100°的姿势，将右上肢停置于身体右侧。

④钩手指端再尽量向外略偏，同时，头略向右上方抬起，双目注视掌心。

练左手时，上述动作相反。

要领：屈膝下蹲时，膝不过足趾，全身重力主要落在后腿，前腿仅负担体重的30%左右。单手上举不要太高，以指尖离开头部约一拳为宜。在练习过程中，五指捏齐，尽量令前臂与外旋指尖指向外侧，并尽力屈腕，将前臂与腕停置在产生酸、胀、痛感觉的位置10秒钟左右，然后，前臂与指尖回到中位停10秒钟左右，再向外旋转，如此反复练习，直至完成规定的练功时间即可

when rotating the arms and generating strength. The beginners of the exercise may practise 1—2 minutes each time and, one week later, add one minute each week till the total time for each session amounts to 7 minutes. Then add one minute every two weeks. Generally, the practitioner should gradually get accustomed to 10—15 minutes for each session of practice.

Note: This exercise can enhance the supporting ability of the lower extremities. It is specially effective in increasing the energy and endurance of the greater pectoral muscle, deltoid muscle, biceps muscle of the arm, circum-lateral muscle of the forearm and the flexor groups of wrist and prolonging the ligament at the back of the wrist joint and the circum-medial muscle of the forearm to improve their reflexibility and anti-tention reaction. It is thus very important for the practitioner to cultivate the supporting ability of his shoulder when hand manipulation is performed, the amplitude and tolerance of his suspended wrist when single-finger meditation is done, the swaying strength and speed of the circum-lateral and circum-medial muscles of his forearm in rolling manipulation as well as his ability of long-time standing. As the exercise takes an important place in basic training of massage, the practitioner should do it perseveringly and repeatedly. However, considering the amount of the exercise, one should do it step by step and should never act with undue haste.

(3) The Posture of Pulling Nine Oxen by the Tails (Fig. 1-9)
Pithy Formula:
The front leg is a bow and the back an arrow,
The lower abdomen is filled with *qi* as if it were hollow,
The strength is directed to the two arms,
And the eyesight is set at the fist.
Movements:
① Preparatory posture: Stand erect.
② Turn the upper body towards the right. Take a big

收势。练习本势时应神志注一，呼吸方法同韦驮献杵，务使呼吸自然，旋臂发力时不得憋气屏息。初练每次 1～2 分钟，1 周后每周每次增加 1 分钟，至 7 分钟后，每两周增加 1 分钟。一般每次练至 10～15 分钟即可。

按语：本势可增强下肢的支持能力，特别对于增加胸大肌、三角肌、肱二头肌，前臂旋外肌及屈腕肌群的力量与持久力，拉长腕关节背侧韧带与前臂内旋肌，提高其柔韧性与抗拉伸力等，均有明显效果。因此，它对培养手法操作时肩部的持久支持力，一指禅推时悬腕的幅度与耐力，滚法时前臂内、外旋摆摆动的力度与速度，以及持久站立操作的能力等，都十分重要。本势在推拿专业练功中占重要地位，学习者一定要持之以恒，反复练习。但由于本势的运动量较大，故应注意循序渐进，不可操之过急。

（3）倒拽九牛尾势（图 1—9）

原文：两骸后伸前屈，小腹运气空松，用力在于两膀，观拳须注双瞳。

动作：①预备姿势：立正。

②上身向右转。右足向前跨出一大步，成右弓步。上身正直，

step forward with the right foot to form a forward lunge, with the upper body upright and falling slightly heavy on the legs, and the angle at the right knee being 90 degrees.

③ Clench one's fists, and stretch one forward not higher than the brows, with the other backward sticking against the lumbosacral portion, both palms facing upwards, the wrists slightly bent and the angle at the elbows being 140—150 degrees. (Fig. 1—10)

④ Set eyes on the centre of the front fist. Do not stretch the elbow forward so hard as to exceed the knee, or protrude the knee so hard as to exceed the toe. Turn the front arm outwards forcefully and the back inwards at the same time as if they were to be twisted into a string (with spiral strength), with the chest tucked in slightly, the back straight and qi gathered in the lower abdomen.

Turn about and change legs, with the upper part of the body toward the left. Carry out the same movements mentioned above.

Essentials: The practitioner should keep the muscles of the shoulder girdle relaxed without raising the shoulders. Strength is exerted at the shoulders intermittently, i. e., when conducting the string-twisting movements, get the "spiral strength" fixed at the location where you feel soreness, distention and pain for about 10 seconds, then relax for about 10 seconds before exerting strength again. Do this exercise for no more than three minutes each time in the first week, then increase one minute each week till 8—10 minutes for each session.

Note: The movements of this form can improve the force, endurance and anti-tension ability of the intorter and extortor of the forearm. They are essential for the training of rolling, pushing and scrubbing manipulations.

(4) The Posture of Three Dishes Falling to the Ground
Pithy Formula:

微向下沉，前腿曲膝90°位，不过足尖。

③两手握拳，前后伸出，拳心向上，两腕略屈，双肘屈曲140°～150°左右，前拳高不过眉，后拳平腰骶处，前后对称。

④双目注视前手拳心，肘不过膝，膝不过足。前臂用力旋外，后臂同时用力旋内，前后两臂成绞绳状（称为螺旋劲）。含胸拔背，胸略内涵，藏气于少腹。

换步时向后转，上身转向左侧，动作左右相同。

要领：肩带肌肉始终保持放松，肩部不要抬起。练功时，两膀反复间歇用力，即双臂在作绞绳状拧旋时，在感到酸、胀、痛的位置停留10秒钟左右后；再间歇10秒钟左右发力。呼吸同上势。初练每次3分钟，1周后每周增加1分钟。一般增至每次8～10分钟即可。

按语：本势主要可发展前臂内、外旋肌的肌力、耐力与抗拉伸力，对㨰法、推法、擦法等动作的训练有很大帮助。

（4）三盘落地势（图1—10）

The tongue is rested on the palate,
The eyes are open and the teeth gnashed.
The legs are bent in a horse stance,
And the hands are pressing firmly as if they were to get
  hold of something.
The palms are turned upwards,
As if a great amount of weight is added.
With the eyes wide open and mouth closed,
The feet are set firm and the body is kept straight.
Movements:

① Preparatory posture: Stand erect. Step out with the left foot to set the feet apart at shoulder-width or a little wider than the shoulders, with the toes slightly turned inward.

② Bend the knees and lower the hips. At the same time, let the palms face upward and elevate them from the sides of the body, along the chest, slowly to the level of the shoulders.

③ Turn the palms upside down and lower them slowly with the fingers separated naturally as if they were pressing something down-ward till they are above the knees. Turn the part between the thumb and the four fingers towards the body as if something, were held with the upper part of the body bending foreward slightly.

④ Set the upper part of the body upright with the chest squared, the back bow-like, and the muscles of the shoulder girdle relaxed. Without raising the shoulders, abduct the shoulder joints at about 50 degrees, with the elbows pointing outward, the forearm rotated inward, the thumbs stretched and the part between the thumb and the index finger turned inward. The neck should be straightened as if it were supporting an object on the head, with the eyes looking straight ahead, the mouth slightly open, the tongue against the palate and the breath (nasal) even.

Essentials: The degree of knee-bending depends on the loading ability and training background of the invididual.

原文：上腭坚撑舌，张眸意注牙，足开蹲似踞，手按猛如拿，两掌翻齐起，千斤重有加，瞪睛兼闭口，起立足无斜。

动作：①**预备姿势**：立正。左足向外横跨一步，两足与肩等宽或略宽于肩，足尖微向内收。

②屈膝，臀部下蹲。同时，两手掌心朝上，自体侧沿胸徐徐上托与肩相平。

③然后，两掌心翻转向下，缓缓下落，五指自然松开，如向下按物，至膝上悬空而驻，虎口朝里如握物状，上身稍向前俯。

④上身转为正直，前胸微挺，后背如弓肩带肌肉放松，肩部不要抬起，肩关节外展约50°，肘尖指向外侧，前臂旋内，拇指外展，虎口向内。头项正直如顶物，双目直视，口唇微开，舌抵上腭，鼻息调匀。

要领：曲膝下蹲的程度，要视各人的负荷能力与练功基础而

The practitioner should assume the high-level horse stance (the angle at the knee being about 160 degrees) at the beginning and change gradually to middle-level horse stance (the angle at the knee being 140—150 degrees or so), or low-level horse stance (the angle at the knee being 100—120 degrees or so). When squatting down, the upper part of the body should be kept straight all the time without bending forward like sitting on a stool, with the knees being within the perpendicular line with the feet. Do this exercise for one minute each time during the first week and add one minute each week after that till the total time comes to five minutes for each session.

Note: The practice of this form will render the axillae and arms more muscular force and endurance and higher anti-tension ability. It is especially important to acquire long-time supporting ability of the lower extremities which makes it easier for the massagist to direct strength and save the energy of the arms when he carries out hand manipulation.

(5) The Posture of the Prone Tiger Pouncing on Its Prey (Fig. 1—11)

Pithy Formula:

Squat with feet apart and incline forward,
Make the left leg bent and the right straight.
Hold up the head and chest to prostrate forward,
Lower the back and waist to get the body stable.
Inhale and Exhale with the breath even and regulated,
Touch the ground with fingertips for support.
Subdue the dragon and tame the tiger a happy thing to do,
And how helpful to health if the skill is learned.

Movements:

① Preparatory posture: Stand erect. Take a big step forward with the left foot, bend the knees at 90 degrees and straighten the right leg with only the toes touching the ground to form a left forward lunge.

② Stretch out the hands to touch the ground with all the

定，初练者可用高档(约屈膝至160°左右)，以后逐渐可选用中档(屈膝至140°～150°左右)，或低档(屈膝至100°～120°左右)。下蹲时，上身始终保持正直，如正身坐在凳子上一样，不可前俯借力。屈膝时膝不可超过足尖。本势初练每次1分钟，以后每周增加1分钟，一般至每次5分钟即可。

按语：通过本势的锻炼，能使腋、臂的肌力与耐力充沛，抗拉伸力增强。特别是对提高下肢的持久支撑力有重要作用，使手法动作时有一个稳固的下盘腿腰力量的支持而便于发力，且节省臂力。

（5）卧虎扑食势(图1—11)

原文：两足分蹲身似倾，屈伸左右腿相更，昂头胸作探前势，偃背腰还似砥平。鼻息调元均出入，指尖着地赖支撑。降龙伏虎神仙事，学得真形也卫生。

动作：①预备姿势：立正。左足向前跨出一大步，屈膝90°，右腿伸直用足尖蹬地，成左弓步。

②两手向前五指撑地，掌心悬空，后腿足跟提起，头向上抬，

fingers, with the centre of the palm suspended. Lift the heel of the right foot and raise the head to get the eyes looking straight ahead.

③ Withdraw the left leg and stretch it backwards to place the back of the left foot on the heel of the right. Tuck in the chest and contract the abdomen slightly to get the body straightened and the head raised.

④ Pull the body backwards, raise the buttocks and straighten the elbows. Then bend the elbows slowly with the head and body lowered to the front as if a prone tiger were ready to pounce on its prey. When the face is lowered about 2 *cun* above the ground, start to straighten the elbows slowly to get the head and body raised upwards to the front; Then pull the whole body backwards and raise the buttocks again to effect wave-like fluctuations.

Essentials: The practitioner should carry out the movements slowly. The fluctuations, which are flexible and suspended with overhanging strength combined with breathing, should be naturally connected. While exhaling, incline the upper part of the body forward slowly. The to-and-fro movement should be balanced and holding of breath should be avoided. The same is required for both left and right forward lunges. At the initial stage of training, the practitioner may support his body with both the fingers and the centre of the palms. When the strength of the arms and fingers is enhanced, he can support himself with the fingers, and so much the better, with only the thumb and the index and middle fingers. Do the exercise step by step according to the adaptability of the individual.

Note: Practising this form of exercise can increase the strength and endurance of the muscles of the shoulder girdle, brachial triceps muscle and biceps muscles of the arm. It is especially beneficial to the persistent supporting power and anti-tension ability of the fingers. Continued practice of it can

双目向前平视。

③前足收回向后伸直，将足背放在后足跟上，胸腹微收，躯干挺直，头向上昂起。

④全身后收，臀部向后突起，两肘挺直。然后，徐徐屈肘，头与躯干向前下方俯伸，如卧虎扑食之势，至头面部离地约2寸时，再缓缓伸肘，使头面与躯干向前上方慢慢抬起，接着全身后收，臀部向后突起，或波浪形起伏往返动作。

要领：全部动作要缓缓进行，昂俯起伏动作过渡要自然，用柔和的悬劲与呼吸密切配合。在呼气时将上身向前慢慢推送，往返动作力求平衡，切勿屏气。换步时，左右相同。本势初练时，也可用五指与掌心同时着地支撑，在臂力与指力增强的基础上，再用五指着地，最后以用拇指、食、中三指着地支撑为最佳。每次练习的次数要量力而行，循序渐进。

按语：本势能增强肩带诸肌、肱三头肌、肱二头肌的力量与耐力，特别是能发展手指的持久支撑力与抗拉伸力，久练还能使手指的关节、韧带、关节囊等组织变得粗壮坚韧。因此，能使术

turn the joints, ligaments and joint capsules sturdy and tensile. These benefits will manifest themselves in form of tremendous and persistent strength of the fingers and the pulling-pushing power of the forearms when the massagist carries out such hand manipulations as pushing, grasping, digital hitting, pressing, scrubbing and rolling. The exercise is also important in prevention of sports injury to the massagist himself when he does massage.

2) *Shaolin* Internal Cultivation Exercise (*Shaolin Nei-gong*)

Shaolin Internal Cultivation Exercise comprises a variety of forms. Introduced here are only basic stances and six common exercises, which can be practised either independently or connectedly and alternately.

(1) Basic Stances

① The Posture of the Up-right Standing

Preparatory Posture: Stand erect.

Movements: Set the feet apart a little wider than the shoulders, with the toes turned in to form inward splayfeet. Set the feet with "hegemonic force" on the ground with the head upright, the eyes looking straight ahead, the breath natural, the shoulders dropped, chest squared to get the scapulae closer to the spinal column, the waist relaxed, the lower abdomen contracted, the buttocks tucked in, and the arms akimbo (fingers in the front and the thumb at the back), to get ready for the exercise (Fig. 1—12).

Essentials: "Hegemonic force" means a force-exerting method which needs the practitioner to get the ten toes clutching at the ground while directing strength to the heels and the thighs which are turned sidewise and tightened.

② The Horse-riding Stance

Preparatory Posture: Stand erect.

Movements: Set the feet apart a little wider than the shoulders in the form of pedes varus. Bend the knees (not

者在进行推、拿、点、按、擦、揉等手法操作时，发挥出强大而持久的指力与前臂的推拉力，并对防止手法操作时自身的运动创伤也有重要作用。

2）少林内功

少林内功的功势很多，这里仅介绍基本裆势与六个常用功势。这些势式可单独进行练习，也可连接起来相互变换进行锻炼。

（1）基本裆势

①站裆势

预备姿势：立正。

动作：两足分开，其间距略宽于双肩，足尖朝里，双足成内八字。下肢用霸力站稳，头端平，目平视，呼吸自然，沉肩，挺胸，两肩胛骨向脊柱靠拢，腰间放松，少腹含蓄，臀部微收，两手叉腰，四指在前，拇指在后。待势（图1--12）。

要领：霸力，即双足以十趾用力抓地，同时，两足跟与大腿发力，使劲外旋、夹紧的用力方法。

②马步势

预备姿势：立正。

动作：两足分开，其间距较肩稍宽，而足成内八字，屈膝下蹲，膝不可向前超过足尖。头端平，目前视，挺胸直腰，臀部下

exceed the vertical line with the feet), with the head set upright, eyes looking straight ahead, chest squared and waist straightened, buttocks dropped (do not stick them backward), and arms akimbo to get prepared for the exercises (Fig. 1—13).

Essentials: The extent of knee-bending can be classified into high-position standing, mid-position standing and low-position standing (see the details in the form "Three Plates Falling on the Ground"). The practitioner may select whatever kind that suits his health status on the basis of his training background.

③ The Posture of the Forward Lunge

Preparatory posture: Stand erect.

Movements: Set one foot in the front and one at the back, with the distance between the feet being about two times as wide as the shoulders. The front leg is bent slightly with the toes inward and the shank being vertical with the ground. The back leg is straightened as much as possible, with the toes being turned slightly outward. The head is set upright with the eyes looking straight ahead, the chest squared and waist relaxed, the abdomen and buttocks contracted or tightened, and arms akimbo to get ready for the exercises (Fig. 1—14).

(2) Common Forms of *Shaolin* Internal Cultivation Exercise

① Stretching the Arms and Supporting the Palms (Fig. 1—15)

Preparatory Posture: Stand as mentioned above.

Movements: After several minutes' standing, get the two palms of the hands which are akimbo facing the floor, with the fingers closed to each other and stretched and the two thumbs abducted forcefully to form a right angle. Dorsiflex the wrist joints, stretch the arms slowly backwards, square the chest, get the scapulae as close to the spinal column as possible, and rotate the forearms forward forcefully with the fingers pointing inward and the palm root pointing outward. Raising of the

沉不要向后突起，两手叉腰，待势（图1—13）。

要领：下蹲的幅度分高档、中档与低档（详见"三盘落地势"），可根据自己的身体与功力情况选择练习。

③弓步势

预备姿势：立正。

动作：两腿一前一后分开，两足之间距离约较肩宽一倍；前腿屈膝，足尖向里，小腿约与地面垂直；后腿用劲挺直，足尖略外展。头端平，目平视，挺胸塌腰，蓄腹收臀，两手叉腰，待势（图1—14）。

（2）少林内功常用功势

①伸臂撑掌（图1—15）

预备姿势：站势。

动作：站势数分钟后，叉腰的两手变俯掌（掌心向下），四指并拢伸直，拇指用力外展与四指约成直角，腕关节尽力背伸，双臂慢慢向后伸直，挺胸，两肩胛骨向脊柱夹紧，前臂用力旋前，使

shoulders should be avoided; the angle between the backward-stretched arm and the trunk should be 30—45 degrees and the elbows should be straight. Breathe naturally and direct *qi* with will to flow through the whole body including the fingers and toes.

Essentials: This is one of the most foundamental standing exercises of Shaolin Internal Cultivation Exercise. During practice, attention should be paid to the "three straightnesses and four levelnesses", i.e., straightnesses of the arms, the body and the legs, and levelnesses of the head, the shoulders, the palms and the feet. The exercise may also be practised in the horse stance or the forward lunge posture. Only one minute is enough at the initial stage of practice. The duration of each session should be prolonged step by step on account of conditions till, as a general rule, the total time of each session comes to ten minutes.

Function: Persistent practice of the exercise will enable the practitioner to direct *qi* with will, train *qi* and transform it into essence, and train essence to improve the vitality, which usually makes the practitioner full of energy and the function of his viscera strong and enables him to transfer *qi* into energy which fills the whole body including the extremities to provide more strength and ability of endurance to the hips, the waist and the legs.

② Pushing Eight Horses Forward (Fig. 1—16)

Preparatory posture: Stand erect or take the horse stance or forward lunge. The elbows are bent at 90 degrees, with palms facing upwards and the thumbs stretched to form a right angle with the fingers.

Movements: Direct strength to the arms and the fingertips. Push the arms forward slowly while turning the palms to get them facing each other, with the thumbs pointing upward. Continue the pushing till the elbows are straight and the arms at the level of the shoulders.

双手指尖向里，掌根朝外。肩部不要抬起，肩关节后伸约30°～45°，肘关节伸直。呼吸自然，以意运气，使气贯全身与四末。

要领：本势是少林内功主要的基础站桩功，练习时要注意"三直四平"（三直，即臂直，身直，腿直；四平，即头平，肩平，掌平，脚平）。本势也可在马步势或弓步势的裆位上进行锻炼。初练从每次1分钟开始，以后据情况慢慢增加练功时间，一般增至每次10分钟即可。

作用：本势久练能以意运气，练气生精，练精全神，使精神充沛，脏腑功能强健，并以气生劲，使劲力充实全身与四肢，增加臂、腰、腿部的力量与耐力。

②前推八匹马（图1—16）

预备姿势：站势。也可作马步或弓步势。两臂屈肘90°，掌心向上，拇指外展伸直与四指约成直角。

动作：蓄劲于双臂及指端，两臂徐徐用力前推。同时，慢慢旋内，使两掌向对，拇指向上，直至肘关节伸直，双臂与肩平齐。

Essentials: Carry out the above-mentioned pushing and pulling for 3—5 times. The pushing-pulling of the arms can also be carried out alternately: the left being pushed while the right. pulling or vice versa. The breathing and strength-exerting of the legs is conducted in the same way as mentioned in the exercise "Stretching the Arms and Supporting the Palms."

Function: This form and those prescribed hereafter are all carried out by continuing strength-directing movements of the upper arms in a state of fixed standing posture. Long-term practice of this type can develop the standing stability and supporting ability of the lower extremities during the movements of the upper extremities and the coordination of the upper and lower extremities to ensure that the strength-directing in the upper extremities and hand manipulations can be smoothly carried out.

③ Pulling Nine Oxen Backward (Fig. 1—17)

Preparatory Posture: See the preparatory posture mentioned in ②.

Movements:

a. Push both arms slowly forward while slowly turning the forearms inward to get the back of the palms facing each other and the thumbs pointing downward at the time when the elbows are straight.

b. Turn palms into tight fists and withdraw the hands while turning the forearms outward as if pulling a strong ox by the tail. When the fists reach the hypochondria, change them into palms which face upward (in the preparatory posture). Stop moving for a minute and then repeat the above back-and-forth movements for altogether 3—5 times.

④ The Overlord Holding-up the Tripod (Fig. 1—18)

Preparatory Posture: See the preparatory posture mentioned in ②.

Movements: With the palms facing upward, raise the arms slowly like holding up a heavy object. When the palms are

要领：锻炼时，可按上述动作，来回推动 3 — 5 次，也可单臂左右交替练习。呼吸与腿部用力方法与伸臂撑掌势同。

作用：本势及以下各势都是在定式裆势下进行的上肢持续性发力动作，久练能发展上肢运动时的下肢稳固的支撑能力与上下配合的协调功能，以利于上肢的发力与手法动作的顺利完成。

③倒拉九头牛（图 1—17）

预备姿势：同上。

动作：

两臂用力缓缓向前推运，同时前臂慢慢内旋，至肘伸直时，两掌心向外，手背向对，拇指向下。

再化掌为拳，用力握紧，并徐徐屈肘收拳，同时前臂外旋，势如向后倒拉犍牛状，至拳达两胁时，变拳为仰掌（还原至预备姿势）。稍作停顿后再重复上势动作，可往返 3—5 次。

④霸王举鼎（图 1—18）

预备姿势：同上。

动作：

两掌心向上，如托重物用力缓缓上举，过肩肘双臂徐徐内旋，

above the shoulders, turn the arms gently inward while stretching them until they are straightened, at the same time, get the fingers of the two hands pointing at each other, palms facing upward, with fingers close to each other and the thumbs as widely apart from them as possible.

b. Hold the "tripod" with force for a minute, then rotate the forearms gently to get the palms facing each other, fingertips pointing upward. Lower the palms with force along the chest until they get to the hypochondria. Stop for a moment and then repeat the movement for 3—5 times.

⑤ The Wind Swaying the Lotus Leaf (Fig. 1—19)

Preparatory posture: See the preparatory posture mentioned in ②.

Movements:

a. With the palms facing upward, stretch the arms slowly forward until the elbows are straight with the palms crossed in front of the chest, the left above the right or vice versa, the space between the two palms being about 1—2 *cun*.

b. Then get the arms apart from each other (the palms still in a pose of holding an object) till an angle of 90 degrees is formed at the shoulder. Then draw the arms towards each other until they are right in front of the chest, with two palms crossed again. Lastly draw the palms back with strength to the sides of the chest. Keep the pose unchanged for a moment and then repeat the above procedures for 3—5 times.

⑥ The Entry of The Black Dragon into the Cave (Fig. 1—20)

Preparatory posture: Take a wide forward lunge with the elbows bent and the hands stretched at the sides of the waist.

Movements:

a. Get the centres of the two palms facing each other and push them slowly forward. While pushing, turn the palms to get them facing downward, with the fingertips pointing forward, the upper body inclining forward and the toes turned inward.

至肘向上挺直时，手指向对，掌心向上，四指并拢，拇指外展伸直。

蓄势片刻后，前臂渐渐旋外，翻掌使掌心与掌面相对，指端向上，自胸前蓄力而下，收回至腰肋两侧。稍待后，仍按上述姿势反复推举 3—5 次。

⑤风摆荷叶（图 1—19）

预备姿势：同上。

动作：

仰掌向前上方徐徐用力推出，至肘伸直时，两掌在胸前交叉，左在右上或右在左上均可，而掌上下相间 1—2 寸。

然后两臂向左右分开，手掌仍保持托物状，至肩关节外展 90°位，再慢慢内收至正前方，两掌交叉，再缓缓用劲收两掌至腰侧。稍待后，再按上势反复练习 3～5 次。

⑥乌龙钻洞（图 1—20）

预备姿势：取大弓档，两臂屈肘，直掌于腰侧待势。

动作：

两直掌掌心相对，徐徐向前推运，边推掌心边向下逐渐化成俯掌，指尖朝前，上身随势前俯，两足尖内扣，用霸力站稳。

Stand firm with "hegemonic force".

b. Push the palms forward until the elbows are straight. Then rotate the arms and palms outward and flex the elbows to pull them back with force and, while getting the palms facing upward slowly, withdraw them to the hypochondria. Keep still for a moment and repeat the movements 3—5 times.

3. Points for Attention during the Exercises

Those who are learning massage should be fully aware of the importance and necessity of basic exercises in the training of professional skills and should be determined to study diligently and train hard. The following points should be kept in mind during the exercises.

1) The exercises should be done orderly and step by step. The duration and the amount of exercise should be arranged reasonably according to one's physiological characteristics and loading ability. The principle of practice should be from simple to complicated, from little to a large amount and from mild to intensified.

2) The practitioner should be assiduous and perseverant. It is advisable to do the exercises for 30—60 minutes daily. Practice by fits and starts should be avoided.

3) The practitioner should concentrate on one form of exercise. This is especially important to the beginners, who should not chop and change. Students of massage should take the Sinew-transforming Exercises and *Shaolin* Internal Cultivation Exercise introduced in this book as the fundamental exercises for practice. Other exercises can be practiced when the above two kinds have been basically mastered and the practitioner has become somewhat skilled in training.

4) During practice, one should concentrate himself, combining mental activities and the movements in one. Joking or holding breath during exercises and forced, reckless practice

向前推至两肘伸直后，即再双臂外旋，两掌外翻，用力屈肘回收，边收掌心边慢慢朝上，收至腰胁两侧。稍待后，再如上势反复3～5次。

3．练功注意事项

推拿学员既要充分认识练功在专业技能训练中的重要性与必要性，下决心勤学苦练，又要在练功时注意以下各点：

1）练功必须循序渐进，并根据各自不同的生理特点与负荷能力，合理安排练功时间与运动量。应掌握从简到繁，从少到多，由弱渐强的原则。

2）练功要持之以恒，以每日坚持练功30分钟至1小时为宜，不可时练时停。

3）选练功法要专一，特别是初练者不可朝此夕彼。推拿学员应以本章介绍的易筋经与少林内功为基本功法进行锻炼，待基本掌握且有一定的功底后，再选练其他功法。

4）练功时要思想集中，心神合一，不开玩笑，不可屏气，不得勉强、蛮干。对练功中出现的异常感觉，如头晕、胸闷、胸痛、

should be avoided. If any abnormal feelings such as dizziness, stuffiness or pain in the chest and fidgetiness occur during the practice, one should consult the massage tutor in time lest exercising deviation or injury should arise.

5) It is necessary for the practitioner to have a quiet, well-lit and will-ventilated place with appropriate temperature. Practising against cold wind should be avoided.

6) It is advisable for the practitioner to wear loose clothes and cloth shoes with soft soles, gym shoes or special exercise shoes. It is not suitable to wear leather shoes or high-heel shoes. Wearing tight or more than enough clothes should be avoided.

7) It is desirable to do the exercises in the morning. The practitioner should not do the exercise when he is quite full or has an empty stomach, or after strenuous exercise or when he is tired. When the practice is over or broken for a rest, the practitioner should wipe the sweat away with a dry towel and put on clothes. Either fanning or cold bath immediately after the exercise is harmful to the health. The proper way is to limber oneself so as to regulate qi and blood, and take some warm tea and nutritious drinks.

8) Female should not do the exercise during the menstrual period or pregnancy.

9) The exercises introduced in this chapter are also therapeutic. However, when the tutor teaches the patient to practise, he should pay special attention to, apart from the above-mentioned aspects, the principle of differential selection of exercises, viz., to select an exercise or a training method that is suitable to the practitioner's health status, age, sex and the severity of his illness, to adjust the amount of exercise with the training method and to practise orderly and step by step. The intensity and duration of the exercise should be adjusted in time on changes of the conditions of the patient. In cooperation with the patient, the massagist may select a specific method of hand manipulation to treat a certain part

烦躁等，要及时求得教师的指导，以免发生练功偏差与损伤。

5）练功的环境要保持安静，室内要光线充足，温度适宜，空气流通，但要避免寒风直接吹到身上。

6）练功者的衣服宜宽松，不要穿得过多或过紧，不宜穿皮鞋或高跟鞋，以穿软底布鞋、球鞋或练功鞋为宜。

7）练功时间最好安排在早晨，练时不宜过饱或空腹，练功前不要做剧烈运动。疲劳时不宜练功。练功完毕或中间休息时，宜用干毛巾将汗擦干，穿好衣服，不可马上吹风或用冷水冲洗。结束后要适当活动身体，以调和气血，并可饮些温热茶水与营养性饮料。

8）女子经期或孕期不宜练功。

9）本章介绍的功法也可作为医疗性练功。但在指导患者锻炼时，除必须注意上述各项外，还要特别注意遵循辨证选功的原则，即根据患者的病情、体质、年龄、性别等具体情况，选择适宜的功法或功式进行锻炼，适当掌握练功的运动量与功式的组合，并强调循序渐进，随着病情的变化，及时调整练功的强度、时间。另外，还可配合一定的功式与功法，在一些特殊的部位应用特定

of the body, for example, the massagist may ask the patient to take a certain training posture and direct his strength to the part to be massaged for effecting a combination of external massage with internal response so that the channel *qi* can be activated and regulated.

Section 4

The Fourteen Channels and Their Commonly-used Points

Shisijing (fourteen channels) is a general term for the twelve regular channels connecting the twelve internal organs, and the *Ren* Channel and the *Du* Channel of the Eight Extra-channels. The theory of the fourteen channels and their commonly-used points is considered as the principal component of the meridian doctrine and the point doctrine and as the most practical and important theoretical rudiment in massage. It is so said because it forms the basis of all the clinical applications, acting as a fundamental guideline in all aspects including the diagnosis of diseases and differentiation of syndromes, determination of treatment methods and prescriptions of the points, and selection of hand manipulations as well as their performing methods such as light, heavy, slow, rapid and orthodromic or antidromic. So, to master massage, one must first learn the massage doctrine.

1. An Outline of the Fourteen Channels

1) The Twelve Channels

The Twelve Channels are generally regarded as the principal part of the channel system, so they are also called "twelve regular channels". They respectively pertain to twelve internal organs, and are named after them. For example, the channel related to the heart is called "the Heart Channel" and

的手法治疗，如采取一定的练功姿势，并令患者运气于接受手法的部位，使治疗内外呼应，以增强对经气的激发与调整作用。

第四节 十四经与常用腧穴

联属十二脏腑的十二经脉与奇经八脉中的任、督二脉，合称为十四经。有关十四经与常用腧穴的理论，是经络学说与腧穴学说的主体内容，也是推拿学实践中最有实用价值、最重要的理论基础。这是因为在推拿临床工作中，从对疾病的诊断、辨证，到治疗配穴处方，手法选择乃至手法动作的轻、重、缓、急与顺逆方向等，无不以经络、腧穴学说为指导。所以欲精推拿者，必须首先学习这些理论。

1．十四经概述

1）十二经脉

十二经脉是经络系统的主体，故又称"十二正经"。它们分属于十二脏腑，并以其所属脏腑而命名。如属于心脏的经络称为"心经"，属于大肠的经脉称为"大肠经"……，属于脏的经脉总称为

that related to the large intestine called "the Large Intestine Channel". Those related to the *zang*-organs are termed "*yin* channel", and to the *fu*-organs, "*yang* channel". They are further divided into three *yin* channels of hand, three *yin* channels of foot, three *yang* channels of hand and three *yang* channels of foot based on the distribution of *yin* channels and *yang* channels in the upper or lower extremities. The details of this part are introduced in the book *Basic Theory of Traditional Chinese Medicine* (I), one of the twelve books of this Library.

The distributing law of the twelve channels on the body surface is: the *yang* channels are mainly distributed on the lateral aspects of the upper and lower limbs and on the back; the *yin* channels mainly on the medial aspects and abdomen (except for the Stomach Channel of Foot-*Yangming* which has its branches of the trunk distributed on the abdomen) the three *yin* channels of hand run from the chest to the hand, the three *yang* channels of hand from the hand to the head, the three *yin* channels of foot from the foot to the abdomen and the three *yang* channels of foot from the head to the foot.

The twelve channels are linked with each other through their branches and collaterals, which constitute six pairs of "interior-exterior" and "pertaining" relations between *zang*-organs and *fu*-organs. Of the twelve channels, the *yin* channels pertain to the *zang*-organs and connect the *fu*-organs while the *yang* channels pertain to the *fu*-organs and connect the *zang*-organs. Through communication with the channels of hand and foot, the twelve channels joint together and form an endless ring, in which *qi* and blood start circulating from the Lung Channel, go through the other channels and finally enter the Liver Channel, and then to the Lung Channel again to restart circulation. *Qi* and blood circulate round and again to nourish the whole body continuously. The names of the twelve channels, their exterior-

"阴经"，属于腑的经脉总称为"阳经"。此外，又根据阴经与阳经在上肢或下肢的分布，又有手、足三阴经和手、足三阳经之分。具体可见本文库《中医基础理论》上册有关部分。

十二经脉在体表的分布规律是：阳经主要分布在上肢与下肢的外侧面以及背部，阴经主要分布在上肢与下肢的内侧面以及腹侧（但足阳明胃经在躯干部的经络例外，分布在腹侧）。手三阴经从胸部起，循行至手部，手三阳经从手部起，循行至头部；足三阴经从足部起，循行至腹部；足三阳经从头部起，循行至足部。

十二经脉通过支脉和络脉的沟通衔接，在脏与腑之间形成六组互为"表里"的"属络"关系。十二经脉阴经属脏络腑，阳经属腑络脏。十二经脉再通过同名手足经的交接，构成了十二经脉的循环传注，即始于肺经，循行诸经而终于肝经，又复始于肺经，如此循环，周而复始，如环无端，从而使人体气血以营运全身，周流不息。十二经的全称、表里关系及流注衔接规律见下表：

interior relations and their flowing order are shown in the following table.

Exterior-Interior Relationship and Flowing Order of the Twelve Channels

The channels of the *zang*-organs are of *yin* channel and belong to the interior.	The channels of the *fu*-organs are of *yang* channel and belong to the exterior.
→ The Lung Channel of Hand-*Taiyin* (1) ⇄	the Large Intestine Channel of Hand-*Yangming* (2)
the Spleen Channel of Foot-*Taiyin* (4) ⇄	the Stomach Channel of Foot-*Yangming* (3) ←
→ the Heart Channel of Hand-*Shaoyin* (5) ⇄	the Small Intestine Channel of Hand-*Taiyang* (6)
the Kidney Channel of Foot-*Shaoyin* (8) ⇄	the Urinary Bladder Channel of Foot-*Taiyang* (7) ←
→ the Pericardium Channel of Hand-*Jueyin* (9) ⇄	the *Sanjiao* Channel of Hand-*Shaoyang* (10)
the Liver Channel of Foot-*Jueyin* (12) ⇄	the Gall Bladder Channel of Foot-*Shaoyang* (11) ←

Note: ←--→ means exterior-interior relationship; ⟶ means flowing order.

The physiological functions of the twelve channels mainly concern three respects: connecting all parts of the body, transporting *qi* and blood and regulating the function of the body.

The channels and collaterals communicate with the viscera and extremities closely, making the five *zang*-organs, six *fu*-organs, extremities, bones, skin, muscles, tendons as well as the five sense organs an organic whole. Channel or "*jing*" in Chinese implies route, which is the main passage in the system of the channel and collateral; while collateral or "*luo*" in Chinese, means "net", which is the branch of the channel in the system. The channels and collaterals spread all over the body and form a criss-cross network, in which *qi* and blood make their circulation and transport various nutrients to the tissues and organs in all parts to maintain the normal physiological functions of the human body. Through the criss-cross connection and overall

十二经脉流注，表里关系表

(←……→示属络表里，→示传注)

| 脏为阴经，属里 | 腑为阳经，属表 |

```
  ┌─► 手太阴肺经①  ◄═══► 手阳明大肠经②─┐
  ├─  足太阴脾经④  ◄═══► 足阳明胃经  ③─┤
  ┌─  手少阴心经⑤  ◄═══► 手太阳小肠经⑥─┐
  ├─  足少阴肾经⑧  ◄═══► 足太阳膀胱经⑦─┤
  ┌─  手厥阴心包经⑨ ───► 手少阳三焦经⑩─┐
  └─  足厥阴肝经⑫  ◄═══► 足少阳胆经 ⑪─┘
```

十二经脉的生理功能，主要体现在沟通内外、运行气血和调节平衡三个方面。

经络内属脏腑，外络肢节，将人体的五脏六腑、四肢百骸、皮肉筋脉及五官等组织、器官紧密地联系成为一个有机的整体。"经"有"途径"之意，是经络系统直行的主要干道；"络"有"网络"之意，是"经"的分支，它们纵横交叉，密布全身。人体的气血就是在这个系统中运行，将各种营养物质传注输布给全身各部的组织、器官，从而维持人体各部的正常生理功能；并通过经络的纵横联系与整体调节，使人体各部相互配合，相互协调，达到抵御

regulation by the channels and collaterals, all parts of the human body cooperate and coordinate with each other to resist invasion of the external pathogenic factors and maintain the normal function of the organism.

Pathogenically, the channels and collaterals are, on the other hand, the reaction system of illness and the transmission routes of diseases. Diseases of the internal organs can be manifested on the body surface by way of channels and collaterals. For instance, some internal diseases often have tenderness and allergic reaction or other manifestations on a certain location of the body surface, as can be seen in waist pain due to kidney disease and pain in the back caused by gastric disorder; while injury and diseases of the body surface can penetrate to affect the internal organs at various depths by way of the system of channel and collateral. Disease of one organ may, if not given timely treatment, affect other organs because of their exterior-interior relationship.

2) The *Ren* Channel and the *Du* Channel

The channels of *Ren*, *Du*, *Chong*, *Dai*, *Yangqiao*, *Yinqiao*, *Yangwei* and *Yinwei* are called, in a general term, the Eight Extra Channels. They are different from the twelve regular channels in that they have neither direct nor exterior-interior relationship with the internal organs. Their main physiological function is to regulate *qi* and blood inside the twelve regular channels according to whether *qi* and blood in the twelve channels are "insufficient" or "overflowing."

The *Ren* Channel runs along the midline of the abdomen and the chest to the mandible. Because it meets all the *yin* channels of the body in its course, it is also named "the sea of the *yin* channels". The *Ren* Channel is able to regulate *qi* in the *yin* channels.

The *Du* Channel runs along the midline of the waist, the back and the nape to the vertex and the face. It meets all the *yang* channels of the body in its course and is so named "the sea

外邪侵袭和维持机体正常功能的目的。

在病理状态下，经络又是病证的反应系统与疾病 的 传 变 途
径。内脏的疾病通过经络可反映到体表，如某些内脏疾病，往往
在体表的某一特定部位出现压痛、过敏点等病理反应，如肾病腰
痛，胃病背痛等；而体表的损伤和疾病又可通过经络系统，由浅
入深地影响到体内各层次的组织器官，某一脏器的疾病如不及时
防治，也可通过经络的表里络属关系，从而使其他的脏器患病。

2）任脉与督脉

任、督二脉与冲脉、带脉、阳跷脉、阴跷脉、阳维脉、阴维
脉总称为奇经八脉。它们与十二正经不同，既不直接属于脏腑，
亦无表里相配关系。其生理功能主要是根据十二经脉气血的盈亏
状况，对其起"蓄"或"溢"的调节作用。

任脉，行于腹、胸正中，上至颏部。全身阴经的经脉均与之
交会，故又称"阴脉之海"，有调节诸阴经经气的作用。

督脉，行于腰、背、项正中，上至头面。全身阳经的经脉均

of the *yang* channels". It has the function of regulating channel *qi* in the *yang* channels.

Traditional Chinese Medicine usually puts the *Ren* and *Du* channels and the twelve regular channels together and calls them "the fourteen channels", mostly because the *Ren* and *Du* Channels have their own points and have important physiological functions as mentioned above.

2. An Outline of the Points

The term Shuxue (points) has several names in Chinese, such as *xuewei, qixue, gukong* and *kongxue*. In Chinese *shu* means transfusion, transmission, conveyance and transportation, while *xue* means hole and pooling. The points are the locations where *qi* and blood of the channels and collaterals and of the viscera come in and go out and pool.

The points are classified as three kinds: "channel points", referring to those that have specific names and locations and are ranged along the course of the fourteen channels; "extra-ordinary points" (extrachannel-points), referring to those which have not been included in the fourteen channels although they have definite locations and names; and "Ashi points" or "*Tianying* points", referring to those that have no specific names and fixed locations and are usually to be decided on the locations of tenderness and other reactions.

All the points, no matter what they are, have close relations with the channels and collaterals. They are closely connected with the viscera and all the tissues of the body by means of channels and collaterals. They can not only manifest the physiological and pathological changes of the viscera and the tissues and organs pertaining to them and provide basis for clinical diagnosis and selection of points and manipulation methods, but also act as the stimulation spots for massage. So, to stimulate the points by hand manipulation may facilitate the readjusting functions of the corresponding

与之交会，故又称"阳脉之海"，有调节诸阳经经气的作用。

由于任、督二脉各有其专属的腧穴，且具有上述重要的生理功能，故中医常将其与十二正经合称为"十四经"。

2．腧穴概述

腧穴，又称输穴、穴位、气穴、骨空、孔穴。"腧"有输注、输送、转输、运输之意；"穴"有孔隙、聚集之意。腧穴是人体经络、脏腑气血输注出入与聚集的部位。

腧穴有以下三种：凡是有特定的名称，一定位置、按十四经循行排列的腧穴，称为"经穴"；虽有明确位置与名称，但未被列入十四经系统的腧穴，称为"经外奇穴"。此外，还有既无具体名称，又无固定位置，而以压痛点或其他反应点定取的穴位，称为"阿是穴"或"天应穴"。

无论何种腧穴，都与经络有密切的关系。腧穴通过经络与脏腑及全身各组织密切相连，它不仅可以反映脏腑及其所属组织、器官的生理或病理变化，作为临床辨证及制定推拿穴位与手法处方的依据，而且还是接受推拿手法的刺激点。因此，对腧穴进行手法刺激，就可进一步调动相应经络的调节作用，以调节脏腑

channels and collaterals, which in turn regulate the function of *qi* and blood in the viscera and activate the resistence of the organism itself to prevent and treat diseases.

Whether the location of a point is right or not may directly affect the effect of massage treatment. And only when one takes a correct locating method, can he find the correct position of a point. The following methods are usually used in point location.

1) Bone-length Measurement

The various regions of the body are given certain length and width and are divided into several equal portions, each division being termed one *cun* and taken as the unit of measurement for locating points. The method is applicable to patients of any age group with any body build. Division of various regions is shown in Fig. 1—21 and the following table.

Regions	Beginning and end	Method of measurement	Length in *cun*	Explanation
Head	Anterior hairline to posterior hairline	Vertical	12	Or 18 *cun* from ophryon to Dazhui (Du14), minus 3 *cun* from ophryon to anterior hairline and 3 *cun* from Dazhui to posterior hairline
Chest and abdomen	Between two nipples	Horizontal	8	For horizontal measurement of chest and abdomen
	From xiphosternal synchondrosis to umbilicus	Vertical	8	

气血的功能，激发机体内在的抗病能力，从而达到防病治病的目的。

取穴正确与否能直接影响推拿治疗的效果。而临诊时，只有采用一定的取穴方法，才能找到穴位的准确位置。常用的取穴法有以下几种：

1）骨度分寸取穴法

将人体各部规定一定的长度与宽度，折成若干等分，每一等分作为1寸，用这种方法来折量取穴的称为"骨度分寸法"。本法适用于任何年龄、任何体型的患者。各部位分寸见下表及 图1—21。

部 位	起 止 点	量法	寸数	说 明
头 部	前发际至后发际	直量	12	如前后发际不明，则可从眉心量至大椎穴作18寸。眉心至前发际为3寸，大椎穴至后发际为3寸。
胸 腹 部	两乳头之间	横量	8	用于胸腹部取穴横寸。
	胸剑联合至脐中	直量	8	

	From umbilicus to upper border of pubic symphysis	Vertical	5		
Back	From two medial borders of scapulae	Horizontal	6	For horizontal measurement of waist and back	
Upper limbs	From anterior axillary fold to transverse cubital crease	Vertical	9	Applicable to measurement of both medial and lateral aspects of upper limbs	
	From transverse cubital crease to transverse carpal crease	Vertical	12		
Lower limbs	From femoral trochanter to centre of patella	Vertical	19	For measurement of thigh	For measurement of anterior, lateral and posterior aspects of lower limbs
	From centre of patella to tip of lateral malleolus	Vertical	16	For measurement of shank	
	From pubis to upper border of internal epicondyle of femur	Vertical	18	For measurement of thigh	For measurement of medial aspect of lower limbs
	From lower border of medial condyle of tibia to top of medial malleolus	Vertical	13	For measurement of shank	

2) Finger-length Measurement

This is a method with which the fingers of the patient are used for measurement to locate points. If the body build of the patient is similar to that of the doctor, the doctor may use

		脐中至耻骨联合上缘	直量	5	
背 部		两肩胛内缘之间	横量	6	用于腰背部取穴横寸
上 肢		腋前横纹至肘横纹	直量	9	上肢内、外侧通用
		肘横纹至腕横纹	直量	12	
下 肢		股骨大转子至膝中	直量	19	用于大腿 · 用于下肢前、外、后侧
		膝中至外踝尖	直量	16	用于小腿
		耻骨平线至股骨内上髁上缘	直量	18	用于大腿 · 用于下肢内侧
		胫骨内侧髁下缘至内踝尖	直量	13	用于小腿

2）指寸法

这是一种以患者手指来测量取穴的方法。如患者身长与医者相仿，也可以医生的手指来量取。一般以中指中节屈曲时两端纹

his own fingers in measurement.   Generally, the distance between the two ends of the interphalangeal joints of the middle finger, when it is flexed, is taken as one *cun*. The breadth of the four fingers (index, middle, ring, and little fingers) close to each other is taken as 3 *cun* (Fig. 1—22)

3) Measurement According to the Anatomical Landmark

To locate a point on the basis of the anatomical landmarks on the body surface is the most fundamental method of point location. The following two approaches are often applied clinically

(1) Fixed Anatomical Landmark

It refers to marks which can not be changed by movement, such as the five sense organs, nipples, umbilicus as well as the prominances or depressions of various bone joints.

(2) Movable Landmark

It refers to marks that appear when a certain posture is assumed in movement, such as the depression or prominance of the muscles, the appearence of the muscle tendon and the creases of the skin.

3. The Course of the Fourteen Channels, Their Commonly-used Points and the Manipulations of Massage

1) The Lung Channel of Hand-*Taiyin* (Fig. 1—23)

It originates in the middle-*jiao* and runs downward to communicate with the large intestine and upward into its pertaining organ, the lung.   It comes transversely and superficially from the pulmonary series (system) to the point Zhongfu (Lu 1) and descends along the radial border of the arm and the radial side of the thumb to Shaoshang (Lu 11). Its branch originating from Lieque (Lu 7), runs to the radial side of the tip of the index finger, where it meets with the Large Intestine Channel of Hand-*Yangming*. The Lung Channel of Hand-*Taiyin* is exteriorly and interiorly related to the Large Intestine Channel.   Located along the Channel are 22 points, of which

头之间或拇指指关节的横度为 1 寸；食指、中指、无名指和小指并拢时的近侧指关节之间的横度为 3 寸(图 1—22)。

3）解剖标志定位法

利用体表各种解剖标志作为定穴依据，是最基本的取穴法。临床常用的有以下两种方法。

（1）定型标志：指不受人体活动影响而固定不移的标志,如五官、乳头、脐及各种骨节的突起或凹陷。

（2）活动标志：指需要采取一定的动作姿势才会出现 的 标志。如活动时的肌肉凹陷或隆起、肌腱显露、皮肤皱襞等。

3．十四经循行、常用腧穴及推拿手法

1）手太阴肺经(图 1—23)

本经起于中焦，下络大肠而上属于肺。其外行线自肺系横行浅出至中府穴，循上肢内侧桡侧缘至拇指桡侧少商穴而终。从列缺分出的支脉，走向食指桡侧端，与手阳明大肠经相联接，互为

the following are used most commonly.

Zhongfu (Lu 1)

Location: 6 *cun* lateral to the midline of the chest, in the interspace between the 1st and 2nd ribs.

Indication: cough with dyspnea, stuffiness in the chest and pain in the chest, shoulder or back.

Manipulation: pushing with one-finger meditation, pressing, kneading and rubbing.

Chize (Lu 5)

Location: in the middle of the cubital crease and the radial side of the tendon of brachial biceps.

Indication: contraction of the elbow and arm, cough with dyspnea, fullness in the chest and hypochondrium.

Manipulation: pressing, kneading, grasping, and pushing with one-finger meditation.

Lieque (Lu 7)

Location: 1.5 *cun* above the transverse crease of the wrist, at the far end of the index finger when the two hands (thumbs) are crossed.

Indication: headache, facial hemiparalysis and hemiplegia.

Manipulation: pressing, nipping.

Yuji (Lu 10)

Location: on the palmar surface, in the middle of the first metacarpal bone at the junction of the "white and red" skin.

Indication: pain in the chest and back, headache, vertigo, sore throat, fever and aversion to cold.

Manipulation: pressing, kneading, nipping.

Shaoshang (Lu 11)

Location: on the radial side of the thumb, about 0.1 *cun* posterior to the corner of the nail.

Indication: sore throat, cough with dyspnea, apoplexy, coma and infantile convulsion.

Manipulation: nipping, nipping-kneading.

2) The Large Intestine Channel of Hand-*Yangming* (Fig.

表里。左右共 22 穴。常用穴如下：

中府

位置：前正中线旁开 6 寸，平第一肋间隙处。

主治：咳喘，胸闷，胸痛，肩背痛。

手法：一指禅推、按、揉、摩。

尺泽

位置：肘横纹中，肱二头肌腱桡侧。

主治：肘臂挛痛，咳喘，胸胁胀满。

手法：按、揉、拿、一指禅推。

列缺

位置：两手交叉，食指尽处，腕上 1.5 寸。

主治：头痛，口眼㖞斜，半身不遂。

手法：按、掐。

鱼际

位置：第一掌骨中点，赤白肉际处。

主治：胸背痛，头痛，眩晕，喉痛，发热恶寒。

手法：按、揉、掐。

少商

位置：拇指桡侧指甲角旁约 0.1 寸。

主治：咽喉肿痛，咳逆，中风昏仆，小儿惊风。

手法：掐、掐揉。

2) 手阳明大肠经（图1-24）

1—24)

It originates from Shangyang (LI 1) on the radial side of the index finger, goes upwards along the radial side of the hand and the arm, passes the anterior margin of the acromion and reaches the point Dazhui (Du 14) or the 7th cervical vertebra where it turns to the supraclavicular fossa. Its interior course descends to communicate with the lung and enter its pertaining organ, the large intestine; its collateral (branch channel) follows the exterior course upwards to the neck, passes through the cheek, enters the lower gum and then winds round the lips and meets with the symmetric branch at Renzhong (Du 26), where the left one turns right while the right turns left, going upwards to the point Yingxiang (LI 20) of both sides to connect with the Stomach Channel of Foot-*Yangming*. The large Intestine Channel of Hand-*Yangming* is exteriorly-interiorly related to the Lung Channel. Along it at each side of the body there are 20 points, of which 6 are used most commonly.

Hegu (LI 4)

Location: the mid-point on a line between the 1st and 2nd metacarpal bones.

Indication: headache, toothache, fever, sore throat, pain in the shoulder and arm, spasm of finger and facial hemiparalysis.

Manipulation: grasping, pressing, kneading and nipping.

Yangxi (LI 5)

Location: on the radial side of the back of the wrist, in the hollow between the tendons of m. extensor pollicis longus and brevis.

Indication: headache, tinnitus, toothache, sore throat, conjunctival congestion and wrist-pain.

Manipulation: pressing, kneading, nipping and grasping.

Shousanli (LI 10)

Location: 2 *cun* directly below the point Quchi (LI 11).

Indication: spasm of elbow with difficulty in extention and flexion, and numbness and aching-pain in the arms.

本经起自食指桡侧之商阳穴，循手及上肢背侧的桡侧缘，向上经肩峰前缘，绕向后面的大椎穴，返回至锁骨上窝处。其内行线入里，络肺属大肠；其外行支脉则上走颈部，经面颊、下齿龈而回绕至上唇，交叉于人中，至对侧迎香穴而终。在鼻旁与足阳明胃经相联接，与肺经相表里。左右共 40 穴。常用穴如下：

合谷

位置：手背第一、二掌骨之间中点处。

主治：头痛，牙痛，发热，咽喉肿痛，肩臂痛，指挛，口眼歪斜。

手法：拿、按、揉、掐。

阳溪

位置：腕背横纹桡侧两筋之间。

主治：头痛，耳鸣，齿痛，咽喉肿痛，目赤，手腕痛。

手法：按、揉、掐、拿。

手三里

位置：曲池直下 2 寸。

主治：肘挛，屈伸不利，手臂麻木酸痛。

Manipulation: grasping, pressing, kneading, and pushing with one-finger meditation.

Quchi (LI 11)

Location: in the depression at the lateral end of the transverse cubital crease when the elbow is flexed.

Indication: fever, hypertension, swelling and pain in the elbows and arms with difficulty in extention and flexion and paralysis.

Manipulation: pushing with one-finger meditation, grasping, pressing and kneading.

Jianyu (LI 15)

Location: in the depression of the acromion when the arm is in full abduction.

Indication: pain in shoulder, dysfunction of the shoulder joints and hemiparalysis.

Manipulation: pushing with one finger meditation, pressing, kneading and rolling.

Yingxiang (LI 20)

Location: in the naso-labial groove, 0.5 *cun* lateral to the nasal ala.

Indication: rhinitis, stuffy-nose and facial hemiparalysis.

Manipulation: nipping, pressing, kneading and pushing with one-finger meditation.

3) The Stomach Channel of Foot-*Yangming* (**Fig.** 1—25)

This channel starts from the side of the nose, ascends to the nose root and meets the Channel of Foot-*Taiyang*. Then it reaches the infraorbital region and the point Chengqi (St 1) and passes downwards the upper gum, round the lips, through the mandible and the point Jiache (St 6), and then ascends along the part in front of the ear and reaches Touwei (St 8) at the corner of the forehead. The branch in the face starts from the mandible and goes along the neck into the supraclavicular fossa. From there it descends through the diaphragm, enters its pertaining organ, the stomach, and communicates with the

手法：拿、按、揉、一指禅推。

曲池

位置：屈肘，当肘横纹外侧头。

主治：发热，高血压，肘臂肿痛，屈伸不利，瘫痪。

手法：一指禅推、拿、按、揉。

肩髃

位置：肩峰外下方，肩外展时呈凹陷处。

主治：肩痛，肩关节活动障碍，偏瘫。

手法：一指禅推、按、揉、㨰。

迎香

位置：鼻翼旁0.5寸，鼻唇沟中。

主治：鼻炎，鼻塞，口眼歪斜。

手法：掐、按、揉、一指禅推。

3）　足阳明胃经（图1-25）

本经起于鼻翼外侧，上行至鼻根部与足太阳经交会后，至眶下缘的承泣穴，向下经上齿龈、唇周围、下颌及颊车穴，再上行耳前达额角处的头维穴。面部支脉从下颌下走颈部进入锁骨上窝，通过横膈，属胃络脾。其外行的支脉从锁骨上窝下行经乳头及

spleen. The external branch descends from the supraclavicular fossa to the medial border of the nipple and the abdomen, then joins the branch which originates from the pylorus at the point Qichong (St 30), goes on to descend along the anterior part of the thigh and the anterolateral aspect of the tibia and reaches the lateral side of the tip of the second toe and the point Lidui (St 45). The branch at the tibia sprouts from the region 3 *cun* below the genu, descends to the lateral side of the middle toe. The branch from the tarsus goes to the radial aspect of the tip of the big toe and connects with the Spleen Channel of Foot-*Taiyin*. The Stomach Channel of Foot-*Yangming* is exteriorly-interiorly related to the Spleen Channel. Along the Channels of both sides of the body there are 92 points, of which the following are the commonly used.

Sibai (St 2)

Location: in the depression at the infra-orbital foramen, directly below the pupil when one is looking straignt ahead.

Indication: facial paralysis, spasm of the facial muscles and conjunctival congestion with pain and itching.

Manipulation: pressing, kneading, and pushing with one-finger meditation.

Dicang (St 4)

Location: 0.4 *cun* lateral to the corner of the mouth.

Indication: facial paralysis and slobbering.

Manipulation: pushing with one-finger meditation, pressing and kneading.

Jiache (St 6)

Location: in the depression one finger-width anterior and superior to the angle of jaw.

Indication: toothache, buccal swelling and facial paralysis.

Manipulation: ditto.

Xiaguan (St 7)

Location: in the depression at the lower border of the zygomatic arch.

腹部与胃下口发出的支脉在腹股沟处的气冲穴会合，再下行循大腿前缘、胫骨前嵴外侧，至足第二趾的厉兑穴。其胫部支脉，从膝下三寸处分出，进入足中趾外侧。其足跗部支脉，从跗上分出，进入足大趾内侧端，与足太阴脾经相联接。与脾经相表里。左右共92穴。常用穴如下：

四白

位置：目正视，瞳孔直下，当眶下孔凹陷中。

主治：口眼歪斜，面肌痉挛，目赤痛痒。

手法：按、揉、一指禅推。

地仓

位置：口角旁0.4寸。

主治：口眼歪斜，流涎。

手法：一指禅推、按、揉。

颊车

位置：下颌角前上方一横指凹陷处。

主治：牙痛，颊肿，口眼歪斜。

手法：一指禅推、按、揉。

下关

位置：颧弓下凹陷处。

Indication: facial paralysis, toothache and temporomandibular joint inflammation.

Manipulation: pushing with one-finger meditation, pressing and kneading.

Touwei (St 8)

Location: 0.5 *cun* above the anterior hairline at the corner of the forehead.

Indication: headache, vertigo and ophthalmalgia.

Manipulation: wiping, pressing, kneading and sweeping.

Renying (St 9)

Location: 1.5 *cun* lateral to the thyroid certilage.

Indication: sore throat, asthma, stuffiness in the chest and hiccup.

Manipulation: grasping, kneading and twining.

Shuitu (St 10)

Location: on the anterior border of m. sternocleidomastoideus, 1 *cun* inferior to Renying (St 9).

Indication: fullness sensation in the chest and cough with dyspnea, sore throat and shortness of breath.

Manipulation: grasping, kneading and twining.

Quepen (St 12)

Location: in the middle of the supraclavicular fossa, on the mammillary line.

Indication: fullness sensation in the chest, cough with dyspnea, inflammation of the throat, numbness and pain in the upper limbs.

Manipulation: pressing, flicking-poking and kneading.

Tianshu (St 25)

Location: 2 *cun* lateral to the umbilicus.

Indication: diarrhea, constipation, abdominal pain and irregular menstruation.

Manipulation: kneading palm-rubbing and pushing with one-finger meditation.

Biguan (St 31)

主治：面瘫，牙痛，颞颌关节炎。

手法：一指禅推、按、揉。

头维

位置：额角发际直上 0.5 寸处。

主治：头痛，眩晕，目痛。

手法：抹、按、揉、扫散法。

人迎

位置：喉结旁开 1.5 寸。

主治：咽喉肿痛，喘息，胸闷，吐逆。

手法：拿、揉、缠。

水突

位置：人迎穴下 1 寸，胸锁乳突肌前缘。

主治：胸满咳喘，咽喉肿痛，气短。

手法：拿、揉、缠。

缺盆

位置：锁骨上缘正中凹陷处，向下直对乳头。

主治：胸满，喘咳，喉痹，上肢痛麻。

手法：按、弹拨、揉。

天枢

位置：脐旁 2 寸。

主治：腹泻，便秘，腹痛，月经不调。

手法：揉、摩、一指禅推。

髀关

Location: in a line between the anterior superior iliac spine and the lateral border of the patella, and at the level of the gluteal groove.

Indication: lumbocrural pain, numbness and flaccidity of the lower limbs and contracture and spasm of muscle with stiffness.

Manipulation: pressing, grasping, kneading, digital hitting, rolling and flicking-poking.

Futu (St 32)

Location: 6 *cun* above the superolateral border of the patella.

Indication: pain and numbness in the knees and paralysis of the lower limbs.

Manipulation: rolling, pressing and kneading.

Liangqiu (St 34)

Location: 2 *cun* above the superolateral border of the patella.

Indication: pain, coldness and numbness in the knees, stomachache and mastitis.

Manipulation: rolling, pressing, digital hitting and grasping.

Dubi (St 35)

Location: in the depression just below the patella, lateral to the patella ligament.

Indication: pain in the knees accompanied with asthenia and stiffness.

Manipulation: digital hitting, pressing and kneading.

Zusanli (St 36)

Location: 3 *cun* inferior to the point Dubi (St 35), one finger-width apart from the anterior crest of the tibia.

Indication: pain and fullness in the abdomen, diarrhea, constipation, coldness and numbness of the lower extremities and hypertension.

Manipulation: pressing, digital hitting, kneading and pushing with one-finger meditation.

位置：髂前上嵴与髌骨外缘连线上，平臀沟处。

主治：腰腿痛，下肢麻木痿软，筋挛急，屈伸不利。

手法：**按、拿、揉、点、掖、弹拨。**

伏兔

位置：髌骨外上缘上6寸。

主治：膝痛麻木，下肢瘫痪。

手法：掖、按、揉。

梁丘

位置：髌骨外上缘上2寸。

主治：膝痛冷麻，胃痛，乳腺炎。

手法：掖、按、点、拿。

犊鼻

位置：髌骨下缘，髌韧带外侧凹陷中。

主治：膝关节疼痛，酸软无力，活动不利。

手法：点、按、揉。

足三里

位置：犊鼻穴下3寸，距胫骨前嵴外1横指处。

主治：腹痛腹胀，腹泻，便秘，下肢冷麻，高血压。

手法：按、点、揉、一指禅推。

Shangjuxu (St 37)

Location: 3 *cun* inferior to the point Zushanli (St 36).

Indication: pain around the navel, diarrhea, appendicitis, pain and numbness in the lower extremities and paralysis.

Manipulation: pressing, grasping, rolling and kneading.

Jiexi (St 41)

Location: on the midpoint of the dorsum of foot at the transverse malleolus crease, between the tendons of m. extensor digitorum longus and hallucis longus.

Indication: sprain of the ankle, numbness in the toes and headache.

Manipulation: pressing, grasping, nipping and digital hitting.

4) The Spleen Channel of Foot-*Taiyin* (Fig. 1—26)

It originates at the point Yinbai (Sp 1), goes along the internal side of the foot and the anterior side of the medial malleolus upwards and ascends along the tibia and the anterior medial aspect of the thigh to the point Chongmen (Sp 12) at the groin. Its external course goes up to the abdomen and ascends along a line 2 *cun* lateral to the ventral line to the chest, and then descends to the point Dabao (Sp 21) at the hypochondrium. Its internal course goes inside and enters its pertaining organ, the spleen, and communicates with the stomach where it ascends along the two sides of the esophagus to reach the root of the tongue and spread over its lower surface. The branch of the channel sprouts from the stomach, goes upwards through the diaphragm, disperses into the heart and connects with the Heart Channel of Hand-*Shaoyin*. This channel is exteriorly-interiorly related to the Stomach Channel. Each side of the body has 21 points along it. The following are the commonly-used points.

Gongsun (Sp 4)

Location: on the medial aspect of the foot, in a depression at the anterior and inferior border of the 1st metatarsal bone.

Indication: diarrhea, abdominal pain, vomiting, swelling and pain in the medial aspect of the foot.

上巨墟

位置：足三里下 3 寸处。

主治：挟脐痛，腹泻，阑尾炎，下肢痛麻，瘫痪。

手法：按、拿、揉、揉。

解溪

位置：足背踝关节横纹中点，当踇长伸肌腱与趾长伸肌腱之间。

主治：踝关节扭伤，足趾麻木，头痛。

手法：按、拿、掐、点。

4）足太阴脾经（图1-26）

本经起于踇趾末端之隐白穴，循足内侧，在内踝前向上，沿胫骨及大腿内侧前缘，至腹股沟之冲门穴。其外行线上腹，循腹中线旁 2 寸上行到胸部，再下行到胁部的大包穴而止；其内行线入里，属脾络胃，上挟食道两旁，联系舌根，分散于舌下；其胃部支脉，向上过膈，流注于心中，与手少阴心经相联接。与胃经相表里。左右共 42 穴。常用穴如下：

公孙

位置：在足跗内侧，第一蹠骨基底部前下缘凹陷处。

主治：腹泻，腹痛，呕吐，足内侧肿痛。

Manipulation: pressing, kneading, digital hitting and pushing with one-finger meditation.

Sanyinjiao (Sp 6)

Location: 3 *cun* above the tip of the medial malleolus, on the posterior border of the medial aspect of the tibia.

Indication: insomnia, enuresis, weakness of the spleen and stomach, uroschesis, nocturnal emission, impotence, irregular menstruation and hypertension.

Manipulation: kneading, pressing and pushing with one-finger meditation.

Yinlingquan (Sp 9)

Location: in the depression on the inferior border of the tibial internal condyle .

Indication: soreness and pain in the knees and dribbling urination.

Manipulation: pressing, kneading, digital hitting, grasping and pushing with one-finger meditation.

Xuehai (Sp 10)

Location: 2 *cun* superior to the medial border of the patella.

Indication: irregular menstruation and pain in the knees.

Manipulation: grasping, pressing and digital hitting.

Daheng (Sp 15)

Location: 4 *cun* lateral to the navel.

Indication: diarrhea of insufficiency-cold type, constipation and pain in the lower abdomen.

Manipulation: pushing with one-finger meditation, rubbing, kneading and grasping.

5) The Heart Channel of Hand-*Shaoyin* (Fig. 1—27)

It starts from the heart, comes out of the cardiac system and descends to connect with the small intestine. The branch of the channel sprouts from the cardiac system, goes upwards along the esophagus, and joins the orbital and brain systems. The original straight channel ascends from the cardiac system to the lung and runs to the point Jiquan (H 1) at the axilla; its exer-

手法：按、揉、点、一指禅推。

三阴交

位置：内踝上3寸，胫骨内侧面后缘。

主治：失眠，遗尿，脾胃虚弱，尿潴留，梦遗失精，阳萎，月经不调，高血压。

手法：揉、按、一指禅推。

阴陵泉

位置：胫骨内侧髁下缘凹陷中。

主治：膝关节酸痛，小便不利。

手法：按、揉、点、一指禅推。

血海

位置：髌骨内上方2寸处。

主治：月经不调，膝痛。

手法：拿、按、点。

大横

位置：肚脐旁开4寸。

主治：虚寒泻痢，大便秘结，小腹痛。

手法：一指禅推、摩、揉、拿。

5）手少阴心经（图1-27）

本经起自心中，出属心系，下络小肠；自心系向上的经脉，挟食道上行，与眼和脑相联系；从心系出的另一条直行经脉，先上行于肺部，再向左右横出于腋窝部的极泉穴，其外行线沿上

nal course travels along the upper arm, the elbow and the ulnar border of the forearm, enters the palm and ends at the point Shaochong (H 9) at the medial aspect of the tip of the small finger, and finally connects with the Small Intestine Channel of Hand-*Taiyang*. This channel is exteriorly-interiorly related to the Small Intestine Channel. Each side of the body has 9 points along the channel. Described here are the commonly-used ones.

Jiquan (H 1)

Location: at the centre of the axilla.

Indication: stuffiness in the chest and hypochondriac pain, pain in the arm and elbow accompanied with coldness and numbness.

Manipulation: grasping and flicking-poking.

Shaohai (H 3)

Location: in the depression at the ulnar end of the transversal cubital crease which appears when the elbow is bent.

Indication: spasm and pain in the elbow and tremor of the hand.

Manipulation: grasping and flicking-poking.

Shenmen (H 7)

Location: in the transversal crease of the wrist, at the radial side of the tendon of m. flexor carpi ulnaris.

Indication: palpitation due to fright, severe palpitation, insomnia, amnesia and arrhythmia.

Manipulation: grasping, pressing and kneading.

6) The Small Intestine Channel of Hand-*Taiyang*(Fig. 1–28)

The channel originates from Shaoze (SI 1) at the ulnar aspect of the tip of the small finger, and follows the ulnar border of the dorsum of the hand and the forearm and passes between the olecranon of the ulna and the medial epicondyle of the humerus. It continues to travel along the posterior border of the lateral aspect of the arm, and out of the shoulder joint. After circling round the shoulder-blade, it meets its symmetric branch at Dazhui (Du 14) and goes foreward to Quepen (St 12) in

臂、肘关节与前臂掌侧的尺侧缘，入掌内，至小指内侧末端的少冲穴而终。与手太阳小肠经相联接。与小肠经相表里。左右共18穴。常用穴如下：

极泉

位置：腋窝正中

主治：胸闷胁痛，臂肘疼痛、冷麻。

手法：拿、弹拨。

少海

位置：屈肘，肘横纹尺侧端凹陷中。

主治：肘关节挛痛，手颤。

手法：拿、弹拨。

神门

位置：在腕横纹上，当尺侧腕屈肌腱的桡侧。

主治：惊悸，怔忡，失眠，健忘，心律不齐。

手法：拿、按、揉。

6) 手太阳小肠经（图1-28）

本经起于小指尺侧端之少泽穴，沿手掌、前臂背侧之尺侧缘，经尺骨鹰嘴与肱骨内上髁之间，沿上臂背侧后缘，出肩关节，绕行肩胛部，交会于大椎穴，再向前至锁骨上窝之缺盆穴

the supraclavicular fossa. From there its internal branch goes inside to connect with the heart and then enters its pertaining organ, the small intestine. Its external branch runs along the neck up to the cheek, enters the ear and ends at the point Tinggong (SI 19). The other branch of the channel, which sprouts from the cheek, ascends to the infra-orbital region, reaches the lateral side of the nose and terminates at the inner canthus where it connects with the Urinary Bladder Channel of Foot-*Taiyang*. The channel is exteriorly-interiorly related to the Heart Channel. Each side of the body has 19 points along the channel. The commonly-used are described as follows.

Shaoze (SI 1)

Location: at the ulnar side of the little finger, about 0.1 *cun* posterior to the corner of the nail.

Indication: fever, apoplectic coma, hypogalactia and sore throat.

Manipulation: nipping.

Xiaohai (SI 8)

Location: in the depression between the olecranon of the ulna and the tip of the medial epicondyle of the humerus when the elbow is flexed.

Indication: toothache, pain in the neck, soreness and pain in the upper extremities.

Manipulation: grasping and kneading.

Bingfeng (SI 12)

Location: in the center of the superior fossa of spina scapula, directly above Tianzong (SI 11).

Indication: pain in the scapular area, difficulty in raising the shoulder and arms with soreness, pain and numbness.

Manipulation: pushing with one-finger meditation, rolling, pressing and kneading.

Jianwaishu (SI 14)

Location: 3 *cun* lateral to the lower border of the spinous process of the 1st thoracic vertebra.

处。其内行分支由此入里，络心，属小肠；其外行线沿着颈部上达面颊，到耳中，至听宫穴而止；其颊部支脉，上行眼眶，抵鼻旁，到目内眦与足太阳膀胱经相联接。与心经相表里。左右共38穴。常用穴如下：

少泽

位置：小指尺侧指甲角旁约0.1寸。

主治：发热，中风昏迷，乳少，咽喉肿痛。

手法：掐。

小海

位置：屈肘，当尺骨鹰嘴与肱骨内上髁之间凹陷中。

主治：牙痛，颈项痛，上肢酸痛。

手法：拿、揉。

秉风

位置：肩胛骨冈上窝中点，天宗穴直上。

主治：肩胛疼痛、抬举不利、酸痛麻木。

手法：一指禅推、拨、按、揉。

肩外俞

位置：第一胸椎棘突下旁开3寸。

Indication: coldness and pain in the shoulder and back, rigidity and spasm in the neck and nape, pain and numbness in the upper extremities.

Manipulation: pushing with one-finger meditation, rolling, pressing and kneading.

Jianzhongshu (SI 15)

Location: 2 *cun* lateral to Dazhui (Du 14).

Indication: cough, asthma, pain in the shoulder and back, and blurred vision.

Manipulation: pushing with one-finger meditation, rolling, pressing and kneading.

Jianzhen (SI 9)

Location: 1 *cun* superior to the posterior axillary fold.

Indication: soreness and pain in the shoulder joint which has difficulty in movement, and paralysis of the upper limb.

Manipulation: rolling, pressing, digital hitting, kneading and grasping.

Tianzong (SI 11)

Location: in the centre of the superior fossa of spina scapula.

Indication: soreness and pain in the shoulder and back, difficulty in shoulder joint movement, rigidity in the neck, pain, numbness or paralysis of the upper extremities.

Manipulation: pushing with one-finger meditation, rolling, pressing, digital hitting and kneading.

Quanliao (SI 18)

Location: directly below the outer canthus, in the depression below the lower border of the zygomatic bone.

Indication: facial hemiparalysis and spasm of the facial muscle.

Manipulation: pushing with one-finger meditation, kneading, pressing and digital hitting.

7) The Urinary Bladder Channel of Foot-*Taiyang* (Fig 1-29)

It comes from Jingming (UB 1) at the inner canthus, ascends to the forehead and joins its symmetrical channel at

主治：肩背冷痛，颈项强急，上肢痛麻。

手法：一指禅推、㨰、按、揉。

肩中俞

位置：大椎穴旁开2寸。

主治：咳嗽，气喘，肩背疼痛，视物不清。

手法：一指禅推、㨰、按、揉。

肩贞

位置：腋后皱襞上1寸。

主治：肩关节酸痛、活动不便，上肢瘫痪。

手法：㨰、按、点、揉、拿。

天宗

位置：肩胛骨冈下窝的中央。

主治：肩背酸痛，肩关节活动不便，项强，上肢痛麻瘫痪。

手法：一指禅推、㨰、按、点、揉。

颧髎

位置：目外眦直下，颧骨下缘凹陷中。

主治：口眼㖞斜，面肌痉挛。

手法：一指禅推、揉、按、点。

7）足太阳膀胱经（图1-29）

本经起自目内眦的睛明穴，上额，交会于巅顶。有一支脉从

the vertex. One of its branches splits off the vertex and goes to the temple. The original channel leaves the vertex for the brain where it re-emerges and runs downward to the nape, and along the medial side of the scapula, it travels parallel to the vertebral column and reaches the lumbar region. From there its internal course enters the body cavity to communicate with the kidney and then goes into its pertaining organ, the urinary bladder. The branch from the lumbar region runs downwards through the gluteal region and into the popliteal fossa. The other branch starts from the nape, passes the medial side of the scapula, runs downwards through the gluteal region and along the lateral side of the thigh, and meets the branch which descends from the lumbar region in the popliteal fossa. From there it makes its way down through the m. gastrocnemius, emerges from the posterior aspect of the external malleolus, runs along the tuberosity of the fifth metatarsal bone and ends at Zhiyin (UB 67) at the lateral side of the little toe, where it descends to connect with the Kidney Channel of Foot-*Shaoyin*. It is exteriorly-interiorly related to the Kidney Channel. Each side of the body has 67 points along the channel, of which the following are the commonly-used.

Jingming (UB 1)

Location: 0.1 *cun* lateral to the inner canthus.

Indication: eye diseases.

Manipulation: pushing with one-finger meditation, pressing and vibrating.

Zanzhu (UB 2)

Location: in the depression proximal to the medial end of the eyebrow.

Indication: headache, insomnia, pain in the supra-orbital bone, conjunctival congestion with swelling and pain.

Manipulation: pushing with one-finger meditation, pressing, kneading, wiping.

Tianzhu (UB 10)

Location: 1.3 *cun* lateral to the point Yamen (Du 15), in

头顶到颞部；其直行的经脉从头顶入里络于脑，又回出下行项后，沿着肩胛骨内侧，挟脊柱到达腰部后，其内行线进入体腔，络肾，属膀胱；自腰部外行的支脉，向下通过臀部，进入腘窝中；后项的另一支脉，通过肩胛骨的内侧缘直下，经过臀部下行，沿大腿外侧，与腰部下来的支脉会合于腘窝中。再向下经小腿肚内，出于外踝后面，沿第五蹠骨粗隆，至小趾外侧的至阴穴而终。向下与足少阴肾经相联接。与肾经相表里。左右共 134 穴。常用穴如下：

睛明

位置：目内眦旁 0.1 寸。

主治：眼病。

手法：一指禅推、按、振。

攒竹

位置：眉头凹陷中。

主治：头痛，失眠，眉棱骨痛，目赤肿痛。

手法：一指禅推、按、揉、抹。

天柱

位置：哑门穴旁开 1.3 寸，当斜方肌外缘凹陷中。

the depression at the external border of the trapezius muscle.

Indication: headache, rigidity in the neck, stuffy nose, pain in the shoulder and back.

Manipulation: pushing with one-finger meditation, pressing, kneading and grasping.

Dashu (UB 11)

Location: 1.5 *cun* lateral to the lower border of the spinous process of the 1st thoracic vertebra.

Indication: fever, cough, rigidity in the neck, and pain in the shoulder and back.

Manipulation: pushing with one-finger meditation, rolling, pressing and kneading

Fengmen (UB 12)

Location: 1.5 *cun* lateral to the lower border of the spinous process of the 2nd thoracic vertebra.

Indication: cold, cough, rigidity in the neck and pain in the shoulder and back.

Manipulation: ditto.

Feishu (UB 13)

Location: 1.5 *cun* lateral to the lower border of the spinous process of the 3rd thoracic vertebra.

Indication: cough and dyspnea, stuffiness or pain in the chest and strain of the muscles of the back.

Manipulation: pushing with one-finger meditation, rolling, pressing, kneading and flicking-poking.

Xinshu (UB 15)

Location: 1.5 *cun* lateral to the lower border of the spinous process of the 5th thoracic vertebra.

Indication: insomnia, amnesia, hemiparalysis, palpitation and irritability.

Manipulation: ditto.

Ganshu (UB 18)

Location: 1.5 *cun* lateral to the lower border of the spinous process of the 9th thoracic vertebra.

主治：头痛，项强，鼻塞，肩背痛。

手法：一指禅推、按、揉、拿。

大杼

位置：第一胸椎棘突下旁开 1.5 寸。

主治：发热，咳嗽，项强，肩背痛。

手法：一指禅推、擦、按、揉。

风门

位置：第二胸椎棘突下，旁开 1.5 寸。

主治：伤风，咳嗽，项强，肩背痛。

手法：同上。

肺俞

位置：第三胸椎棘突下旁开 1.5 寸。

主治：咳嗽气喘，胸闷胸痛，背肌劳损。

手法：一指禅推、擦、按、揉、弹拨。

心俞

位置：第五胸椎棘突下旁开 1.5 寸。

主治：失眠，健忘，半身不遂，心悸，心胸烦乱。

手法：同上。

肝俞

位置：第九胸椎棘突下旁开 1.5 寸。

Indication: hypochondriac pain and distention due to diseases of the liver and gallbladder, eye diseases, gastric disorder and pain in the waist and back.

Manipulation: ditto.

Danshu (UB 19)

Location: 1.5 *cun* lateral to the lower border of the spinous process of the 10th thoracic vertebra.

Indication: hypochondriac pain and distention due to diseases of the liver and gallbladder, bitter taste in the mouth, jaundice, and pain in the waist and back.

Manipulation: ditto.

Pishu (UB 20)

Location: 1.5 *cun* lateral to the lower border of the spinous process of the 11th thoracic vertebra.

Indication: distention and pain in the gastric region, indigestion and chronic infantile convulsion.

Manipulation: pushing with one-finger meditation, digital hitting, pressing, kneading and rolling.

Weishu (UB 21)

Location: 1.5 *cun* lateral to the lower border of the spinous process of the 12th thoracic vertebra.

Indication: gastric diseases, vomiting of milk in infants and indigestion.

Manipulation: ditto.

Sanjiaoshu (UB 22)

Location: 1.5 *cun* lateral to the lower border of the spinous process of the 1st lumbar vertebra.

Indication: intestinal gargling and distention, vomiting, rigidity and pain in the waist and back.

Manipulation: pushing with one-finger meditation, pressing, kneading, digital hitting and rolling.

Shenshu (UB 23)

Location: 1.5 *cun* lateral to the lower border of the spinous process of the 2nd lumbar vertebra.

主治：肝脏及胆囊病症之胁肋胀痛，目疾，胃病，腰背痛。

手法：同上。

胆俞

位置：第十胸椎棘突下旁开 1.5 寸。

主治：肝脏及胆囊病症之胁肋胀痛，口苦，黄疸，腰背部疼痛。

手法：同上。

脾俞

位置：第十一胸椎棘突下旁开 1.5 寸。

主治：胃脘胀痛，消化不良，小儿慢脾风。

手法：一指禅推、点、按、揉、擦。

胃俞

位置：第十二胸椎棘突下旁开 1.5 寸。

主治：胃病，小儿吐乳，消化不良。

手法：同上。

三焦俞

位置：第一腰椎棘突下旁开 1.5 寸。

主治：肠鸣腹胀，呕吐，腰背强痛。

手法：一指禅推、按、揉、点、擦。

肾俞

位置：第二腰椎棘突下旁开 1.5 寸。

Indication: deficiency of kidney, lumbago, seminal emission and irregular menstruation.

Manipulation: ditto.

Qihaishu (UB 24)

Location: 1.5 *cun* lateral to the lower border of the spinous process of the 3rd lumbar vertebra.

Indication: lumbago and hemorrhoid.

Manipulation: pushing with one-finger meditation, pressing, kneading and rolling.

Dachangshu (UB 25)

Location: 1.5 *cun* lateral to the lower border of the spinous process of the 4th lumbar vertebra.

Indication: pain in the waist and legs, lumbar muscle strain, and enteritis.

Manipulation: ditto.

Guanyuanshu (UB 26)

Location: 1.5 *cun* lateral to the lower border of the spinous process of the 5th lumbar vertebra.

Indication: lumbago, diarrhea.

Manipulation: pushing with one-finger meditation, pressing, rolling, kneading and digital hitting.

Baliao

Location: a collective term for Shangliao (UB 31), Ciliao (UB 32), Zhongliao (UB 33) and Xialiao (UB 34), located in the 1st, 2nd, 3rd and 4th posterior sacral foramina respectively.

Indication: pain in the waist and legs, diseases of the urogenital system.

Manipulation: digital hitting, pressing, rolling, scrubbing and striking.

Zhibian (UB 54)

Location: 3 *cun* lateral to the inferior border of the 4th sacral process.

Indication: pain in waist and buttocks; flaccidity of the lower extremities, difficulty in micturition and constipation.

主治：肾虚，腰痛，遗精，月经不调。

手法：同上。

气海俞

位置：第三腰椎棘突下旁开 1.5 寸。

主治：腰痛，痔。

手法：一指禅推、按、揉、擦。

大肠俞

位置：第四腰椎棘突下旁开 1.5 寸。

主治：腰腿痛，腰肌劳损，肠炎。

手法：同上。

关元俞

位置：第五腰椎棘突下旁开 1.5 寸。

主治：腰痛，泄泻。

手法：一指禅推、按、擦、揉、点。

八髎

位置：在第一、二、三、四骶后孔中（分别称为上髎、**次髎、**中髎、下髎）。

主治：腰腿痛，泌尿生殖系疾患。

手法：点、按、擦、擦、击。

秩边

位置：第四骶椎棘突下旁开 3 寸。

主治：腰臀痛，下肢痿痹，小便不利，便秘。

Manipulation: rolling, grasping, pressing, kneading, digital hitting and flicking-poking.

Yinmen (UB 37)

Location: 6 *cun* inferior to the midpoint of the gluteal fold.

Indication: sciatica, paralysis of the lower extremities, pain in the waist and back.

Manipulation: rolling, digital hitting, heavy pressing and grasping.

Weizhong (UB 40)

Location: the exact midpoint of the popliteal transverse crease.

Indication: lumbago, difficulty in knee joint movement and hemiparalysis.

Manipulation: rolling, grasping, pressing, kneading, and pushing with one-finger meditation.

Gaohuangshu (UB 43)

Location: 3 *cun* lateral to the lower border of the spinous process of the 4th thoracic vertebra, in the depression of the medial border the scapula.

Indication: cough, asthma, hectic (tidal) fever, mania, amnesia and nocturnal emission.

Manipulation: rolling, pressing, kneading and pushing with one-finger meditation.

Zhishi (UB 52)

Location: 1.5 *cun* lateral to the point Shenshu (UB 23).

Indication: seminal emission, impotence, irregular menstruation, enuresis and chronic lumbago.

Manipulation: ditto.

Chengshan (UB 57)

Location: the top of the depression between the two gastrocnemius muscles.

Indication: pain in the waist and legs, systremma and diarrhea.

Manipulation: rolling, grasping, pressing, kneading and

手法：擦、拿、按、揉、点、弹拨。

殷门

位置：臀沟中央下 6 寸。

主治：坐骨神经痛，下肢瘫痪，腰背痛。

手法：擦、点、压、拿。

委中

位置：腘窝横纹中央。

主治：腰痛，膝关节屈伸不利，半身不遂。

手法：擦、拿、按、揉、一指禅推。

膏肓俞

位置：第四胸椎棘突下旁开 3 寸，当肩胛骨脊柱缘的凹陷中。

主治：咳嗽，哮喘，潮热，发狂，健忘，梦中失精。

手法：擦、按、揉、一指禅推。

志室

位置：肾俞穴旁开 1.5 寸。

主治：遗精，阳痿，月经不调，遗尿，慢性腰痛。

手法：擦、按、揉、一指禅推。

承山

位置：腓肠肌两肌腹之间凹陷的顶端。

主治：腰腿痛，腓肠肌痉挛，腹泻。

手法：擦、拿、按、揉、擦。

scrubbing.

Kunlun (UB 60)

Location: in the depression between the posterior border of the lateral malleolus and the medial aspect of the tendon calcaneus.

Indication: headache, stiff neck, lumbago and sprain of the ankle.

Manipulation: pressing, grasping and digital hitting.

8) The Kidney Channel of Foot-*Shaoyin* (Fig. 1—30)

The Kidney Channel of Foot-*Shaoyin* starts from the plantar surface of the little toe, and runs obliquely towards the point Yongquan (K 1) in the centre of the sole. Emerging from the interior aspect of the tuberosity of the navicular bone, it goes behind the medial malleolus and reaches the heel. Then ascending along the medio-posterior aspect of the shank, the popliteal fossa and the thigh, it runs into the vertebral column, where it enters its pertaining organ, the kidney, and communicates with the urinary bladder. Then it re-emerges from the pubic bone, goes along the abdomen and ends at the point Shufu (K 27) which is located inferior to the clavicle. Its direct branch re-emerges from the kidney, runs straight up through the liver and diaphragm and enters the lung, from which it travels along the throat and terminates at the two sides of the root of the tongue. The other branch exits from the lung, connects with the heart and spreads over the thoracic cavity to meet the Pericardium Channel of Hand-*Jueyin*. The Kidney Channel of Foot-*Shaoyin* is interiorly-exteriorly related to the Urinary Bladder Channel. There are fifty-four points along its two sides, of which the following are used most commonly.

Yongquan (K 1)

Location: at junction between anterior 1/3 and posterior 2/3 of the sole (the length of the toe is not included), the depression formed when the toes make plantar flexion.

Indication: migraine headache, hypertension, infantile

昆仑

位置：外踝与跟腱之间凹陷中。

主治：头痛，项强，腰痛，踝关节扭伤。

手法：按、拿、点。

8）足少阴肾经（图1-30）

本经起于足小趾下，斜向足心的涌泉穴，出于舟骨粗隆下，沿内踝后进入足跟，再向上行于小腿、腘窝与大腿的内侧后缘，然后入里通向脊柱，属肾络膀胱，再从横骨处浅出，循腹上行，到胸部锁骨下的俞府穴而止。从肾脏向上直行的经脉，通过肝和横膈，进入肺，沿喉咙，挟于舌根两侧；另外，由肺部发出的支脉，联络心脏，流注于胸中，与手厥阴心包络相联接。与膀胱经相表里。左右共54穴。常用穴如下：

涌泉

位置：于足底（去趾）前1/3与后2/3的连接处，足趾跖屈时呈凹陷处。

主治：偏头痛，高血压，小儿发热，吐泻，失眠。

fever, vomiting and diarrhea, and insomnia.

Manipulation: scrubbing, pressing, kneading, and grasping.

Zhaohai (K 6)

Location: in the depression on the inferior border of the medial malleolus.

Indication: irregular menstruation, pain in the lower abdomen, dryness in the throat, aphasia and retention of urine.

Manipulation: pressing and kneading.

9) The Pericardium Channel of Hand-*Jueyin* (Fig. 1—31)

The channel commences from the chest where it exits from its pertaining organ, the pericardium. Then it descends through the diaphragm and links with the three-*jiao* in turn from the chest to the abdomen. One of its branches runs along the chest, emerges from the point Tianchi (P 1) which is located on the hypochondrium, and travels transversely to the axilla. Along the middle line of the medial side of the upper arm, it makes its way downward to the forearm, between the tendons of m. palmaris longus and m. flexorcarpi, and enters the palm, where it continues its way along the middle finger to the point Zhongchong (P 9) at the tip of the finger. Its other branch leaves Laogong (P 8), runs along the ring finger to its tip to connect with the Sanjiao Channel of Hand-*Shaoyang*.

The Pericardium Channel of Hand-*Jueyin* has the exterior-interior relationship with the Sanjiao Channel. Each side of the channel has 9 points, and the following are used most often.

Quze (P 3)

Location: in the middle of the transverse cubital crease, at the ulnar side of tendon of m. biceps brachii.

Indication: angina pectoris, aching-pain in and trembling of the upper extremities.

Manipulation: grasping, pressing and kneading.

Neiguan (P 6)

Location: 2 *cun* above the transverse carpal crease, be-

手法：擦、按、揉、拿。

照海

位置：内踝下缘凹陷中。

主治：月经不调，小腹痛，咽干，失语，尿潴留。

手法：按、揉。

9）手厥阴心包经(图1—31)。

本经起自胸中，发出后属心包，再向下过横膈，从胸至腹依次联络三焦。其胸部的支脉，沿着胸中，浅出于胁部的天池穴，再横行至腋下，抵腋窝，向下沿上肢内侧正中，行于前臂掌长肌腱与桡侧腕屈肌腱的中间，进入掌内，至中指端之中冲穴。其掌中支脉，从劳宫穴分出沿着无名指端与手少阳三焦经相联接。与三焦经相表里。左右共 18 穴。常用穴如下：

曲泽

位置：肘横纹中，肱二头肌腱尺侧缘。

主治：心绞痛，上肢酸痛颤抖。

手法：拿、按、揉。

内关

位置：腕横纹上 2 寸，当掌长肌腱与桡侧腕屈肌腱之间。

tween the tendon palmaris longus and the mediocarpal tendon.

Indication: stomachache, vomiting, palpitation, angina pectoris, hypertension, asthma and mental diseases.

Manipulation: pushing with one-finger meditation, pressing, kneading and grasping.

Laogong (P 8)

Location: at the midpoint of the transverse palmar crease, between the 2nd and 3rd metacarpal bones.

Indication: mental disorder, palpitation, heatstroke and vomiting.

Manipulation: pressing, nipping and grasping.

Zhongchong (P 9)

Location: at the tip of the middle finger.

Indication: Coma, fever, heatstroke, stiff tongue with difficulty in speaking.

Manipulation: nipping and nipping-kneading.

10) The Sanjiao Channel of Hand-*Shaoyang* (Fig. 1—32)

It starts from the point Guanchong (SJ 1) at the tip of the ring finger, runs upwards between the 4th and 5th metacarpal bones to the dorsal side of the forearm and travels between the two bones or the radius and ulna. It goes on to ascend through the olecranon, along the lateral aspect of the upper arm and reaches the shoulder, where it continues its ascent to reach the supraclavicular fossa. From the fossa its inward branch descends and spreads itself into the chest to communicate with the pericardium. Descending through the diaphragm, it communicates with the three-*jiao* in succession. One of its branches originates from the chest and ascends to the supraclavicular fossa. Going along the nape and the posterior border of the ear, it makes a direct ascent through the superior aspect of the auricula and the temple, curves down round the cheek and reaches the infraorbital region. The other branch which originates from the postauricular region [enters the ear and comes out in front of the ear. It crosses the above-mentioned branch at the cheek

主治：胃痛，呕吐，心悸，心绞痛，高血压，哮喘，精神病。

手法：一指禅推、按、揉、拿。

劳宫

位置：手掌心横纹中第二、三掌骨之间。

主治：精神病，心悸，中暑，呕吐。

手法：按、掐、拿。

中冲

位置：中指尖端。

主治：昏迷，发热，中暑，舌强不语。

手法：掐、掐揉。

10）手少阳三焦经（图1-32）

本经起于无名指末端之关冲穴，向上沿第四、五掌骨间，循前臂背侧尺、桡骨之间，经肘尖，上行于臂外侧达肩部，再向前至锁骨上窝处，其内行线入里分布于胸中，络心包，向下过横膈，从胸至腹历属三焦；其从胸中发出的支脉向上又返出于锁骨上窝，上走项部，沿耳后直上，出于耳上方，再经颞部下行面颊，止于眼眶下；其后的支脉从耳后入耳中，出走耳前，与前脉交叉于面颊，达目外眦之丝竹空穴。并向下与足少阳胆经相联接。与心包

and reaches the point Sizhukong (SJ 23) at the outer canthus, where it connects with the Gall Bladder Channel of Foot-*Shaoyang*. This channel has the exterior-interior relationship with the Pericardium Channel. Each side of it has 24 points, of which the commonly-used are described below.

Zhongzhu (SJ 3)

Location: on the dorsum of the hand, between the small ends of the 4th and 5th metacarpal bones, in the depression posterior to the metacarpophalangeal joint when the hand is in a fist.

Indication: migraine, pain in the palm or finger with difficulty in stretching or flexing and pain in the elbow and arm.

Manipulation: digital hitting, pressing, kneading and pushing with one-finger meditation.

Waiguan (SJ 5)

Location: 2 *cun* above the transverse crease of dorsum of wrist, between the radius and the ulna.

Indication: headache and pain in the elbow, arm and fingers with difficulty in stretching and flexing.

Manipulation: pushing with one-finger meditation, nipping, pressing and kneading.

Jianliao (SJ 14)

Location: lateral and inferior to the acromion, in the depression about 1 *cun* posterior to the point Jianyu (LI 15).

Indication: aching pain in the shoulder and arm, difficulty in shoulder joint movement.

Manipulation: pushing with one-finger meditation, pressing, kneading, rolling and grasping.

11) The Gall Bladder Channel of Foot-*Shaoyang* (Fig. 1—33)

The channel starts from Tongziliao (GB 1) at the outer canthus of the eye, runs upwards to the temple and curves downwards to the post-auricular region. Then it descends along the side of the neck to the shoulder and enters the supraclavicular fossa. One of its branches originates in the post-auricular

经相表里。左右共48穴。常用穴如下：

中渚

位置：握拳，第四、五掌骨小头后缘之间凹陷中。

主治：偏头痛，掌指疼痛、屈伸不利，肘臂痛。

手法：点、按、揉、一指禅推。

外关

位置：腕背横纹上2寸，桡骨与尺骨之间。

主治：头痛，肘臂手指疼痛、屈伸不利。

手法：一指禅推、掐、按、揉。

肩髎

位置：肩峰外下方，肩髃穴后寸许凹陷中。

主治：肩臂酸痛，肩关节活动不便。

手法：一指禅推、按、揉、掖、拿。

11) 足少阳胆经(图1-33)

本经起于目外眦的瞳子髎穴，向上到颞部，从耳后下行，经

颈部到肩上，再向前下行进入锁骨上窝。耳后的支脉入耳中，再

region, passes through the ear, re-emerges in front of the ear and reaches the posterior aspect of the outer canthus. Another branch leaves the outer canthus downwards for the point Daying (St 5) and meets the Channel of Hand-*Shaoyang* in the infraorbital region, where it descends through Jiache (St 6), reaches the neck and meets with the original channel which enters the supraclavicular fossa as mentioned above. Then it continues to travel across the chest and the diaphragm to enter its pertaining organ, the gallbladder, and communicate with the liver. It then travels along the inside of the hypochondrium to the inguinal region, passes through the vulva and goes transversely to the hip joint. The third straight branch descends from the supraclavicular fossa to the front of the axilla. Along the lateral aspect of the chest and through the hypochondrium it continues its descent to meet with the above-mentioned branch at the hip joint. From the meeting point, it goes down along the lateral side of the thigh and knee and the anterior aspect of the fibula, through the lateral malleolus, directly to Qiaoyin (GB 44) which is located at the lateral side of the tip of the 4th toe. The fourth branch originates in the dorsum of the foot and communicates with the Liver Channel of Foot-*Jueyin*. The channel has an exterior-interior relationship with the Liver Channel. There are 45 points along each side. The commonly-used are described below.

Tongziliao (GB 1)

Location: lateral to the outer canthus, at the lateral border of the orbital bone.

Indication: migraine, conjunctivitis, myopia and optic atrophy.

Manipulation: kneading, pressing and pushing with one-finger meditation.

Yangbai (GB 14)

Location: 1 *cun* superior to the midpoint of the eyebrow, directly above the pupil when looking straight ahead.

出耳前到外眦的后方，从外眦部发出的支脉，下走大迎穴，与手少阳经会于眼眶下，下经颊车穴，到颈部与上述进入锁骨上窝的支脉相会，然后进入胸中，过横膈，络肝属胆，再沿胁肋里面，下出于腹股沟部，经外阴，横入髋关节处；另一条从锁骨上窝直行的经脉，下走腋窝前面，沿着人体侧面的胸胁部，与上述入髋部的经脉会合，向下沿着大腿与膝的外侧、腓骨前面，经外踝前至第四趾外端的窍阴穴而止。从足跗发出的支脉与足厥阴肝经相联接。与肝经相表里。左右共90穴。常用穴如下：

瞳子髎

位置：在目外眦外侧，当眶骨的外缘。

主治：偏头痛，结膜炎，近视，视神经萎缩。

手法：揉、按、一指禅推。

阳白

位置：目平视，眉毛上1寸，直对瞳孔处。

Indication: facial paralysis, headache and prosopalgia.

Manipulation: pressing, wiping, lateral pushing and kneading.

Fengchi (GB 20)

Location: between the sternocleidomastoid muscle and the trapezial muscle, at the same level of Fengfu (Du 16).

Indication: headache, migraine, cold, neurosism, mental diseases, myopia and hypertension.

Manipulation: pushing with one-finger meditation, pressing, kneading, digital hitting and grasping.

Jianjing (GB 21)

Location: at the midpoint of the line connecting Dazhui (Du 14) and the acromion at the highest point of the shoulder.

Indication: stiff neck, aching of the shoulder and back, mastitis and difficulty in raising the arm.

Manipulation: grasping, kneading, pushing with one-finger meditation and rolling.

Juliao (GB 29)

Location: at the mid-point of the line between the anterosuperior iliac spine and the highest point of the greater trochanter of femur.

Indication: pain in the loins and legs, soreness and pain in the hip joint, sacro-iliilis.

Manipulation: rolling, pressing, digital hitting and heavy pressing.

Huantiao (GB 30)

Location: at the junction of the external one third and the internal two thirds of the distance between the highest point of the greater trochanter of femur and the hiatus of sacrum.

Indication: pain in the waist and legs and paralysis of the lower extremities.

Manipulation: rolling, digital hitting, pressing and heavy pressing.

Fengshi (GB 31)

主治：面瘫，头痛，三叉神经痛。

手法：按、抹、偏峰推、揉。

风池

位置：在胸锁乳突肌与斜方肌之间，平风府穴。

主治：偏正头痛，感冒，神经衰弱，精神病，近视，高血压。

手法：一指禅推、按、揉、点、拿。

肩井

位置：大椎穴与肩峰连线的中点。

主治：项强，肩背酸痛，乳腺炎，手臂上举不利。

手法：拿、揉、一指禅推、按。

居髎

位置：髂前上棘与股骨大转子连线的中点。

主治：腰腿痛，髋关节酸痛，骶髂关节炎。

手法：按、按、点、压。

环跳

位置：股骨小转子与骶管裂孔连线的外1/3与内2/3交界处。

主治：腰腿痛，下肢瘫痪。

手法：按、点、按、压。

风市

位置：在大腿外侧中线，腘横纹上 7 寸处。

Location: on the lateral midline of the thigh, 7 *cun* superior to the popliteal transverse crease.

Indication: soreness and pain in the knee joint, paralysis of the lower extremities and neuritis of lateral cutaneous nerve of the thigh.

Manipulation: rolling, digital hitting, pressing and scrubbing.

Yanglingquan (GB 34)

Location: in the depression anterior and inferior to the small head of the fibula.

Indication: soreness and pain in the knee joint, hypochondriac pain, paralysis of the lower extremities and cholecystitis.

Manipulation: grasping, pressing, kneading and digital hitting.

Juegu (GB 39)

Location: 3 *cun* above the lateral malleolus, at the posterior border of the fibula.

Indication: headache, stiffness of nape, soreness and pain in the lower extremities, paralysis, and diseases of the ankle joint.

Manipulation: grasping, pressing and kneading.

Qiuxu (GB 40)

Location: anterior and inferior to the external malleolus, in the depression on the lateral side of the tendon of the m. extensor digitorum longus.

Indication: pain in the ankle, paralysis of the lower extremities, pain in the chest and hypochondria.

Manipulation: pressing, digital hitting, grasping and kneading.

12) The Liver Channel of Foot-*Jueyin* (Fig. 1—34)

The channel originates from Dadun (Liv 1) at the tip of the big toe and passes the dorsum of the foot and the anterior border of the medial malleolus. Ascending along the shank, knee and the medial side of the thigh, it reaches the pubisure region where it goes round the external genitalia to enter the lower

主治：膝关节酸痛，下肢瘫痪，股外侧皮神经炎。

手法：㨰、点、按、擦。

阳陵泉

位置：腓骨小头前下方凹陷处。

主治：膝关节酸痛，胁肋痛，下肢瘫痪，胆囊炎。

手法：拿、按、揉、点。

绝骨

位置：外踝上3寸，腓骨后缘。

主治：头痛，项强，下肢酸痛，瘫痪，踝关节疾患。

手法：拿、按、揉。

丘墟

位置：外踝前下方，趾长伸肌腱外侧凹陷中。

主治：踝关节痛，下肢瘫痪，胸胁痛。

手法：按、点、拿、揉。

12）足厥阴肝经（图1-34）

本经起自踇趾端的大敦穴，沿足跗经内踝前向上循小腿、膝及大腿内侧，再进入阴毛中，环绕过阴器上达腹部。其外行线斜

abdomen. Its external branch goes obliquely to the point Qi-men (Liv 14) between the two ribs inferior to the nipple; its internal branch goes into the abdomen, runs along the side of the stomach and enters its pertaining organ, the liver, and communicates with the gall-bladder. Further upward, it passes through the diaphragm, spreads into the hypochondrium, and ascends along the posterior aspect of the larynx to the nasopharynx, where it connects with the surrounding tissues of the eye. Then emerging from the forehead upwards, it meets the *Du* Channel at the vertex. The branch originating in the surrounding tissues of the eye goes upwards into the cheek and curves round the lips. The branch from the liver goes upwards into the lung, where it connects with the Lung Channel of Hand-*Taiyin*. The channel is exteriorly-interiorly related to the Gall Bladder Channel. The two sides have altogether 28 points, of which the commonly-used are introduced below.

Taichong (Liv 3)

Location: on the dorsum, in the depression distal to the articulation of the 1st and 2nd metatarsals.

Indication: headache, vertigo, hypertension, hypochondriac pain, infantile convulsion, mental diseases, swelling and pain in the dorsum of the foot.

Manipulation: pressing, digital hitting, kneading and pushing with one-finger meditation.

Zhangmen (Liv 13)

Location: at the free end of the 11th rib.

Indication: distention and pain in the chest and hypochondrium, chest stuffiness and cholecystitis.

Manipulation: pressing, kneading and rubbing.

Qimen (Liv 14)

Location: directly below the nipple, in the intercostal space between the 6th and 7th ribs.

Indication: distention and pain in the chest and hypochondrium, mastitis and diseases of the gall-bladder tract.

至乳头下二肋间的期门穴；内行线则入腹挟行于 胃 旁，属 肝 络胆，上膈分布于胁肋，再向上沿着喉咙后，进入鼻咽部联接于目系，并经额向上，在头顶处与督脉相交会。从目系分出的支脉还下行颊里，环绕口唇。另外，从肝分出的支脉，向上流注 于 肺，与手太阴肺经相联接。与胆经相表里。左右共28穴。常用 穴 如下：

太冲

位置：足背第一、二跖骨结合部前的凹陷处。

主治：头痛，眩晕，高血压，胁痛，小儿惊风，精神病，足背部肿痛。

手法：按、点、揉、一指禅推。

章门

位置：第十一肋端。

主治：胸胁胀痛，胸闷，胆囊炎。

手法：按、揉、摩。

期门

位置：乳头直下，第六肋间。

主治：胸胁胀痛，乳腺炎，胆道疾患。

Manipulation: rubbing, pressing and kneading.

13) The *Ren* Channel (Fig. 1—35)

The *Ren* Channel originates in the lower abdomen, comes out from the perineum and goes upwards along the midline of the abdomen and chest to reach the throat, where it continues its way up to Chengjiang (Ren 24). It then curves the lips, passes through the cheek, and goes into the infraorbital region. The *Ren* Channel is named "the sea of all the *yin* Channels". There are 24 points altogether. The commonly-used are introduced below.

Zhongji (Ren 3)

Location: 4 *cun* below the umbilicus, on the midline of the abdomen.

Indication: pain in the lower abdomen, enuresis, urine retention, irregular menstruation and pelvic inflammation.

Manipulation: pushing with one-finger meditation, rubbing, kneading, digital hitting and pressing.

Guanyuan (Ren 4)

Location: 3 *cun* inferior to the umbilicus.

Indication: irregular menstruation, dysmenorrhea, seminal emission, impotency, enuresis, chronic diarrhea and general health care.

Manipulation: rubbing, kneading, pressing, digital hitting and pushing with one-finger meditation.

Qihai (Ren 6)

Location: 1.5 *cun* below the umbilicus.

Indication: seminal emission, impotency, dysmenorrhea, diarrhea, enuresis, irregular menstruation and general health care.

Manipulation: rubbing, kneading, pressing, vibrating, and pushing with one-finger meditation.

Shenque (Ren 8)

Location: in the centre of the umbilicus.

Indication: abdominal pain and diarrhea.

手法：摩、按、揉。

13) 任脉（图1-35）

本经起于小腹内，下出会阴，沿腹直上，经腹、胸部正中线，到达咽喉，再上行承浆穴。其经线上行环绕口唇，经过面部，进入眼眶下。任脉为阴脉之海。全径共24穴。常用穴如下：

中极

位置：前正中线上，脐下4寸。

主治：少腹痛，遗尿，尿潴留，月经不调，盆腔炎。

手法：一指禅推、摩、揉、点、按。

关元

位置：脐下3寸。

主治：月经不调，痛经，遗精，阳痿，遗尿，慢性腹泻，亦可用于保健。

手法：摩、揉、按、点、一指禅推。

气海

位置：脐下1.5寸。

主治：遗精，阳痿，痛经，腹泻，遗尿，月经不调，亦可用于保健。

手法：摩、揉、按、振、一指禅推。

神阙

位置：肚脐正中。

主治：腹痛，泄泻。

Manipulation: rubbing, pressing, kneading and vibrating.

Zhongwan (Ren 12)

Location: 4 *cun* above the umbilicus.

Indication: stomachache, abdominal distention, vomiting and indigestion.

Manipulation: rubbing, pressing, kneading and vibrating.

Tanzhong (Ren 17)

Location: on the anterior median line at the level of the 4th intercostal space, and at the midpoint between the two nipples.

Indication: cough with dyspnea, chest stuffiness, chest pain, hiccup, mastitis and angina pectoris.

Manipulation: pushing with one-finger meditation, rubbing, pressing and kneading.

Tiantu (Ren 22)

Location: at the centre of the suprasternal fossa.

Indication: cough with dyspnea, difficulty in coughing up sputum, aphasia and hiccup.

Manipulation: kneading, pressing, nipping and digital hitting.

Lianquan (Ren 23)

Location: Superior to the laryngeal protuberance, in the depression of the superior border of the hyoid bone.

Indication: aphasia, stiff tongue, dysphagia and laryngopharyngitis.

Manipulation: pressing, kneading, digital hitting and flicking-poking.

Chengjiang (Ren 24)

Location: at the midpoint of the mentolabial sulcus.

Indication: facial paralysis, prosopalgia and toothache.

Manipulation: pressing, kneading and nipping.

14) The *Du* Channel (Fig. 1—36)

The channel originates in the lower abdomen and emerges from the perineum. It goes backwards to Changqiang (Du 1), ascends through the spinal column, reaches Fengfu (Du

手法：摩、按、揉、振。

中脘

位置：脐上4寸。

主治：胃痛，腹胀，呕吐，消化不良。

手法：摩、按、揉、振。

膻中

位置：前正中线，平第4肋间隙，两乳间正中点。

主治：咳喘，胸闷，胸痛，呃逆，乳腺炎，心绞痛。

手法：一指禅推、摩、按、揉。

天突

位置：胸骨上窝正中。

主治：喘咳，咯痰不畅，失语，呃逆。

手法：揉、按、掐、点。

廉泉

位置：在喉结上方，舌骨上缘凹陷中。

主治：失语，舌强，吞咽困难，咽喉炎。

手法：按、揉、点、弹拨。

承浆

位置：在颏唇沟正中。

主治：面瘫，三叉神经痛，牙痛。

手法：按、揉、掐。

14）督脉（图1-36）

本经起于小腹内，下出会阴，向后至长强穴，上行于脊柱内，

16) and enters the brain.   It then passes through the vertex and goes down along the forehead to the tip of the nose. Through Renzhong (Du 26) or the groove of the upper lip it reaches Yinjiao (Du 28) at the upper labial frenum. The *Du* Channel is termed "the sea of all the *yang* channels'. There are altogether 30 points. Those commonly-used are described below.

Changqiang (Du 1)

Location: 0.5 *cun* inferior to the tip of the coccyx.

Indication: diarrhea, constipation, anus prolapse and pain in the waist and spine.

Manipulation: pressing and kneading.

Yaoyangguan (Du 3)

Location: inferior to the spinous process of the 4th lumbar vertebra.

Indication: pain in the waist and spine and paralysis of the lower extremities.

Manipulation: rolling, pushing with one-finger meditation, pressing, kneading and scrubbing.

Mingmen (Du 4)

Location: inferior to the spinous process of the 2nd lumbar vertebra.

Indication: pain in the waist and spine, seminal emission, impotency, chronic diarrhea, irregular menstruation and dysmenorrhea.

Manipulation: rolling, pushing with one-finger meditation, pressing, kneading and scrubbing.

Shenzhu (Du 12)

Location: inferior to the spinous process of the 3rd thoracic vertebra.

Indication: cough and pain in the back.

Manipulation: rolling, pressing, kneading and pushing with one-finger meditation,

Dazhui (Du 14)

上达风府，进入脑内，上行巅顶，沿前额下行到鼻柱，并经人中沟至口中上唇系带的龈交穴。督脉为阳脉之海。全经共 30 穴，常用穴如下：

长强

位置：尾骨尖下 0.5 寸。

主治：腹泻，便秘，脱肛，腰脊疼痛。

手法：按、揉。

腰阳关

位置：第四腰椎棘突下。

主治：腰脊疼痛，下肢瘫痪。

手法：揉、一指禅推、按、揉、擦。

命门

位置：第二腰椎棘突下。

主治：腰脊疼痛，遗精，阳痿，慢性腹泻，月经不调，痛经。

手法：揉、一指禅推、按、揉、擦。

身柱

位置：第三胸椎棘突下。

主治：咳嗽，背痛。

手法：揉、按、揉、一指禅推。

大椎

Location: inferior to the process of the 7th cervical vertebra.

Indication: cold, fever, stiff neck, cough, asthma and pain in the neck and back.

Manipulation: rolling, pressing, kneading, fist-striking and pushing with one-finger meditation.

Fengfu (Du 16)

Location: 1 *cun* above the midpoint of the posterior hairline.

Indication: stiffiness and pain in the nape and head, mental diseases and sequel of apoplexy

Manipulation: pushing with one-finger meditation, pressing, kneading and digital hitting.

Baihui (Du 20)

Location: 7 *cun* above the posterior hairline, midway on the line connecting the apex of both ears.

Indication: headache, dizziness, coma, hypertension, prolapse of anus and mental diseases.

Manipulation: pressing, kneading, pushing with one-finger meditation and vibrating.

Renzhong (Du 26)

Location: at the junction of the upper one-third and lower two-thirds of the midline of the nasolabial groove.

Indication: infantile convulsion, facial paralysis, mental diseases and acute sprain of the waist.

Manipulation: nipping and kneading.

4. Common Extraordinary Points and the Manipulations of Massage

Yintang (Extra 1)

Location: at the midpoint of the line connecting the medial ends of the two eyebrows.

Indication: headache, rhinitis and insomnia.

Manipulation: pushing with one-finger meditation, wiping, pressing and kneading.

位置：第七颈椎棘突下。

主治：感冒，发热，落枕，咳嗽，哮喘，项背痛。

手法：擦、按、揉、拳击、一指禅推。

风府

位置：后发际正中直上 1 寸。

主治：头项强痛，精神病，中风后遗症。

手法：一指禅推、按、揉、点。

百会

位置：后发际直上 7 寸，当两耳尖联线的中点。

主治：头痛，头晕，昏厥，高血压，脱肛，精神病。

手法：按、揉、一指禅推、振。

人中

位置：人中沟正中线上1/3与下2/3交界处。

主治：惊风，口眼歪斜，精神病，急性腰扭伤。

手法：掐、揉。

4. 常用奇穴及推拿手法

印堂

位置：两眉头连线的中点。

主治：头痛，鼻炎，失眠。

手法：一指禅推、抹、按、揉。

Taiyang (Extra 2)

Location: in the depression about 1 *cun* lateral to the line connecting the lateral end of the brow and the outer canthus.

Indication: headache, cold and eye diseases.

Manipulation: pressing, kneading, wiping and pushing with one-finger meditation.

Yuyao (Extra 3)

Location: in the middle of the eyebrow.

Indication: pain in the superciliary ridge, conjunctival congestion with swelling and trembling of the eyelids.

Manipulation: wiping, pushing with one-finger meditation, and pressing.

Yaoyan (Extra)

Location: in the depression of 3 *cun* lateral and inferior to the spinous process of the 3rd lumbar vertebra.

Indication: sprain of the waist and soreness in the waist and back.

Manipulation: rolling, pressing, grasping and scrubbing.

Huatuo Jiaji (Extra 21)

Location: the line 0.5 *cun* lateral to the inferior border of each spinous process from the 1st thoracic vertebra to the 5th lumbar vertebra.

Indication: pain and stiffness in the spinal column, pain in the waist and abdomen, diseases of the internal organs, and health promotion.

Manipulation: rolling, scrubbing, heavy pressing, pushing and pushing with one-finger meditation.

Shiqizhuixia (Extra 19)

Location: inferior to the spinous process of the 5th lumbar vertebra.

Indication: pain in the waist and leg.

Manipulation: digital hitting, rolling and pressing.

Shixuan (Extra 30)

Location: at the tips of the ten fingers, 0.1 *cun* from the nail.

太阳

位置：眉梢与目外眦之间向后约1寸处凹陷中。

主治：头痛，感冒，眼病。

手法：按、揉、抹、一指禅推。

鱼腰

位置：眉毛的中点。

主治：眉棱骨痛，目赤肿痛，眼睑颤动。

手法：抹、一指禅推、按。

腰眼

位置：第三腰椎棘突下旁开3寸凹陷处。

主治：腰扭伤，腰背酸楚。

手法：㨰、按、拿、擦。

华佗夹脊

位置：第一胸椎至第五腰椎，各椎棘突下旁开0.5寸。

主治：脊椎疼痛、强直，胸腹诸痛，脏腑疾患，并有强壮作用。

手法：㨰、擦、压、推、一指禅推。

十七椎下

位置：第五腰椎棘突下。

主治：腰腿痛。

手法：点、㨰、按。

十宣

位置：十手指尖端，距指甲0.1寸。

Indication: coma.

Manipulation: nipping.

Heding (Extra 31)

Location: in the depression at the center of the upper border of the patella.

Indication: swelling and pain in the knee joint.

Manipulation: pressing, kneading and digital hitting.

Lanwei (Extra 33)

Location: 2 *cun* inferior to Zusanli (St 63).

Indication: appendicitis and abdominal pain.

Manipulation: pressing, grasping, kneading, digital hitting.

Jianneiling (Extra)

Location: midpoint of a line connecting the upper end of the anterior axillary fold and the point Jianyu (LI 15)

Indication: soreness and pain in the shoulder joint with difficulty in movement.

Manipulation: pushing with one finger meditation, rolling, grasping, pressing, kneading.

Qiaogong (Extra)

Location: the line posterior to the ear connecting Yifeng (SJ 17) and Quepen (St 12).

Indication: hyperactivity of the liver-*yang* manifested as headache, distension of the eye, hypertension.

Manipulation: pushing with one-finger meditation, pressing, and kneading.

主治：昏厥。

手法：掐。

鹤顶

位置：髌骨上缘正中凹陷处。

主治：膝关节肿痛。

手法：按、揉、点。

阑尾穴

位置：足三里穴下2寸。

主治：阑尾炎，腹痛。

手法：按、拿、揉、点。

肩内陵

位置：腋前皱襞顶端，与肩髃穴连线中点。

主治：肩关节酸痛、运动障碍。

手法：一指禅推、㨰、拿、按、揉。

桥弓

位置：耳后自翳风到缺盆一线。

主治：肝阳上亢，头痛，目胀，高血压。

手法：一指禅推、按、揉。

Chapter Two

Adult Massage

In ancient Chinese massage there were not such terms as adult massage or child massage. In order to make it different from the child massage which has been confirmed and developed ever since the Ming Dynasty, modern scholars put forward the academic terminology — "adult massage". Adult massage refers to the massage therapies used for the prevention and treatment of various diseases of adults. Compared with child massage, it has the following characteristics: ① its manipulation movement has a greater range with heavier strength; ② its chief manipulated portions are the superficial routes of the fourteen channels and collaterals, points on the regular channels (*Jing* points), channel tendons, skin areas, extra-ordinary points, and specific areas on the trunk and limbs; ③ it has an extensive adaptable sphere with indications in the departments of internal medicine, surgery, gynecology, traumalogy, nerves, rehabilitation and the five sense organs. In addition, because it has various manipulations and its effective intensity can be readjusted with a great elasticity, we can also use it to treat the common diseases of infants so long as we follow the principles of determining manipulation according to differentiation of syndromes and keeps uitable stimulation.

Section 1

Commonly-used Manipulations

"Manipulation" is the importa~t means of massage treatment. Its manipulating quality · ~ of its clinical dif-

第 二 章

成 人 推 拿

中国推拿在古代并无成人与小儿之分。近代学者为了有别于自明代以来确立、发展起来的小儿推拿,遂提出了"成人推拿"这一专业名称。成人推拿是指主要用于防治成年人各种病证的推拿方法,与小儿推拿相比,其特点:一是手法动作幅度较大、用力较深重;二是施术部位以十四经络外行经线、经穴、筋经、皮部、经外奇穴及躯干、四肢的特定部位为主;三是适应范围广,适应症遍及内科、外科、妇科、骨伤科、神经科、康复科及五官科等临床各科。而且,由于其手法种类多,作用强度可调范围大,故在临床实用时,只要遵循辨证施术的原则,掌握好适宜的刺激量,这种方法同样也可用于治疗儿科的各种常见病证。

第一节 常用手法

"手法"是推拿治病的主要手段,手法操作的质量及临诊辨证

ferentiation can directly affect the curative result of massage. Therefore, in order to become a qualified massage doctor, one must also work hard at the technical theory of the manipulations and their movement principles so as to have a good command of the standardized skills of various manipulations besides the conscientious studies of the TCM theory and constant improvement of the diagnosis and differentiation.

Massage manipulations refer to the manipulating skills with standardized movement structure for the treatment done by the massagers with their hands, limbs or other parts of the body at the specified locations of the patients. The operation structure or appearance of the manipulation is called movement structure consisting of the following two aspects: ① The characteristics of the movement shown by the time and the space features of the manipulation movement, i.e. kinematic features of the manipulation; ② the phenomena and features of the mutual-acted forces which determine the movement style of the manipulation, also known as the mechanic features of the manipulation. In the concrete operation, it is chiefly related to the support and cooperation of the operator's posture, carriage, breath and activities of his will; The manipulation's preparatory posture, the stages of operation, operation style and the essentials of operation include the angles of various links of the movement, trace and speed of the movement, frequency, rhythm, period, labour-division of acting muscles and their interrelations and so on. Traditional massage strongly emphasized the standardization of operating structure because the manipulating technique based on the standardized structure of operation can not only create specified dynamic effect on the human body so as to give an excellent therapeutic effect, but also have great significance for the professional massagers themselves to prevent prefessional injury.

Traditional massage requires that manipulation should be permanent, forceful, even and soft so as to be deep and tho-

施术的水平，可直接影响推拿的医疗效果。因此，要想成为一名合格的推拿医生，除认真学习中医理论，不断提高诊病与辨证本领外，还必须努力钻研手法技术理论与动作原理，并通过刻苦练习，娴熟地掌握好各种手法规范的操作技能。

以医疗为目的，术者用手或肢体其他部分，在受术者身体特定部位，进行的各种具有规范化动作结构的操作技术，称为推拿手法。手法动作的方式与外形称为手法的动作结构，主要包括两个方面的内容：一是手法动作的时间和空间特征所表现出来的动作形式上的特点，即手法的运动学特征；二是决定着手法动作形式的诸力相互作用的情况和特点，即手法的动力学特征。在具体操作时，主要涉及术者的体位、姿势、呼吸、意念活动的支持与配合；手法的预备姿势、动作阶段、动作方法与动作要领，包括术者各运动环节的角度、运动轨迹与速度、频率、节律、周期以及动作肌肉的分工及相互关系等各个方面。传统推拿学十分强调动作结构的规范化，这是因为建立在规范化动作结构基础上的手法技能，不但对人体可产生具有特定动力形式的作用力，从而发挥良好的医疗效果，而且对防止推拿专业工作者自身的职业性损伤具有重要意义。

传统推拿学对手法动作技术要求持久、有力、均匀、柔和，

rough. The so-called "permanence" is that manipulation should last for a certain period of time according to the requirement, that is, the structure of manipulation keeps unchanged within a certain period of time and has a steady dynamic form; "forcefulness" is that manipulation must have a certain force which should be strengthened or weakened according to the patient's constitution, state of illness, age, therapeutic portions, etc; so-called "evenness" is that manipulation should be rhythmical, with the same frequency and pressing force all the time; "softness" is that the manipulation should be light but not superficial, heavy but not retained, not rough and hard, and the shift of the movements should be natural and smooth; "deepness and thoroughness" means that the manipulation must keep a certain direction of force in addition to the requirements above in order to achieve a deep effect on the affected part of the patient's body and create curative effect. The aspects above are closely interrelated. These are the operating essentials of all kinds of manipulations, which guide in practice the technical training of the manipulation and clinical operation. However, because of the variety of manipulations and different structures of operation, the requirement for each concrete manipulation may vary, and each manipulation has its distinctive emphasis. For example, the pushing with one-finger meditation and rolling manipulation require "softness" with strength residing in but with emphasis on "softness"; digital hitting manipulation requires accurate resolute, rapid and forceful hitting "with softness residing in", but emphasizing "strength"; rubbing technique requires that the operation should be "neither rapid nor slow, neither mild nor forceful, and be proceeded in a moderate manner," and the operator should also concentrate on "the moderate manner". Therefore the operator must not only have a good command of the basic requirements of the operating technique, but also try to fathom carefully the distinctive cha-

从而达到深透的目的。所谓"持久"，是指手法能按要求持续运用一定时间，亦即在一定间时内手法动作结构保持不变，且具有稳定的动力形式；所谓"有力"，是指手法必须具有一定的力量，这种力量应该根据受术者的体质、病情、年龄、部位等不同情况而增减；所谓"均匀"是指手法动作要有节奏性，操作频率不要时快时慢，压力不要时轻时重；所谓"柔和"，是指手法要轻而不浮，重而不滞，用力不可生硬粗暴，动作变换要自然、流畅。"深透"，是指在上述要求的基础上，手法操作还必须掌握一定的用力方向，从而使作用力深入受术者体内直达病所，而发挥治疗作用。以上是对各种手法动作要领的总结，在实践中指导着手法的技能训练和临床施术。但是，由于手法种类多，动作结构不完全一样，故对于每一种具体的手法来说，要求并不完全一致，而是各有侧重。如一指禅推法，㨰法要求以"柔和为贵"，要柔中寓刚，突出一个"柔"字；击点法则要求击点准确，用力果敢快速而刚强，要"刚中带柔"，强调一个"刚"字；而摩法又要求操作时"不宜急，不宜缓，不宜轻，不宜重，以中和之义施之"，又立意在"中和"。所以，学者不但要从总体上把握好手法技术的基本要求，而且还必

racteristics of every manipulation, so that he can understand the principles of the manipulation thoroughly, moreover, through hard practice, he can improve his operation to an ideal realm of "once in clinic, touching outside with the skillful force inside; changing the manipulation with the mind concentrated, and getting principles from the concentration of mind".

Massage in China goes back to the ancient times. In its long development, ancient and modern medical scientists have created many effective manipulations. Up to now, more than 300 kinds of massage have been recorded in writing. Twenty basic manipulations will be briefly introduced as follows:

1. Pushing Manipulation with One-finger Meditation

Pushing with one-finger meditation refers to the manipulation of operator's using the tip of the thumb, or the whorled surface of the thumb to push the region to be treated with the shoulder relaxing, the elbow dropping, wrist hanging, elbow flexing and stretching cyclically to power the forearm and wrist joint to swing inward and outward, with the combination of thumb's flexion and extension (Fig. 2—1).

STRUCTURE OF OPERATION

In operation, the operator is in a regular sitting position or upright standing position. When the sitting position is used, the operator should draw in his chest and pull up the back with the lumbar region straightened in order to keep the upper part of the body in upright sitting posture, but he should not arch his back and collapse his waist. The operator sets his feet on the ground steadily with a slight separation, just the same width as that of his shoulders. In standing position, the operator's feet take a T-shaped posture.

The preparatory posture of the operating upper limb is as follows: relaxing muscles of the shoulder girdle in a naturally dropping position, slightly stretching the shoulder joints out-

须细心揣摩每种手法各自的特点，才有可能对手法技术的原理有全面的理解，并在此基础上，通过刻苦练习，使手法达到"一旦临诊，机触于外，巧生于内，手随心转，法从心出"的高超境界。

中国推拿源远流长，在漫长的发展过程中，古今医学家创造了许多行之有效的手法，至今可见之于文字记载的就有三百多种。现将最常用的二十种基本手法简要介绍如下：

1. 一指禅推法

用大拇指指端或罗纹面或偏峰着力于治疗部位，沉肩、垂肘、悬腕，以周期性的肘关节屈伸，带动前臂与腕关节作内、外摆动，与拇指关节屈伸的联合动作，即谓一指禅推法(图2-1)。

【动作结构】

本法在操作时，术者取端坐位或直立位。坐势时，要含胸拔背，腰部挺起以保持上身正直，不要弓背塌腰。双足放平踏稳，并略分开与肩等宽；站势时取丁字步。

施术上肢的预备姿势为：肩带部肌肉放松，呈自然下垂，肩

wards and forwards about 15 to 30 degrees so as to have a space of a fist in the axillary fossa (dropping shoulders); under the condition that the elbow joint is suspended at the shoulder region and sustained by the powered thumb, lowering the elbow joint without outward lifting-up and keeping flexion between 90 to 100 degrees, with the forearm in prone position and the palm facing downward and keeping it even (dropping elbow); the wrist joint is suspended and dropped to form an angle of 90 to 110 degrees at the wrist joint region between the lower end of the radius and the first metacarpal bone (suspending wrist); making a hollow fist with the index finger, middle finger, ring finger and the little finger naturally flexed, but never pinch tightly and forcefully (empty palm); stretch straightly the thumb to cover the fist center, solidly and steadily press the finger tip or the whorled surface against the part to be treated to make a angle of 90 degrees between the longitudinal line of the thumb and the region to be treated.

The manipulation can be divided into two stages: outward swinging and inward swinging. In operation, beginning from the preparatory posture as mentioned above, the operator extends outward the elbow joint with the power from his brachial triceps muscle which makes the forearm, wrist and thumb swing 30°—45° outward, and then, with the brachial triceps muscle relaxed, contracts the brachial biceps muscle of the arm to cause a reverse change of the elbow joint from outward extension to inward flexion and make his forearm and wrist move from outward swinging position through the preparatory posture to the inward swinging position of about 30 degrees; meanwhile, the thumb joint has also changed from the extending position in outward swinging position to the flexing position. The range of the elbow joint's extension and flexion during the whole movement of swinging is about 10 to 20 degrees. Moreover, the operator, with the surface of the thumb as the sustaining point, contracts and excites his

关节略向前外方伸出约在 15°～30°左右，使腋窝有一约能容一拳大小的空间（沉肩）；肘关节在肩部悬吊与着力指支撑的条件下，顺势下沉，不要向外抬起，并保持在屈曲90°～120°之间，前臂则在旋前位掌面朝下放平（垂肘）；腕关节屈曲向下悬垂，使桡骨下端与第一掌在腕关节处的夹角在90°～110°之间（悬腕）；食、中、无名、小指呈自然屈曲状，使手握空拳，不要用力捏紧（掌虚）；而拇指伸直盖住拳眼，以指峰或罗纹面着力，稳实地支撑在治疗部位，使拇指的纵轴线与治疗部位垂直，呈90°直角。

本法整个动作过程，可分为外摆与内摆二个阶段，操作时，从上述预备位开始，先以肱三头肌发力，使肘关节外伸，并带动前臂、腕部与拇指向外摆动30°～45°；接着肱三头肌放松，肱二头肌开始收缩，使肘关节由外伸逆转向内屈，并带动前臂、腕部从外摆位向内经过预备位，再向内摆动30°左右，此时，拇指关节也从外摆时的伸展位过渡到屈曲位。肘关节在整个摆动中的伸屈范围在10°～20°左右。如此，以拇指着力面为支撑点，由肱

brachial triceps muscle and biceps muscle of his arm alternatively, which causes the forearm, the wrist and thumb at the two sides of the preparatory posture to proceed back and forth the inward and outward swinging movement lastingly, evenly and rhythmically. This kind of manipulation is called pushing with one-finger meditation.

Among them, operating with the power from the tip of the thumb is called finger-tip pushing; in which the interphalangeal joint of the thumb is fixed at the back-stretching position, operating with the force from the whorled surface is called whorl-pushing; operating with the force from the Shaoshang (Lu 11) point at the side of the thumb-radius is called lateral pushing, in this operation, the operator slightly flexes his wrist joint with index finger, middle finger, ring finger and little finger naturally stretching forward in the finger-separating pattern. The frequency of the three types of pushing is about 120—160 times per minute. There is another manipulation, in which the operator pushes with the force from the finger tip, with a narrow range and quick frequency of more than 240 times per minute. That kind of manipulation is called quick vibrating-pushing manipulation or quick pushing manipulation.

In operating with this technique, first, the principle of exerting force naturally is emphasized, as a result of the weight of the upper limb and the interracted force in the operation, enough applied force will be created in the thumb's longitudinal direction, and the force will be transmitted and permeated in an undulating manner into the part to be treated through the contacting point of the thumb so as to exert the therapeutic effect. Therefore, the operator should avoid pressing forcefully and deliberately to increase the force of the manipulation in case the applied force is stagnant, heavy, stiff or even causing injury; then during the process of manipulation, the power-app'ying point of the thumb should be constantly "fixed"

二头肌与肱三头肌交替兴奋、收缩，并带动前臂、腕与拇指在起始位的两侧，往复地以均匀节律持久进行的内、外摆动的动作即为一指禅推法。

其中，以拇指端峰为着力点操作的称指峰推；操作时，拇指指间关节固定在背伸位，以罗纹面为着力点的称罗纹推；以拇指桡侧少商穴处为着力面的又叫偏峰推，此法操作时腕关节略屈，食、中、无名、小指向前自然伸开，成散手状。以上三种推法频率均在 120～160 次/分左右。还有一种以指峰着力，摆幅小，频率快达每分钟 240 次以上者，称缠推法或缠法。

本法操作时，首先要强调自然着力原则。因为，由于上肢自身的重量及动作过程中诸力相互作用的结果，会自然地向拇指纵轴所指的方向产生足够的作用力，并以波动的形式通过拇指着力点向治疗部位传递与深透，从而发挥手法的治疗作用，所以，不要采用故意用力向下按压的方法，来增加手法的力度，以免所产生的作用力滞重、生硬, 甚或发生损伤；其次，在施术过程中, 拇指的着力点要始终"吸定"在治疗穴点上，不得在皮肤表面滑移或

on the point for treatment, and slipping or rubbing on the surface of the skin should be avoided. In the swinging process, the shift of manipulation should be natural, steady and not in a jumping manner, so that the manipulation is soft.

For the dynamic type resulted from the standardized one-finger meditation, refer to the dynamic curve diagram of pushing manipulation with one-finger meditation (Fig. 2—2, 2—3, 2—4, 2—5) recorded live during the operation by the contemporary disciples of one-finger pushing manipulation Zhu Chunting, Wang Jisong, etc. themselves.

CLINICAL APPLICATION

The characteristics of this technique is that the area of power-applying point is small but the applied force has great pressure and deepness and thoroughness, and the stimulating intensity can be adjusted at will according to the specified requirement, and the stimulus is lasting, rhythmical and soft. This technique is applied to the operation on all the channels and collaterals and points all over the body. It can be used to treat various kinds of common diseases in departments of internal medicine, gynecology, traumatology, five sense organs and pediatrics. Whorl-pushing is applied best to the abdominal regions to treat the diseases of gastrointestinal alimentary system and the common diseases in the department of gynecology; finger-tip pushing is good at treating the miscelaneous diseases in the internal medicine department such as headache, dizziness, insomnia, hypertension, stagnation of the liver-qi, arthralgia-syndrome; quick pushing manipulation has special therapeutic effect on the laryngological diseases, carbuncle, furuncle and so on; lateral pushing, because of its light stimulation, is suitable for the operation on the craniofacial region and the regions around the five sense organs; it is commonly used to treat myopia, monochromatism, rhinorrhea with turbid discharge, facial paralysis, headache, tinnitus, toothache, etc.

摩擦，摆动时，要做到动作过渡自然、平稳，不得跳动，以使手法柔和。

由规范的一指禅推法动作所产生的动力形式，可见由当代一指禅推拿的传人朱春霆、王纪松等亲自操作时所实录的一指禅推法动态曲线图（图2-2,2-3,2-4,2-5）。

【临床应用】

本法的特点是着力点面积小，作用力压强大，深透性强，刺激量的大小可根据需要随意调节，是一种持续的节律性的柔和刺激。该法适用于在全身各部经络、穴位操作，可治疗内、妇、骨伤、五官及儿科各种常见病证。其中，罗纹推适用于腹部，以治疗胃肠消化系统及妇科病证见长；指峰推善于治疗头痛、头晕、失眠、高血压、肝郁、痹症等内科杂病；缠推法则对喉科病证以及痈疖等证有特效；偏峰推刺激量小，适用于在头面和五官周围操作，故常用于治疗近视、色盲、鼻渊、面瘫、头痛、耳鸣、牙痛等病证。

2. Rolling Manipulation

With the minor thenar eminence and dorsoulnar used as the force-applying surface, the practitioner lowers his shoulder and drops his elbow with his arm erected and his palm set upright, proceeds cyclical flexion, extension and inward and outward arm-rotating swinging with the elbow joint and his forearm accompanied with extension and flexion of the wrist joint to roll the round back of the hand to and fro on the region to be treated. Such manipulation is called rolling manipulation (Fig. 2—6).

STRUCTURE OF OPERATION

In the operation, the operator is usually in a standing position. The posture of sitting on a tall stool can be adopted when it is necessary. When the standing position is adopted, the operator should separate his lower limbs and keep them as wide as or slightly wider than his shoulders, set his feet on the ground steadily and relax the popliteal fossae; forward lunge can also be adopted, the posture of which should be adjusted at any time to a suitable height according to the requirement, and the operator should keep the upper part of his body upright with slight forward bending so as to make it easy for his upper limbs to generate force.

The preparatory posture of the manipulation is as follows: the operator lowers his shoulder and drops his elbow with the wrist joint straightly stretched and his forearm in moderately erecting position (arm-erecting), setting his palm upright, pressing the minor thenar eminence against the part for treatment with his palm and phalangeal joints naturally flexed.

Beginning from the preparatory posture, the operator slightly extends his elbow with the force from the brachial triceps muscles, and at the same time, co-operatively contracts

2. 𢷬法

以小鱼际及手背尺侧为着力面，**沉肩、垂肘、立臂、竖掌**，肘关节与前臂做周期性的屈、伸与内、外旋臂摆动，并带动腕关节伸、屈，使弓成圆形的手背在施术部位上作来回滚动的手法即谓𢷬法(图2-6)。

【动作结构】

本法在操作时，术者一般取站位，必要时可用高凳坐位。站势时，两下肢分开与肩等宽，或略宽于肩，双足踏稳、两腘空松，或取弓步势，步势要根据需要随时调节至适当的高度，上身保持正直，略向前倾，以利于上肢的发力。

施术的预备姿势为：沉肩、垂肘、腕关节伸直，前臂于中立位(立臂)，手掌竖起，以小鱼际肌肌腹按贴在治疗部位，手掌与手指关节呈自然屈曲状。

动作从预备位开始，首先由肱三头肌发力，使肘略伸，同时

the supinator muscle of his forearm and biceps muscle of his arm to cause his forearm to supinate to outward swinging position of about 45 degrees. At this moment, the lower end of his radius intersects in front of the ulna to cause the wrist joint to flex forwards and make his rounded hand back accomplish a half circle ontward rolling on the part for treatment, along the sustaining surface, from minor thenar eminance to 1/3—1/2 of the ulnar; then he relaxes the brachial triceps muscle, biceps muscle of his arm and supinater muscle group, and contracts pronator group to cause his forearm to proceed with inward rotation of his arm in the pronator manner and go on to swing inward from moderately erecting position to the inward swinging position with about 15° pronation. At this moment, the radius is rotated back again to the back of the ulna, and the wrist joint is also changed from flexion to extension; the force-applying surface of his hand back on the treating region also returns to minor thenar eminance from the portion at 1/3—1/2 of the ulnar region, so that a half-circle rolling has been accomplished in the inward swinging process.

When the manipulation is used continuously from inward swinging to outward swinging, and vice versa, the following should be carefully observed: the operator's hand back should be kept close to the skin of the operated region, scrubbing to and fro and slipping on it should be avoided; the intensity of the force and rhythem should be even, never be quick one moment and slow the next, or light one moment and heavy the next, and stiff push is not allowed; the operating hand should not be lifted up away from the therapeutic region between the swinging periods in case tapping will be caused; the metacarpophalangeal and interphalangeal joints keep in natural flexing position without any active pinching or closing or extending; the transition of the wrist joints' flexion and extension should be natural without any jerk. The frequency of this manipulation is 120—160 times per minute.

前臂旋后肌与肱二头肌协同收缩，使前臂旋后转臂至约45°的外摆位。此时，桡骨下端交叉到尺骨前方，并带动腕关节向前折屈，使弓成圆形的手背，沿着其支撑面，从小鱼际到尺侧1/3～1/2处，在施术部位上完成向外半周的滚动，接着，肱三头肌、肱二头肌与旋后肌群放松，旋前肌群收缩，使前臂向内作旋前转臂，经过中立位再向内摆动至旋前约15°的内摆位。此时，桡骨又回旋至尺骨的后方，腕关节亦随之由屈过渡到伸，手背的着力面在施术部位上，也从尺侧1/3～1/2处返回至小鱼际，完成了内摆阶段的半周滚动。

本法在连续操作时，内摆至外摆，外摆又复内摆，周而复始连绵不断，要特别注意，手背着力面须始终紧贴治疗部位的皮肤，不能在上面来回拖擦与滑移，力度与节律要均匀，不能忽快忽慢、时轻时重，或用重力硬顶，在摆动周期之间，术手不要抬起离开治疗部位，以免造成上、下起落的敲击动作，手的掌指与指间关节一直保持自然屈曲的姿势，无任何主动捏拢与伸展的动作，腕关节的屈伸交替要过渡自然，不要引起跳动。本法的频率在每分钟120～160次之间。

Rolling manipulation is the main therapeutic manipulation of the rolling-massage school. For the dynamic type produced by the standardized rolling manipulation, refer to the dynamic curve diagram of rolling manipulation recorded live while the founder of rolling manipulation Professor Ding Jifeng, was doing this manipulation (Fig 2—7, 2—8, 2—9).

CLINICAL APPLICATION

Rolling manipulation which has a large area of stimulation with strong effect, evident deepness and thoroughness, is one of the most commonly-used manipulations. This manipulation can be performed on all the points except the craniofacial regions, anterior cervical part and thoracico-abdominal region, and it is especially suitable for the operation on the lumbodorsal region, lumbo-buttock region and thick muscle regions of the limbs. In operation, if the stimulation needs strengthening, then the operating hand can be erected to operate with the force from the second, third, fourth and fifth metacarpophalangeal joints. This manipulation has the following effects: reflexing the muscle and tendon and dredging the channel, expelling pathogenic wind and cold, warming the channel, expelling pathogenic dampness, promoting blood circulation to remove blood stasis, relieving spasm and pain, relaxing adhesion, lubricating joint, etc. and it is good at treating the diseases in motor system and nerve system.

3. Kneading Manipulation

This is a manipulation performed by kneading slowly and softly the therapeutic region to-and-fro with fingers, the bottom of the palm, major thenar eminance or the tip of the elbow. According to the different parts to be operated, it can be divided into middle-finger kneading manipulation, thumb-kneading manipulation, palm-root kneading manipulation, major-thenar kneading manipulation, elbow-kneading manipulation, etc. (Fig. 2—10).

滚法是滚法推拿流派的主治手法，由规范的滚法动作所产生的动力形式，可见由滚法推拿创始人丁季峰教授操作时实录的滚法动态曲线图(图2-7,2-8,2-9)。

【临床应用】

滚法刺激面积大，作用力强，深透作用明显，是临床最常用的手法之一。本法除头面、前颈及胸腹部外,其他部位均可使用，特别适用于腰背、腰臀及四肢肌肉较为丰厚的部位。治疗时，如需加大刺激量，可将术手立起来，以第2、3、4、5掌指关节处着力来进行操作。本法具有舒筋通络、祛风散寒、温经胜湿、活血化瘀、解痉止痛、松解粘连、滑利关节等功效，尤以治疗运动系统与神经系统疾病见长。

3. 揉法

以指、掌根、大鱼际或肘尖为着力点，在治疗部位做轻柔缓和的回旋动作即为揉法。其中，根据着力部位的不同，可分为中指揉法、拇指揉法、掌根揉法、大鱼际揉法和肘揉法等(图2-10)。

STRUCTURE OF OPERATION

In this manipulation, the operator can be either in sitting position or standing position. He presses the operated region with his middle finger, thumb-tip, palm-root or the end of his elbow, and, with the cooperation of his shoulder, elbow, forearm and wrist joint, does annulospiral rotation within a narrow range, which causes the skin of the treated region to rotate slowly and softly so that the soft, light and slow internal rubbing is produced between the skin and the internal soft tissue. The whole manipulation emphasizes softness, and the range of kneading and rotating should be gradually extended, and the force gradually increased. The operating hand should be fixed on the treated region without any rubbing or slipping on the skin surface. The frequency is about 100—160 times per minute.

CLINICAL APPLICATION

The effect of kneading manipulation is light, soft and slow but deep and thorough. Warm effect can be created in the deep layer of the tissue by the internal rubbing caused by kneading. This manipulation can be applied to all parts of the body, and is one of the commonly-used manipulations of clinical massage. Among the kneading manipulations, major thenar kneading manipulation is frequently applied to the craniofacial and, thoracico-abdominal regions and the swelling or aching parts of the limbs caused by acute sprain and contusion; palmar-bottom kneading manipulation is frequently applied to the lumbodorsal region, buttock region and the thick muscular regions of the limbs; finger-kneading manipulation can be operated on all the channel points throughout the body and the regions that need digital stimulation; elbow-kneading manipulation is suitable for treating the deep layer of the tissue. Kneading manipulation has the following effects: soothing the chest oppression and regulating the flow of qi, strengthening the spleen and regulating stomach, promot-

【动作结构】

应用本法，术者可取坐位或站位。以中指端面，或拇指端面，或掌根，或肘尖部着力按压在治疗部位，在肩、肘、前臂与腕关节的协同下，做小幅度的环旋转动，并带动施术处的皮肤一起婉转回环，使之与内层的软组织之间产生轻柔缓和的内摩擦。整个动作贵在柔和，揉转的幅度要由小而大，用力应先轻渐重，术手要吸定在操作部位上，不得在皮肤表面摩擦与滑动，频率在每分钟100～160次之间。

【临床应用】

揉法作用力轻柔缓和而深透，通过揉动形成的内摩擦，可在组织深层产生温热作用。本法适用于在全身各部操作，是推拿临床常用手法之一。其中，大鱼际揉法多用于头面部、胸腹部及四肢由急性扭伤所致的局部肿痛处；掌根揉法多用于腰背、臀部及四肢肌肉丰厚处；指揉法可用于全身各部经穴以及需要做点状刺激的部位；肘揉法则适宜于对深层组织的治疗。揉法有宽胸理气、

ing blood circulation to remove blood stasis, subducing swelling and alleviating pain, expelling pathogenic wind and cold, promoting the flow of *qi* by warming the channel, tranquilizing the mind and relieving convulsion, etc. It is commonly used to treat headache, dizziness, insomnia, facial paralysis, fullness and pain in the epigastric region, oppressed feeling in the chest and pain in the hypochondrium, constipation and diarrhea, the injuries of lumbodorsal and extremital soft tissue, etc.

4. Rubbing Manipulation

The manipulation performed by rhythmically rubbing the therapeutic part in a circular motion with the palm or the palmar side of the operator's fingers close to the therapeutic region is called rubbing technique. Rubbing with the operator's palm is called rubbing manipulation with the palm; rubbing with the palmar side of the fingers is called rubbing manipulation with fingers (Fig. 2—11).

STRUCTURE OF OPERATION

The operator is in a sitting position. He lowers his shoulder and drops his elbow with his forearm in a prone position and his palm facing downwards. In palm-rubbing manipulation, the operator slightly flexes his wrist with the whole palm pressing on the therapeutic part; in finger-rubbing manipulation, he flexes his wrist about 160 degrees, lifts up his palm with the fingers combining together, uses the palm as the power-applying surface. In the operation, with the cooperative motion of his shoulder, elbow, etc., the palmar surface as the power center continuously proceeds circular rotation in either clockwise direction or counter-clockwise direction. Its frequency should be moderate, even and steady, about 100—120 circles per minute.

CLINICAL APPLICATION

Rubbing technique is mainly applied to operating on

健脾和胃、活血散瘀、消肿止痛、祛风散寒、温经通络、安神镇惊等功效。常用于治疗头痛、眩晕、失眠、面瘫、脘腹胀痛、胸闷胁痛、便秘、泄泻以及腰背、四肢软组织损伤等病证。

4. 摩法

用手掌或食、中、无名、小指掌面附着在治疗部位上，以一定的节律做环形抚摩的手法称为摩法。其中，以手掌着力者谓掌摩法；以四指掌面着力操作者称指摩法(图2-11)。

【动作结构】

术者取坐位。沉肩，垂肘，前臂旋前，掌面朝下。掌摩时，腕略屈以全掌按放在治疗部位；指摩时，屈腕约160°,手掌抬起,四指并拢以其掌面着力。操作时，在肩、肘等运动环节的协力下，着力面朝顺时针或逆时针方向，沿圆形轨迹回旋运行,周而复始。频率应平稳适中，一般在每分钟 100～120 周左右。

【临床应用】

摩法主要适用于胸胁、脘腹部，具有疏肝理气、温中和胃、健

the chest, hypochondrium and the epigastric region, and it has the effects of relieving the depressed liver and regulating the circulation of *qi*, warming the middle-*jiao* and regulating the stomach, invigorating the spleen, promoting digestion and removing stagnant food, regulating gastrointestinal peristalsis, etc. It is commonly used to treat such diseases as cold of insufficiency type in the middle-*jiao*, fullness in the epigastric region, borborygmus and pain in the abdomen, oppressed feeling in the chest and stagnation of the flow of *qi*, distending pain in the hypochondrium, injury of the chest and hypochondrium, constipation and diarrhea, cold of insufficiency type of the lower-*jiao*. In the clinical operation, according to the different intensities, frequencies and directions of the manipulation, the invigorating or purging effect can be added. For example, "slow rubbing is used to invigorate; quick rubbing to purge"; in the operation on the lower abdomen region, clockwise rubbing can have the effect of removing stagnant food in the intestines and relieving constipation by purgation; counterclockwise rubbing can have the therapeutic effect of warming the middle-*jiao* to stop diarrhea and warming and recuperating the lower-*jiao*.

5. Scrubbing Manipulation

The manipulation of rubbing and scrubbing the therapeutic part to and fro along a straight line with the operator's palmar face, minor or major thenar eminance is called scrubbing manipulation. According to the different operating parts, this manipulation can be divided into three types: palm-scrubbing, minor-thenar scrubbing and major-thenar scrubbing (Fig. 2—12).

STRUCTURE OF OPERATION

In the operation of this manipulation, the operator is usually in a standing position. The preparatory posture is as follows: the operator lowers his shoulder, drops his elbow.

脾助运、消积导滞及调节肠胃蠕动等功效。常用于治疗中焦虚寒、脘腹胀满、肠鸣腹痛、胸闷气滞、胁肋胀痛、胸胁迸伤、泄泻、便秘、下元虚冷等病证。临床使用本法时，根据操作的力度、频率与方向的不同,可起到或补或泻的作用。例如,"缓摩为补,急摩为泻";又如，在小腹部操作时，顺时针方向摩运可通调肠腑积滞，起到泻热通便的作用；而逆时针方向摩运则能温中止泻，发挥温补下元的功效。

5. 擦法

以手掌掌面、小鱼际或大鱼际为着力面，在治疗部位沿直线进行往返摩擦的方法，谓之擦法。根据着力部位不同，本法可分为掌擦法、小鱼际擦法和大鱼际擦法三种(图2-12)。

【动作结构】

本法操作时，术者多取站势。预备姿势为：沉肩、垂肘，掌

In palm-scrubbing manipulation, with the medial aspect of his forearm facing the therapeutic part, he extends his wrist, palm, thumb and fingers straightly with his whole palm pressing closely on the therapeutic part; in minor-thenar scrubbing manipulation, his forearm is in a moderately erecting position, he extends his wrist, palm and fingers straightly and puts his fingers together, and rubs the therapeutic part with minor thenar force; in major-thenar scrubbing manipulation, his forearm is in the prone position, with his palm facing downwards, his thumb and first metacarpal bone abducted, and the protuberant muscular belly of major thenar eminance closely applied to the therapeutic part.

In operation, the operator rectilinearly rubs and scrubs the therapeutic part with the coordinative motion of the procurvation and backward extension of his shoulder joint with extension and flexion of his elbow joint. This manipulation should be operated within a large range, and the operator should try to lengthen the distance of pushing and scrubbing. During the operation, the operating part should be kept close to the skin of the therapeutic region, and the rubbing force should be even and moderate.

CLINICAL APPLICATION

This manipulation has strong rubbing force with a large range of movement, so it has evident warming effect and the function of removing obstruction. It can be applied to all parts of the body. Palm-scrubbing manipulation is suitable for the operation on large regions such as chest and back, the abdominal region, and it can create soft warming effect; minor-thenar scrubbing manipulation is mainly applied to the lumbosacral Baliao points, Jiaji points and sacrospinal muscle; because of its small effect area, concentrated high heat effect can be created; major-thenar scrubbing manipulation is mainly applied to the limbs, by which the moderate warming effect can be created. The manipulation has the

擦时，前臂内侧与治疗部位相对，腕、掌与五指伸直，以全掌附着在治疗部位；小鱼际擦时，前臂取中立位，腕、掌与手指用力伸直，五指并拢，以小鱼际着力；大鱼际擦时，前臂取旋前位，掌面朝下，拇指与第一掌骨内收，以隆起的大鱼际肌肌腹附着在治疗部位。

操作时，以往复进行的肩关节前屈、后伸与肘关节伸展、屈曲的联合运动，使着力面在治疗部位，沿直线来回摩擦。本法的动作幅度要大，使推擦的距离尽量地拉长。在操作过程中，着力面要始终与受术部位的皮肤贴紧，用力均匀、适中。

【临床应用】

本法的摩擦力强、动作幅度大，故具有明显的温热效应与推荡消散作用。适用于全身各部位施术。其中，掌擦法宜在胸背与腹部面积较大的部位操作，可产生较缓和的热效应；小鱼际擦法，主要用于腰骶部八髎穴、夹脊穴及骶棘肌，由于其作用面积小，故可产生较为集中的高热效应；大鱼际擦法，主要用在四肢部，可

following effects: relieving chest stuffiness and regulating the circulation of *qi*, warming the channels and alleviating pain, expelling pathogenic wind and cold, relieving swelling and removing obstruction of the channels, promoting flow of *qi* and blood circulation, relieving arthralgia and removing dampness, etc.

In operation, the affected part should be exposed fully. The operator starts rubbing softly and slowly, then a bit more quickly. Each treatment is accomplished when the operated part becomes warm. It should not be operated for too many times, and the time should not be too long in case the therapeutic region becomes so hot that scald blisters will be caused. About 10 times is usually suitable to each treatment. In order to prevent the skin from being abraded, produce greater warmth and enhance therapeutic effect, a certain medium is often used in this manipulation.

6. Grasping Manipulation

Grasping manipulation is performed by symmetrically and slowly lifting and squeezing the therapeutic part and meanwhile holding and twisting, foulaging, kneading and pinching it with the operator's thumb and, index finger and middle finger or with five fingers. Operating with the operator's thumb and index finger and middle finger is called the manipulation of three-fingers grasping; the manipulation with five fingers is called five-fingers grasping (Fig. 2—13).

STRUCTURE OF OPERATION

In using this manipulation, the operator is often in standing position, and lowers his shoulder with his shoulder joint abducted 30 degrees to 45 degrees and protruded about 30 degrees, flexes his elbow about 90 to 110 degrees with his wrist joint slightly flexed, and extends the interphalangeal joints of his thumb and other two fingers or four fingers with the metacarpophalangeal joints flexed about 110 to

产生中等的温热作用。有宽胸利气、温经止痛、祛风散结、行气活血、蠲痹胜湿等功效。

本法在操作时，受术部位要充分暴露，开始几次推擦宜缓和稍慢，以后速度可稍快。每次治疗以局部发热为度，操作次数不宜太多，时间也不应过长，以免造成局部过热、发烫起泡。一般每次以 10 次左右为宜。为防止擦破皮肤并有助于产热与增强疗效，施用本法时，一般要使用介质。

6. 拿法

以拇指与食、中二指或其他四指，缓缓地对称用力，将治疗部位挟持、提起，并同时捻搓揉捏的手法称为拿法。其中，以拇指与食、中二指操作的称三指拿法；与其他四指操作的谓五指拿法(图2-13)。

【动作结构】

本法施术时多取站势，沉肩，肩关节外展30°～45°，前伸30°左右，屈肘约90°～110°，腕关节略屈，拇指与其余二指或

120 degrees. Then he holds the tendon or muscle bundle of the therapeutic part, lifts it up and meanwhile twirls and kneads it, and releases it after stimulating it several times. The operation is done repeatedly.

During the operation, every movement should be coordinated and operated rhythmatically. The part being lifted and grasped is chiefly the cord tissue such as tendon, ligament and muscle bundle of deep layers of the body, so holding the epiderm or even digging and nipping the operated part with finger nails should be avoided in case discomforts such as pain will be caused.

CLINICAL APPLICATION

This manipulation is deep and heavy but soft stimulation. It is chiefly applied to the cord soft tissues such as the muscles and tendons of the neck, shoulder, back, lateral abdomen, upper and lower limbs, etc. It has the following effects: inducing resuscitation and restoring consciousness, relieving superficies syndrom by means of diaphoresis, expelling pathogenic wind and cold, relaxing muscles and tendons to promote blood circulation, relieving spasm and pain, etc. In clinical application, one-hand grasping or both-hand grasping can be adopted according to the different requirements. In both-hand grasping manipulation, the operator should grasp and let go the operated part alternatively with both hands.

7. Pressing Manipulation

Pressing is the manipulation performed by pressing the therapeutic region continuously with the operator's finger-tip, palm, palm-root or the tip of his elbow, from lightly to heavily, shallowly to deeply. According to the different manipulating parts, it can be divided into thumb-pressing manipulation, middle-finger-pressing manipulation, phalangeal-joint-pressing manipulation, palm-root-pressing manipulation, palm-pressing ma-

四指各指间关节伸直，掌指关节屈曲约 110°～120°,以指面挟持住治疗部位的肌腱或肌束，然后提起，并同时捻揉，刺激数次后再放下，如此反复操作。

操作过程中，各动作环节要协调，并富于节律。提拿的部位主要是人体深层的肌腱、韧带与肌束等条索状组织，故不要仅挟持表皮，更不能用指甲着力抠掐治疗部位，以免引起疼痛等不适感。

【临床应用】

本法刺激深重而柔和。主要用于颈项、肩背、侧腹部及四肢部肌肉、肌腱等条索状软组织部位。具有开窍醒神、发汗解表、祛风散寒、舒筋活血、解痉止痛等功效。临床使用时,根据需要,可单手拿或双手拿。双手拿时，两手要交替地做提拿与放松动作。

7. 按法

以指端、掌、掌根或肘尖着力，先轻渐重、由浅而深地反复按压治疗部位的手法称按法。根据其着力部位不同，可分为拇

nipulation, elbow-pressing manipulation, etc. (Fig. 2—14).

STRUCTURE OF OPERATION

In order to generate force easily, the operator can adopt sitting posture in light pressure manipulation, and standing posture in heavy pressure manipulation. In operation, the operator should breathe in a normal way (never hold his breath) and press steadily from light to heavy till a certain deepness is achieved. When the patient has experienced evident sensations such as soreness, distention, numbness and radiation, the operator should retain his hand on the operated part for about 5 to 10 minutes, then slowly lift his hand up. If the manipulation is required to carry great force and needs operating continuously for many times, the superposed kneading manipulation can be adopted, that is, the operator superposes his thumbs or palms (he presses the operated region with his one thumb or palm and puts another thumb or palm on it). He presses the operated region naturally and repeatedly with his forearms slightly extended and the upper part of his body slightly inclined forwards. In this manipulation, the operator presses the operated part with the pressure from his own gravity, and his hand or arm does not need to generate force actively, so the manipulation saves the operator a lot efforts of strength but has great effect.

CLINICAL APPLICATION

Pressing manipulation is a traditional manipulation which dates back to the ancient times, it has many indications and can be applied to operating on all the points over the body. Finger-pressing manipulation is applied to all the channel-points and it can achieve acupuncture effect "with the finger instead of needle"; so it is also called "finger-pressure therapy";palm-pressing manipulation is chiefly applied to the abdominal region; palm-root-pressing manipulation is suitable for the operation on the regions of large and thick muscles such as the lumbodor-

指按法、中指按法、指节按法、掌根按法、掌按法与肘按法等（图 2—14）。

【动作结构】

为了便于发力，轻按时术者可取坐势；重按时则应取站势。施术时，术者要呼吸自然，不得屏气，用力平稳，由轻而重逐渐加力，当达到一定深度，患者有明显的疼、胀、麻、放射等"得气感"时，停留约 5～10 秒钟左右，再将手慢慢抬起。本法在需要较大力度与反复多次操作时，宜用叠揉法，即以双手拇指或双掌重叠（一手拇指或手掌按放在治疗部位上，另一手拇指或手掌重叠按放在其背侧），双臂伸直，上身向前略倾，在治疗部位反复做自然支撑样的按压。此法利用自身重力来施加压力，手或臂无需主动用力，故作用力强而术者省力。

【临床应用】

按法是一种古老的传统手法，其适用范围很广，可在全身各部操作施术。指按法适用于全身各部经穴，可"以指代针"发挥针刺样的治疗作用，故又有"指针法"之称；掌按法主要用于腹部；掌根按适用于腰背及臀部面积较大肌肉又丰厚的部位；肘按法又

sal region and the buttock region; elbow-pressing manipulation is frequently used when great stimulation is required. This manipulation has the following effects: tranquilizing the mind and allaying excitemint, relieving spasm and pain, inducing resuscitation, relaxing muscles and tendons and promoting blood circulation, relieving arthralgia and removing obstruction in the channel, strengthening the tendon and muscles, etc. It is commonly used to treat headache, insomnia, epigastralgia, arthralgia syndrome, numbness of the limbs, aching and paralysis, etc.

8. Flat-pushing Manipulation

Flat-pushing is the manipulation performed by rectilinearly pushing and scrubbing the operated part to and fro with the operator's palm and thumb radial border, with his thumb abducted at a right angle with the other fingers. It is also called palmpushing manipulation (Fig. 2—15).

STRUCTURE OF OPERATION

The operator is usually in standing posture. The preparatory posture is as follows: the operator lowers his shoulder girdle with his shoulder joint abducted 30 degrees, stretch his arm forword about 30 to 45 degrees, and flexes his elbow about 90 to 120 degrees with his forearm in moderately erecting position and its internal side facing the operated part; and he extends straightly his wrist and metacarpophalangeal joints with his fingers kept together, abducts his thumb to make a right angle with his palm, and keeps his whole palm (including his palm, the surface of his fingers and his thumb's radial border) close to the operated part.

In operation, first, the operator protrudes his shoulder, meanwhile extends his elbow joint outwards, and pushes the operated part rectilinearly with his palm and, with his thumb pushing and mopping forcefully along 'it, his thumb is changed from abduction to being close to the index fingers'

称肘压法，需作重力刺激时常用此法。本法具有安神镇静、解痉止痛、开通闭塞、舒筋活血、蠲痹通络与壮筋养肌等作用，常用以治疗头痛、失眠、胃脘痛、痹证、肢体麻木、酸痛瘫痪等证。

8. 平推法

拇指外展，与四指垂直，以手掌及拇指桡侧缘着力，在施术部位上沿直线作来回推擦的手法，称平推法，亦称掌推法（图2-15）。

【动作结构】

术者多取站势。预备姿势为：肩带下沉，肩关节外展30°并前伸30°～45°左右，屈肘90°～120°左右，前臂取中立位，内侧面与治疗部位相对，腕与掌、指伸直，四指并拢，拇指外展与掌垂直，以全掌（包括掌、四指掌面与拇指桡侧缘）着力紧贴在治疗部位上。

操作时，首先肩向前伸，同时肘关节顺势伸出，使手掌沿直线向前推去，拇指也在所经过的部位上用力向前推荡，并由外展位过

radial border; then he extends his shoulder backwards, flexes his elbow and uses his palm to push and rub along the original trace back to the initial position, and his palmar posture is returned to its original one.

The following should be emphasized in this manipulation: in pushing forwards a strong force should be used and in pushing back to the original position a weak force; the movement should be smooth, and the operation route should be long; in generating force, the operator should breathe normally and avoid holding his breath; in addition, the operated region should be exposed, and a certain medium can be used in operation in order to make the operation easy and protect the skin. Its frequency manipulation is about 100 times per minute.

Flat-pushing is the chief manipulation of internal exercise massage. For its typical dynamic type you can refer to the dynamic curve diagram of flat-pushing manipulation recorded live when Mr. Li Xijiu, the contemporary disciple of internal exercise massage, was doing this manipulation (Fig. 2—16).

CLINICAL APPLICATION

This manipulation is a combination of "warmth and force", so it has a good effect on warming and dredging the channels and collaterals, promoting circulation of blood and qi, etc. It is suitable for the operation on the thoracodorsal region and lumbo-abdominal region. When it is applied to the thoraco-dorsal region, it has the effect of relieving the chest stuffiness, promoting circulation of qi, relieving cough and asthma; when it is applied to the gastric and hypochondriac regions, it functions in invigorating the spleen and regulating the stomach, and relieving depressed liver and regulating the circulation of qi; when it is applied to the lumbosacral and the lower abdomen regions, it has the effect of invigorating the loins and strengthening the kidney. It is commonly used to cure oppressed feeling in the chest, chest pain, angina pectoris, pulmonary emphysema, asthma, chronic cough, distension and pain in the epigastric region, stagna

度到向食指桡侧靠拢的位置。然后，肩再后伸，同时屈肘，使手掌沿原来的轨迹轻轻地推擦到起始的位置，并恢复到原来的掌式。

应注意，本法在向前推去时用实力，而往回推至原位时用虚劲。整个动作要舒展，操作路线要拉长，在发力动作时，呼吸要自然，切忌屏气。另外，受术部位要暴露，为便于操作与保护皮肤，操作时要用介质。平推法的频率每分钟 100 次左右。

平推法是内功推拿的主治手法。其典型的动力形式，可见由当代内功推拿的传人李锡九老先生操作时实录的平推法动态曲线图（图2-16）所示。

【临床应用】

本法是一种"温、力"并行的方法，故有良好的温经通络、行气活血等治疗作用。适宜于在胸背及腰腹部操作。施术于胸背部时，有开胸利气、止咳平喘之功；用于上腹与两胁时，具健脾和胃、疏肝理气之效；用于腰骶及下腹部时，则能壮腰健肾。常用以治疗胸闷、胸痛、心绞痛、肺气肿、哮喘、气短、久咳、脘腹

tion of the liver-*qi*, lumbago, deficiency of the kidney, etc.

9. Digital-pressing Manipulation

Digital pressing is the manipulation performed by heavily pressing the deep layer tissue with the operator's thumb or his middle finger tip or the protrusive part of the proximal interphalangeal joints of his flexed middle finger, index finger and thumb. According to the different operating parts, it can be divided into thumb-pressing manipulation, middle-finger-pressing manipulation and phalangeal joint-pressing manipulation (Fig. 2—17, 2—18).

STRUCTURE OF OPERATION

This manipulation is developed from pressing manipulation, and its operation structure is similar to that of pressing manipulation. The difference is that this manipulation has strong stimulation, so special attention should be paid to helping and protecting the operating finger in operation. For example, in middle-finger-pressing, the operator should flex the metacarpophalangeal joint of his middle finger and straightly extend his phalangeal joint with his index finger and thumb held and protecting it at the front and back part of its distal interphalangeal joint to reinforce his middle finger so as to strengthen its firmness and solidness in forcefull digital pressing manipulation and avoid the sprain caused by sudden tiredness and softness of the joint. In thumb-pressing manipulation, the fingers nearby should be used to help and protect and strengthen the thumb in order to secure the operation and make the manipulation stable, solid and effective.

This is a manipulation with strong stimulation. In operation, the operator should frequently produce stronger arm force, so he should not hold his breath to generate force in case symptoms such as oppressed feeling and pain in the chest should be caused with the time passing on. Pressing force should change gradually from light to heavy, and specified intensity

胀痛、肝气郁滞、腰痛、肾虚等病证。

9. 按点法

用拇指或中指指峰，或中指、食指、拇指屈曲后的近侧指间关节的突起部为着力点，用重力按压人体深层组织的手法，谓之按点法或称点法。其中，按其着力部位不同，又分别称为拇指点法、中指点法和指节点法（图2-17，2-18）。

【动作结构】

本法是由按法演化而来，其动作结构与按法基本相同。所不同的是，本法的刺激量强，故操作时要特别注意对着力指的护持，如中指点时，中指掌指关节屈曲，指关节伸直，要用食指与拇指指面分别护持在其远侧指间关节的前、后方，以加固中指，使之在用力按点时增强稳固性与坚挺力，避免在发力时关节突然瘫软而发生扭伤。在施用拇指点时，也要注意用周围的手指来护持、加固，以保证其安全操作，并使手法作用力稳实而有效。

本法是一种强刺激手法，施术时，术者往往要用较强的臂力，故要注意不可常用屏气发力的方法，以免日久招致胸闷、胸痛等

and deepness must be achieved in order to bring intense sensory effect on the patient.

CLINICAL APPLICATION

This manipulation has small and concentrated acting area, and the acting layer is deep with evident stabbing pain effect, and it is applied to the indurated tissue of muscles or between bones or tenderness points, and it has a good effect of "treating pain with pain". It is chiefly used to cure the contractive pain in epigastric region, pertinacious numbness of the limbs, pain of old injury, numbness and paralysis.

10. Digital-striking Manipulation

Digital-striking technique is a manipulation performed by striking the therapeutic region with the operator's middle finger tip, or tip of thumb, fore and middle fingers, or the tips of his five closed-up fingers. According to the different operating parts, it can be divided into three types: middle-finger striking, three-finger striking, five-finger striking (Fig. 2—19).

STRUCTURE OF OPERATION

In light digital striking manipulation, the operator can be in a sitting posture; in heavy digital striking manipulation, the operator is frequently in a standing posture. The operation structure of middle-finger striking manipulation is similar to that of middle-finger pressing manipulation; in the three-finger striking manipuation, the operator keeps the tips of his thumb, index finger and middle finger at the same level, holds them together, and strikes the operated part with the three tips; in five-finger striking, the operator keeps the tips of his thumb and fingers at the same level, holds them together, and strikes the operated part with the tips of his thumb and fingers. In light digital striking manipulation, the operator lowers his shoulder and drops his elbow with the motions centering on the wrist joint, and he extends his wrist and lifts his hand up, then, lowers his wrist joint with the help of gravity, and strikes the operated point with elastic force. In moderate digital

症的发生。用力要由轻渐重，务必达到一定的强度与深度，使受术者产生强烈的感觉效果。

【临床应用】

本法的作用点小而集中，作用层次深，刺痛效应明显，常用于肌肉或骨缝深处的硬结组织或压痛点，具有良好的"以痛止痛"效果。临床主要治疗脘腹挛痛、肢体顽痹、陈伤疼痛、麻痹瘫痪等病症。

10. 击点法

以中指端，或拇、食、中三指，或五指捏拢后的指端，在施术部位进行击打点穴的方法，称为击点法或点法。其中，根据着力部位不同，又分别称为中指点、三指点与五指点(图2—19)。

【动作结构】

轻点时，术者可取坐势；重点时，多取站势。中指击点时的手式与中指按点法相同；三指击点时，拇、食、中三指指端对齐并拢并捏紧，以三指指端着力；五指击点时，五指指端对齐并拢并捏紧，以五指指端着力。轻度点击时，以腕关节为中心，沉肩，垂肘，先伸腕将手抬起，接着腕关节用力顺势下落，以一种富有

striking, the whole motion is centered on the operator's elbow joint and the operator lowers his shoulder with his elbow flexed about 90 to 100 degrees. In the operation, he lifts his forearm up and extends his wrist, then quickly lowers it with his forearm and wrist force aided by gravity, and strikes the operated point with the finger tips. In heavy digital striking, its motion is centered on the operator's shoulder joint. First the operator lifts up his upper arm at the shoulder joint and his hand can be above his head. He flexes his elbow about 90 degrees with his dorsal carpal region extended to about 30 degrees, then lowers his upper limb with a great force. In the whole operation, the operator's forearm is in prone position with his palm facing downwards, and his wrist joint is also changed from extension to flexion. When the operator strikes the operated region with his fingers, he flexes his wrist about 30 to 45 degrees. In the operation of these striking manipulations above, the fingers should be "bounced up" away from the operated part as soon as they touch the operated region.

Digital-striking technique can be divided into two types: single-digital striking and rhythm-digital striking. In single-digital striking, one single striking motion is marked as a stimulation unit, its frequency is 2 to 3 times per second, and the intensity each time should be kept the same. In rhythm-digital striking, a group of rhythmical digital strikings are marked as one stimulation unit. Its commonly-used patterns are as follows: one weak striking followed by two strong ones, two weak strikings followed by two strong ones, three weak strikings followed by two strong ones or five weak strikings followed by two strong ones, etc. The force in weak strikings should be light and quick; the force in strong striking should be heavy and slow.

Digital-striking is the chief manipulation of digital point massage. For its typical dynamic type you can refer to the typical dynamic curve diagram recorded when Jia Lihui, the digital point master in Laoshan, operates with the technique (Fig. 2—20).

弹性的力,对准施术穴点做点状叩击;以中等力度击点时,整个动作要以肘关节为中心环节,沉肩并屈肘 90°～100° 左右。操作时,先将前臂抬起,并同时伸腕,然后,使前臂与腕用力,快速地顺势下落,以着力指端对准治疗穴点击打;重力型击点时,动作以肩关节为中心,先将整个上肢在肩关节处向上举起,手可高达头以上。此时,屈肘 90° 左右,腕背伸约 30°,接着用力使上肢下落,在这个过程中,前臂在旋前位掌面朝下,腕关节由伸展位顺势向屈曲位过度,当着力指击打在受术部位时屈腕约 30°～45° 左右。在进行上述各式击点法时,手指击打到治疗穴点后,要随即"弹起"离开施术部位。

击点法有单点法与节律点法二种。单点法是以一次击点动作为一个刺激单元,一般每秒钟点 2～3 次,每次的力度基本一致。节律点是以一组有固定频率与力度变化的节律性点击为一个刺激单元的手法,常用的有一虚二实、二虚二实、三虚二实、或五虚二实等几种形式,虚点时用力轻、速度快,实点时用力重而速度慢。

击点法是点穴推拿的主治手法,其典型动力形式,可见由崂山点穴大师贾立惠氏操作时,所录的击点法动态曲线图(图2—20)所示。

CLINICAL APPLICATION

This technique is developed from the motion in striking technique of traditional Chinese *Wushu* such as digital point, grasping point, beating point, kicking point. Its motion is swift with quick and vigorous force, strong penetration and great stimulation. Especially in heavy digital striking, the striking force can in stantaneously reach about 60 to 70 kg., so its effect can be transmitted swiftly to the deep layer of the patient's tissue and the patient's limb's distalis and intense reaction of organism is created. Clinically, the doctor should pay more attention to using different manipulations according to different syndromes; generally speaking, the slow and soft rhythm digital striking and light single digital striking are suitable for infants, women, weak patients or first visit patients, and the doctor can gradually increase the manipulation force when the patients are accustomed to the striking, and he should avoid vigorous digital striking from the very beginning in case injury should be caused. This technique has the following effects: exciting the mind, relieving stagnation, promoting the kidney-*yang*, activating functional activities of *qi* and treating arthralgia and relieving pain. It is chiefly used to cure the intractable diseases such as neurosism, insomnia, traumatic paraplegia, cerebral palsy, hysterical paralysis, commenorative sign caused by poliomyelitis, peripheral neuritis, infectious polyradicaulitis, hemiparalysis, prolapse of lumbar intervertebral disc.

11. Patting Manipulation

The manipulation of patting-beating with empty palm on the body surface is called patting manipulation or patting-hitting manipulation (Fig. 2—21).

STRUCTURE OF OPERATION

The doctor can be either in sitting or in standing position. While operating, the doctor's fingers are closed-up and straightly-stretched. The metacarpophalangeal joints are slightly

【临床应用】

本法由中国传统武术中的点穴、拿穴、打穴、踢穴解等击技性动作演化而来，动作速捷，劲力迅猛，深透性强，刺激量大，尤其是重型击点法在其施术的瞬间，叩击力可达 60～70 公斤左右，故作用力可迅速地传递到人体组织的深层与体肢远端引起强烈的机体反应。临诊时应注意辨证施术，一般对儿童、妇女、体弱者或初次受术者，宜先选用比较缓和的节律点与轻型单点法，待其适应后再慢慢加大手法的力度，切不可一开始就用强力猛然点击，以免造成损伤。本法具有振奋精神、开达郁闭、发散壅阻、激发元阳、活跃气机与蠲痹镇痛的功效。主要用于治疗神经衰弱、失眠、外伤性截瘫、脑性瘫痪、癔病性瘫痪、小儿麻痹后遗症、末梢神经炎、感染性多发性神经炎、偏瘫、腰椎间盘突出症等顽固性病证。

11. 拍法

用虚掌拍打体表的手法，称为拍法或拍打法(图 2—21)。

【动作结构】

术者可取坐位或站势。操作时五指并拢，手指伸直，掌指关

flexed as to concave the palm to form an empty palm. The doctor lifts up the operating hand, and pat down the therapeutic region with elastic and skillful strength, then the hand bounces up right away, and restores to its initial position for operation so as to perform the next patting. The stimulus of this therapy can be divided into light, intermediate and heavy types. The structure of this operation is similar to that of digital strikig manipulation.

CLINICAL APPLICATION

This manipulation is mainly used on the shoulder and back, lumbosacral portion and the thigh. Light patting can also be used on thoracico-abdominal region and the head. Lasting and strong patting has the effect of sedation, analgesia, promoting blood circulation and removing blood stasis, spasmolysis, strengthening the body, etc.; short and light patting has cephalocathartic and neurotonic effect and the effects of exciting the nerve, regulating the function of the stomach and intestine, soothing the chest oppression, regulating the flow of qi, etc. This manipulation is frequently used to treat various kinds of diseases such as arthralgia due to pathogenic wind-dampness, old trauma and internal injury causd by over-strain, new trauma and blood stasis, myophagism, hypoesthesia, enteroparalysis, stuffiness and pain in the chest, dizziness, heavyness in the head, involuntary movement caused by the deviation of qigong.

12. Tapping Manipulation

The manipulation of using the back of fist, palmar root, palmar center, minor thenar eminence, or the stick made of mulberry twigs to pound and hit the body surface is calld tapping manipulation or striking manipulation (Fig. 2—22).

STRUCTURE OF OPERATION

Fist-hitting manipulation: The operator lowers his shoulder, drops the elbow, with his forearm in a backward rotating position,

节略屈，使掌心凹成"虚掌"，先将术手抬起，对准治疗部位以一种富有弹性的巧劲向下拍打后，随即"弹起"，并顺势将术手抬起到动作开始的位置，以便于进行下一个拍打动作。本法的刺激量也有轻、中、重之分，其动作结构与击点法相似。

【临床应用】

本法主要用于肩背，腰骶与大腿部，轻拍也可用于胸腹部与头部。强而长时间的拍打具有镇静止痛、活血祛瘀、解痉及强壮等作用；轻而短时间的拍打有清脑醒神、兴奋神经、调理肠胃、宽胸理气等功效。本法常用于治疗各种风湿痹痛、陈伤劳损、新伤血瘀、肌肉萎缩、感觉减退、肠麻痹、胸闷胸痛、头昏头沉以及气功偏差所致的大动不已等病证。

12. 叩击法

用拳背、掌根、掌心、小鱼际，或桑枝棒叩击体表的手法，称为叩击法或击法(图2-22)

【动作结构】

拳击法：沉肩、垂肘，前臂呈旋后位，外侧面对向受术者，

and its lateral side facing the patient, the operating hand turned into an empty fist, the wrist joint straightened, and the fist back facing the location to be tapped. In operating, the doctor first lifts up his arm, flex the elbow and wrist, keeps a certain distance between the back of his hand and the region to be tapped, then, taps this region with force.

Palm-tapping manipulation includes palm-center-striking and palm-root-tapping. In case of palm-root-tapping, the doctor keeps the fingers combined, with the thumb abducted in a natural flexed position, the wrist joint stretched backwards for 45 degrees, and the protruding palmar root directed at the treated region; in case of palm-center-striking, the doctor keeps the fingers combined, with the thumb abducted and the wrist, 'metacarpophalange, and all manual interphalangeal joints sligtly flexed so as to turn the palm into a shallow arc to fit the operated part — the vertex. The operation structure of this manipulation is the same as that of patting manipulation.

Minor thenar-hitting is also called "side-hitting" or "cut-beating". In operating, the doctor straightly stretches his joints of fingers, palm and wrist, with the thumb in a natural abduction; keeps the fingers combined and the forearm and the palm in a neutral position; pounds the operated region rhythmically and alternatively either with one hand or two hands, using the ulnar surface of minor thenar eminance to apply force.

Stick-striking is a manipulation by using the treating stick made of mulberry twigs to strike the therapeutic region of the body surface.

When the tapping manipulation is operated, the force given in tapping should be in a decisive and swift manner, and the doctor should lift up the operating hand at once after tapping. The tapping should be very short. In tapping, the doctor

术手握成空拳，腕关节伸直，以拳背对准待击部位。操作时，先抬臂、屈肘、屈腕，使手背离开待击部位一定距离，然后，用力朝治疗部位击打。

掌击法包括掌心击法与掌根击法二种。掌根击时，四指并拢，拇指外展呈自然屈曲状，腕关节背伸约45°，使掌根突起对准待击部位；掌心击时，四指并拢，拇指外展，腕、掌指与各指间关节略曲，使整个手掌弯成一浅圆弧形，以与治疗部位——头顶——相适应。本法的动作方式与拍法同。

小鱼际击法，又称"侧击法"或"切打法"。操作时，手指、掌及腕关节伸直，拇指自然外展，四指并拢，前臂与手掌取中立位，用小鱼际的尺侧面着力，以单手或双手有节律地交替叩击治疗部位。

棒击法，是用桑枝制成的治疗棒，击打体表治疗区的方法。

各种叩击法操作时，用力应果断、快速，击打后将术手立即抬起，叩击的时间要短暂。击打时，手腕既要保持一定的姿势，

should not only keep the wrist in a certain posture, but also relax it, and tap with a controlled elastic force so that the manipulation can have a specified dynamic force and the patient can feel relaxed and comfortable. Violent tapping should be avoided to keep the patient away from unnecessary injury and pain.

CLINICAL APPLICATION

Fist-back-hitting manipulation is mainly applied to Dazhui (Du14) and the lumbosacral portion; palm-hitting, the anterior fontanelle of the vertex and Baihui (Du 20); minor thenar-hitting, lumbodorsal portion and limbs region. When the tapping with much force is operated, in order to make it safe and effective, not only should the doctor master the correct structure of operation and the suitable stimulating force, but also the patient should adopt a specified posture depending on the treated regions. For example, in the case of hitting the vertex, the patient should be in standing posture of *Shaolin* internal exercise, or in the sitting posture with the tongue against the palate, his teeth clenched, his vital *qi* directed through concentration to the Baihui (Du 20) of the vertex or the anterior fontanelle; when the stick-striking manipulation is operated on the shank, the patient should adopt a forward half-squatting posture and so on. This manipulation has the effects of relaxing muscles and tendons and activating the flow of *qi* and blood in the channels and collaterals, promoting blood circulation to remove blood stasis, regulating *qi* and blood, etc. And it has an evident effect on the symptoms such as hypertension, arthralgia due to wind and dampness, numbness, muscular spasm, paralysis of extremities, and myophagism.

NOTE: The method of making mulberry-twig stick.

Strip off the bark of 12 thin mulberry twigs (about 0.5 cm thick), remove the peel and dry them. Roll each twig up tightly with mulberry paper, tightly tie it with a thread, and bundle the twigs up. Again tie them tightly with a thread,

又要放松，以一种有控制的弹性力进行叩击，使手法既有一定的力度，又使受术者感觉缓和舒适。切忌用暴力打击，以免给受术者造成不应有的伤痛。

【临床应用】

拳背击法主要用于大椎穴及腰骶部；掌击法常用于头顶前囟与百会穴；小鱼际击法适用于腰背与四肢部；棒击法可用于头顶、肩背、腰骶及四肢部。在施用重型叩击法时，为使手法操作安全、有效，除术者要掌握好正确的动作结构与适宜的刺激量外，受术者还要根据受术部位采用特殊的体位，如击打头顶时，受术者要取少林内功站裆势，或正坐势，并舌抵上腭，咬紧牙关，运气于头顶百会穴或前囟穴；又如棒击小腿时，受术者要取弓步势等。本法具有舒筋通络、活血祛瘀、调和气血等作用，对高血压、风湿痹痛、麻木不仁、肌肉痉挛、肢体瘫痪、肌肉萎缩等病证有明显的疗效。

【附】 桑枝棒的制法

用细桑枝十二根（粗约0.5厘米），去皮阴干，每根用桑皮纸卷紧，并用线扎紧，然后把桑枝合起来，先用线扎紧，再用桑皮

then roll them up tigntly with mulberry paper layer upon layer, and then tie it with thread and wrap it with a piece of cloth and sew it. Moderate hardness, elasticity and combination of thick and thin twigs are required. It is about 4.5—5 cm in diameter and about 40 cm long.

13. Vibrating Manipulation

Vibrating manipulation is performed by using the forearm to stretch-flex the muscle group with the tip of the middle finger or the palm as the force-giving points; and contracting in a narrow range, swiftly and alternatively to cause soft vibration which keeps effecting on the treated region on the body surface. It is also called "vibrating trembling manipulation". The manipulation with the middle finger as the force-giving point is called "finger-vibrating manipulation"; that with the palm as the force-giving point is called "palm-vibrating manipulation" (Fig. 2—23).

STRUCTURE OF OPERATION

The doctor is in a sitting or standing position. In operation, the doctor relaxes the muscles of his upper limb, with the shoulder joint abducting for about 30 degrees, upper limb naturally stretching out forwards, and the forearm in forward rotating position. With the palm facing downwards, the doctor naturally presses his middle finger or his palm on the therapeutic region and the elbow joint is flexed for about 90–100 degrees. In palm-vibrating manipulation, the palm is pressed close to the treated region, and the elbow should be slightly lower to the wrist. In finger-vibrating manipulation, the doctor straightly stretches his middle finger with the metacarpophalangeal joint flexed for about 100 degrees, vertically puts the tip of the finger on the point with the wrist joint slightly flexed. In operation, the wrist of the forearm's flexing and stretching muscle groups are continuously and alternatively contracted and relaxed to make the movements of flexing and stretching of the hand reverse swiftly after each

纸层层卷紧并用线绕好，外面用布裹紧缝好即成。要求软硬适中，具有弹性，粗细合用，直径约4.5～5厘米，长约40厘米。

13.振法

以中指端或手掌面为着力点，用前臂伸、屈肌群小幅度、快速地交替收缩所产生的轻柔振颤，持续地作用于体表治疗部位的手法，称为振法或振颤法。以中指着力者称指振法；以手掌着力者称掌振法(图2-23)。

【动作结构】

术者取坐势或站势。操作时，上肢肌肉放松，肩关节外展约30°，上肢向前方自然伸出，前臂呈旋前位，掌面朝下，将中指或手掌自然地按放在治疗部位上，肘关节屈曲至90°～100°左右。掌振时，手掌与治疗部位贴平，肘略低于腕，中指振时，指伸直，掌指关节屈曲100°左右，指端垂直放置于穴点上，腕关节略屈。动作时，前臂的腕屈肌群与腕伸肌群持续地交替收缩与放松，使手的屈、伸动作在每一次短促的振动终了时，迅速地发生逆转，于是就产生了

short vibration, so that vibration and quiver are caused. Its frequency is about 8–12 times per second. The operation of vibrating can be divided into two types: calming type and undulating type. When the operating hand vibrates, the pressing force of the upper limb keeps steady, this is called calming vibrating; if it is accompanied by regular and rhythmical pressing, the undulating type of vibrating is caused. The standard power type can be refered to Fig. 2–24 and 2–25.

In operating this manipulation, the doctor should concentrate his attention, regulate his breath evenly, direct his *qi* through concentration down to *Dantian* and direct the flow of *qi* up from *Dantian* by his will, and direct the flow of *qi* from the in side of the operating hand to Laogong (P 8) point of the palm or the tip of the middle finger. The operation should direct his strength through concentration by his will, produce force with the flow of *qi* and vibration with the force. The operation should be accomplished naturally, fluently, harmoniously and uniformly. Vibration by holding his breath strongly is prohibited, for the manipulation can not remain for a long time, and in the course of time, it would destroy the vital-*qi* resulting in autolesion. This manipulation can be handled skillfully only after a long time training. A skillful doctor can remain vibrating and quivering with ease for half an hour and even 1–2 hours within a single *gong*-exertion.

CLINICAL APPLICATION

This manipulation can be applied to all the points on the body, especially to the craniofacial region and the thoracico-abdominal region. It has the effects of tranquilizing and allaying excitement, improving vision and intelligence, warming the middle-*jiao* and regulating the flow or *qi*, promoting digestion and removing stagnated food, regulating enterogastric peristalsis, etc. It has evident effects on insomnia, amnesia, anxiety, vegetative nerve functional disturbance, gastrointes-

振颤。频率约为每秒钟 8 ～ 12 次。振法的动作形式有平直型与起伏型二种。当术手振动时，上肢的按压力量保持稳定，为平直型振法；如果同时伴有规则的节律性按压动作时，则为起伏型振法，其典型的动力形式，可见图2-24与图2-25所示。

本法在操作过程中，术者要精神集中，呼吸调匀，气沉丹田，并用意念将气从丹田提起，沿术手内侧运引至掌中劳宫穴或中指端，做到以意引气，以气生力，以力发振，动作自然、流畅协调、统一。切不可闭气用强力"硬屏"而发振，这样不但手法不能持久，而且，久之必损正气造成自伤。本法需经长期训练方能运用自如。技能娴熟者，一次发功可持续振颤半小时乃至 1～2 小时而轻松自如。

【临床应用】

本法可用于全身各部经穴，尤其适用于头面部与胸腹部。具有镇静安神、明目益智、温中理气、消积导滞、调节肠胃蠕动等功能。对失眠、健忘、焦虑、植物神经功能紊乱、胃肠功能失调、

tinal dysfunction, tension of athletes before match, etc.

14. Foulage Manipulation

Two palms facing each other rapidly roll-knead the held part of the body with relative force and move upwards and downwards repeatedly. This manipulation is called Foulage (Fig. 2–26).

STRUCTURE OF OPERATION

The doctor is in half-squatting position, with upper body slightly inclining forwards; holds the operated limb with symmetric force by two forward-stretching hands. In foulaging, the frequency of the hands should be rapid, and amplitude should be even; but the up and down moving ought to be slower. The entire operation demands "rapid foulaging and slow moving".

CLINICAL APPLICATION

Foulage is one of the supplimentary manipulations that are used in massage. It is used mainly as an ending therapy of upper limbs and costal regions, also of waist and lower limbs. It has the function of regulating *qi*, blood and tissues, relaxing muscle and tendons and removing obstruction in the channels.

15. Holding-twisting Manipulation

Holding the operated parts such as fingers and toes with the thumb and the forefinger and rolling-kneading to and fro with relative force is called holding-twisting (Fig. 2–27).

STRUCTURE OF OPERATION

There are three ways of pinching fingers and toes of the patient: with palmar sides of the thumb and the index finger; with palmar sides of the thumb, index and middle fingers; with the palmar sides of the thumb and radial surface of the middle joint of the first index finger which is flexed into the shape of a bow. The holding-twisting should be dexterous and quicker. A tacit agreement is needed between the acts of the holding thumb and fingers. And the force used should be a bit greater,

运动员赛前紧张等有显效。

14. 搓法

用双手掌相对用力，对被挟持的肢体做快速的来回搓揉，并同时作上下往返移动的手法，称为搓法（图2-26）。

【动作结构】

术者取马步，双腿下蹲，上身略向前倾，双手向前伸出，对称用力挟持住治疗肢体。搓动时，双手来回搓动的频率要快，幅度要均匀；但上下移动的行进速度则宜稍慢，整个动作要求做到"快搓慢移"。

【临床应用】

本法是推拿常用的辅助手法之一，主要用于上肢、胁肋部、也可用于腰与下肢，作为治疗最后的结束手法。具有调和气血、理顺组织、舒筋通络与放松肌肉的作用。

15. 捻法

用拇指与食指挟持住受术者的指、趾等治疗部位，并相对用力做来回搓揉动作，称为捻法（图2-27）。

【动作结构】

本法挟持住受术者的指、趾的手势有三种：一是用拇、食指指面；二是用拇指指面与食、中二指指面；三是用拇指指面与屈曲成弓形的食指中节桡侧面。捻动时，动作要灵活、稍快，相对指

but even and moderate.

CLINICAL APPLICATION

This manipulation is primarily applied to small joints of fingers and toes, and finger-tips. It has the function of lubricating joints, subduing swelling, alleviating pain, and relaxing muscles and tendons to promote blood circulation, and is mainly used to treat symptoms of aching pain, swelling, inconvenient flexing and stretching, and sprain of finger and toe joints. It may also be used as a supplementary manipulation to treat cervical spondylopathy, paralysis and numbness of extremities. It can be done by operateing repeatedly around the joints or moving slowly from the finger roots to tips while holding-twisting.

16. Shaking Manipulation

A manipulation by which the doctor holds the distal end of the patient's affected upper or lower limbs and makes a constant, narrow range, up and down shaking (Fig. 2—28).

STRUCTURE OF OPERATION

The doctor is in a half-squatting position. His two upper limbs are naturally extended forwards and elbows are flexed for 130—160 degrees. He holds the patient's wrist or ankle with two hands, and pulls the affected limb into a natrural straight position; fixes the affected limb in a abducted position of 45—60 degrees while shaking the upper limbs; raises the affected limb to form a 30 degree angle with the bed while shaking lower limbs, and then shakes it up and down slowly, constantly, in a narrow range. Be careful that the two hands fixing the affected limbs should not be held too tightly. Do not pull the shaken limbs too straight and the range of shaking should be from narrow to wide. Rapid frequency is needed.

CLINICAL APPLICATION

This manipulation is mainly applied to extremities and mostly after foulage as an endling manipulation of therapy, which has the function of regulating *qi*-blood and tissues, and

的搓捻动作要配合默契，用力稍重但要均匀而适度。

【临床应用】

本法主要用于手指、脚趾小关节及指端末梢,具有滑利关节、消肿止痛、舒筋活血的功效,主治指、趾关节酸痛、肿胀、屈伸不利与扭伤等病证；也可作为辅助手法治疗颈椎病、肢体瘫痪、麻木等。可在关节周围反复操作,也可自指根边捻边向指端慢慢移动。

16. 抖法

用双手握住患者的上肢或下肢远端,用力做连续的小幅度上下颤动的手法,称为抖法(图2-28)。

【动作结构】

术者取马步势,上身略向前倾,两上肢自然向前伸出,屈肘约130°~160°之间,两手握住腕部或踝部,将患肢牵引至自然伸直位。抖上肢时,将患肢固定在外展45°~60°位；抖下肢时,将患肢抬起至约离床面30°处,再缓缓做连续不断的小幅度上下抖动。应注意固定患肢的双手不要捏得太紧,不要将抖动的肢体牵拉得太紧,颤动的幅度要由小而大,频率要快。

【临床应用】

本法主要用于四肢,常在搓法之后使用,作为治疗的结束手

relaxing muscles. It's also applied to the waist. In operation, raise the two lower limbs of the patient simultaneously and pull-shake powerfully to get the vibrating force directly to the waist. Thus it is also called "shaking-pulling manipulation", used primarily to treat prolapse of lumbar intervertebral disc, which can enlarge the interspace of lumbar vertebrae to help reduce projecting pulpiform nucleus, relax adhesion between the projection and nerve roots to remit or release its pressure upon nerve roots. Over 10 times are needed in one operation to shake limbs; 3—4 times in one operation for shaking-pulling lumbar vertebrae.

17. Wiping Manipulation

A manipulation of massage, performed by softly rubbing the skin of the affected part with the surface of one thumb or surfaces of two thumbs up and down, or right and left, straightly. (Fig. 2—29).

STRUCTURE OF OPERATION

In two-hand-wiping, if in one direction, the two hands should operate along a straight line, and up and down alternatively; if in two directions, the two hands operate simultaneously. Frequency should be even, about 100—120 times per minute. The force used should be moderate, not too great so as to avoid stagnating and astringent operation; nor too light so as to prevent superficial operation. To avoid skin scratches, mediums such as talc powder can be used in operation.

CLINICAL APPLICATION

Wiping is a manipulation of lighter stimulus, mainly applied to head, face, five sense organs, and cervical part, which has the function of inducing resuscitation, tranquilizing the mind, restoring consciousness, improving vision, alleviating pain, and relaxing muscles and tendons to promote blood circulation. It is also curative for symptoms of headache, dizziness, facial paralysis, prosopalgia, myopia, and stiffness and pain of the nape.

法，具有调和气血、放松肌肉与理顺组织的作用。本法也可用于腰部。操作时，将受术者双下肢同时提起，用强力牵拉抖动，使产生的振动力直达腰部，故此法又称"抖拉法"。该法主要用来治疗腰椎间盘突出症，能拉宽椎间隙，促使突出髓核还纳；松解突出物与神经根粘连，以缓解或解除对神经根的压迫。用抖法抖动肢体时，每次操作十几次；抖拉腰椎时，每次做 3～4 次即可。

17.抹法

用双手或单手拇指指面，紧贴于治疗部位，沿直线轻轻地做上下或左右反复摩擦的手法，称为抹法(图2-29)。

【动作结构】

双手抹时，如果朝一个方向操作，双手要沿直线一起一落地交替进行；如向左右分抹时双手要同时操作，频率要均匀，每分钟在100～120次左右；用力要适中，不可太重以免动作滞涩；又不可太轻而使动作飘浮。为防止擦破皮肤，施术时，可用滑石粉等介质。

【临床应用】

本法是一种刺激量较轻的手法，主要用于头面、五官及颈项部，具有开窍镇静、醒脑明目、安神止痛、舒筋活血等作用。对头痛、头晕、面瘫、三叉神经痛、近视及颈项强痛等病证有较好的治疗作用。

18. Rotating Manipulation

Hold the proximal and distal ends of the affected joint with both hands respectively and move the joints with forward and backward flexion-extention, right and left lateral flexion, or rotation, within the limit of its physiological movement along the joint moving axis (Fig. 2—30).

STRUCTURE OF OPERATION

With one hand, the doctor holds the upper proximal end of the patient's rotated joint to fix it and holds its lower distal end with the other hand. The doctor rotates the joint with force in different directions and within different ranges according to structures of the joint moving axis. Rotations of shoulders, elbows, wrists, fingers and toes fall into this operation.

But if the distal end of the operated joint is fixed by an asistant or with the help of the body of the patient himself, the doctor may hold the distal end to rotate the joint with both of his hands. So are the rotations of joints such as cervical vertebrae, knee, hip, ankle, etc.

In course of operations, the two hands should be well coordinated; the force used smooth and moderate; rotation range from narrow to wide, and not beyond the moving limit of the joints. If the operated joints are in pathological states such as adhesion and its degree of moving is distinctly decreased, the rotation scope should be within the patient's permissible limit. It should be finished step by step. Haste is forbidden.

CLINICAL APPLICATION

Rotation is one of manipulations of passive articular moving, which may be applied to joints all over the body such as the neck, lumbar vertebrae, and extremities. It has the function of lubricating joints, releasing adhesion, relaxing muscles and tendons, relieving spasm, strengthening and renewing articular

18. 摇法

用双手分别握住治疗关节的近侧端与远侧端，在关节的生理运动范围内，顺着关节运动轴的方向，使关节做前后伸屈、左右侧屈或环转等被动运动的手法，称为摇法（图2-30）。

【动作结构】

术者一手握在受术者被摇关节近侧上端，使受术关节固定，另一手握在受术关节远侧下端，根据关节运动轴的不同结构，用力使受术关节做各个不同方向与幅度的被动摇动。如肩、肘、腕、指、趾等关节的摇法，即是如此操作。

但是，如果受术关节的远侧端由助手来固定，或可以由其自身的躯干起固定作用的，那么术者的双手可一同握住受术关节的远端作环转摇动。如颈椎、膝、髋、踝等关节摇法的操作方法即是。

在施术过程中，双手的动作要互相协调。用力要平稳缓和，摇动幅度要由小渐大，不得超越关节的生理运动范围。如果受术关节处在粘连等病理状态而运动幅度明显缩小时，摇动的幅度应以病人能够耐受为度，循序渐进，切勿操之过急。

【临床应用】

本法是关节被动运动类的手法之一。可用于颈、腰椎及四肢等全身关节。具有滑利关节、解除粘连、舒筋解痉、增强与恢复

moving ability. It is also curative for cervical spondylopathy, prolapse of lumbar intervertebral disc, lumbar vertebral hyperplasia, and symptoms of articular adhesion, stiffness, inconvenient flexion and extension, swelling and pain which are caused by articular inflammation or sprain of extremities.

19. Pulling Manipulation

A manipulation peformed with both hands pulling the two articular ends of the limbs with force in opposite directions.

STRUCTURE OF OPERATION

In application of this manipulation, one must master the features of sports anatomy of human body and apply corresponding operations to the affected joints of different structures, fol lowing the theories of sports biomechanics and making full use of mechanical effect of lever so as to make the operation reasonable, effort-saving, safer, painless and effective. The following is a brief introduction of the operation structure of pulling manipulations which are often used in the clinics:

1) Pulling of the Neck

(1) Obliquely-pulling of the Cervical Vertebrae

The patient sits up straight, with his head flexed forwards for 30 degrees. One hand proping and holding the occiput of the patient, the other hand holding his lower chin, the doctor makes the head have a maximum lateral rotation of about 45 degrees (or just the maximum degrees that the neck rotation can reach if the neck of the patient is in a pathological state and the degree of the neck rotation is decreased). Pull the cervical vertebrae tightly with the two hands in opposite directions (Fig 2—31).

(2) Obliquely-pulling after localizing cervical vertebrae

The patient sits up straight, with his head flexed forwards for 30 degrees. Standing behind the patient, the operator props the lower chin of the patient with the cubital fossa of his own flexed elbow of one upper limb, and holds the occiput with the palm crossing behind the opposite ear; meanwhile, with the

关节运动功能的功效。对颈椎病、腰椎间盘突出症、腰椎增生及四肢关节炎症或损伤所致的关节粘连、强直、屈伸不利、肿胀疼痛等病症有较好的治疗作用。

19．扳法

用双手在治疗关节的两端做相反方向用力扳动肢体的 手 法，称为扳法。

【动作结构】

在应用本法时，必须掌握人体运动解剖学特征，并按照运动生物力学原理，充分利用杠杆的机械效益，对各种结构不同的受术关节，采用相应的操作方法，以使动作合理、省力、安全、无痛与有效。现将临床常用的几种扳法的动作结构简介如下：

1）颈部扳法

（1）颈椎斜扳法

受术者端坐，头略向前屈约30°。术者一手抵握住受术 者 的枕部；另一手托握住下颌部。使头向一侧旋转至最大限度约为45。左右（如果病理状态下，受术者的转颈范围减小，则旋至其 能 够达到的最大幅度即可）。再两手同时做相反方向的用力，扳动颈椎（图2-31）。

（2）颈椎定位斜扳法

受术者端坐，头向前倾约30°。术者在其背后取站 位。术 者一上肢屈肘，将受术者的下颌支托在其肘窝内，手掌绕过对侧耳后扶握住枕骨部；同时用另一手的拇指顶按住受术颈椎棘突向着

thumb tip of the other hand presses the lateral of the spinous process of the patient's operated cervical vertebra that faces the doctor; then slowly and powerfully rotates the head of the patient to the maximum degree in the direction of the operator; then gives a rapid, narrow range rotating-pulling. At the same time, the other thumb pulls with force in the opposite direction (Fig. 2—32).

2) Pulling of Chest and Back

(1) Chest-Expansion Pulling

This manipulation is mainly applied to sternocostal joints. The patient sits up straight, and his two hands grasp each other by the thumbs and fingers, which are put on the neck part. The doctor, standing behind the patient, holds the patient's elbows with two hands, and holds out one of his knees against the center of the patient's back. The patient is asked to throw out and expand the chest by pulling his two elbows backwards. When his active movement is in the functional position, the doctor pulls the two elbows backwards with two hands in a slight and rapid way; at the same time the knee pushes forwards against the patient's back, thus ending the manipulation (Fig. 2—33).

(2) Counter-reduction of Thoracic Vertebrae

In sitting position, the patient puts up both of his hands for 180 degrees. The doctor stands behind the patient, with Hand A holding the lower end near the elbow joint of the upper limb and the thumb of Hand B pressing the affected spine near the back neck. The doctor first tells the patient to throw out his chest, then pulls his upper limbs backwards with Hand A and push-presses the spinous process of the affected cervical vertebrae foreward for its reduction (Fig. 2—34).

3) Pulling of the Waist

(1) Obliquely-Pulling of the Lumbar Vertebrae

① Obliquely-pulling of the lumbar vertebrae with the patient in a lateral position.

术者自身的一侧。然后，用力将受术者的头向自身站立 的 方 向慢慢旋转至最大限度，再作一个快速的小幅度旋转牵拉动作；同时，另一手的拇指朝相反方向用力扳动（图2-32）。

2）胸背部扳法

（1）扩胸牵伸扳法

本法主要作用于胸肋关节。受术者端坐，令其两手手指相交叉扣住，置于项部。术者在其背后，用双手握住受术者两 肘 部，并用一侧膝部顶在其背后正中。先嘱受术者自行挺胸并两肘后伸作扩胸动作，待其自主动作至功能位时，术者两手作一小幅度的快速动作，将两肘向后扳动，同时，膝稍用力向前顶推其后背而完成扩胸牵伸扳动作（图2-33）。

（2）胸椎对抗复位法

受术者取坐位，两上肢上举至180°。术者站其身后，甲手在前握住其上臂下端，近肘关节处；乙手拇指在后顶按住患部脊柱。先嘱受术者挺胸，同时，术者顺势用甲手向后扳动其双上肢，乙手向前用力推按患椎棘突，使其复位（图2-34）。

3）腰部扳法

（1）腰椎斜扳法

①侧卧位腰椎斜扳法

The patient is in lateral-lying position with the leg below stretching straight, the leg above flexing the hip and knee. The upper limb above is put behind the body and upper limb below is naturally put before the body. The doctor props the anterior shoulder of the patient with Hand A; and hip or anterior superior spine with Hand B. In operating, Hand A push-lugs the shoulder in the patient's back direction; Hand B rotates the pelvis in the direction of his lateral abdomen. After rotating the lumbar vertebrae in such a manner to a maximum degree, the doctor with two hands operates a rapid pushing-dashing by heaving in opposite directions and thus ends the operation (Fig. 2—35).

② Long-handle obliquely-pulling of lumbar vertebrae with the patient in a supine position

The patient is in supine position with his left upper limb abducted and left lower limb flexing the hip (for 90 degrees) and knee; his right upper limb naturally put on the side of the body and right lower limb stretching straight. The doctor who stands to the right lateral of the patient presses the left shoulder of the patient with his left hand and grasps the left knee with right hand. In the operation, the operator's left hand presses the left anterior shoulder against the bed and right hand pulls the left leg of the patient to the right to make his pelvis rotate to the right to a maximum degree (at this moment the patient's thigh is parallel to bed surface). At this moment, the right hand makes the lower limb of the patient have a downward, rapid, and narrow range pushing-dashing. So is the obliquely-pulling of lumbar vertebrae (Fig 2—36). In obliquely-pulling to the left, the doctor stands to the left of the patient. And the directions of the operation are opposite to the above-mentioned.

③ Obliquely-pulling of lumbar vertebrae with the patient in a sitting position

The patient sits up straight with two legs set slightly apart.

受术者侧卧位，在下面的腿伸直，上面的腿屈髋屈膝；上面的上肢放在身后，下面的上肢自然地放在身前侧。术者用甲手抵住受术者肩前部，乙手抵住臀部或髂前上棘部。动作时，甲手将肩部向其身后方向推拉；乙手将骨盆朝其腹侧方向推转，如此把腰椎旋转至最大限度后，再双手同时相反用力，做一个小幅度快速的推冲动作，即完成本法（图2-35）。

②仰卧位长柄式腰椎斜扳法

受术者仰卧位，左侧上肢外展，同侧下肢屈髋90°，并屈膝；右侧上肢自然放在体侧，下肢伸直。术者站在受术者的右侧，左手按压住受术者左侧肩前部，右手握住其左膝部。动作时，术者左手将其左肩紧压在床面，右手将其左腿向右侧牵拉，使其骨盆随之向右侧旋转，旋转至最大限度时（此时，受术者的大腿约与床面平行），右手将所握住的受术者的下肢向下做一快速小幅度的推冲动作，即可完成对腰椎的斜扳动作（图2-36）。向左侧斜扳时，术者站在受术者的左侧，其动作、手势的方向均与上述相反。

③坐位腰椎斜扳法

受术者端坐，两腿略分开。术者站在其一侧，用腿挟住其一

The doctor who stands to one side of the patient seizes the patient's lower limb of one lateral with his legs, one hand proping the posterior shoulder that is close to the doctor, the other hand entering from under the axillary region of the opposite lateral to hold the anterior shoulder, then two hands giving force simultaneously in opposite directions to cause rotation of the upper body for the pulling of lumbar vertebrae (Fig. 2—37).

2) Rotating Reduction of Lumbar Vertebrae

The operator sits on a square stool. Take the rotation-pulling of the right lateral for example: the assitant fixes the left lower limb of the patient with his two knees and hands. The operator who stands to the right back of the patient press-props near the right of the operated spinous process of the lumbar vertebrae with the left thumb, and, the right hand, crossing from under the right axillary region, to hold the patient's cervical part. In operation the patient is asked to bend his back and bow the body forwards to the maximum degree; the doctor pulls the patient's upper body with force to the right with his right hand and rotates to the right when the lumbar vertebrae is in forward-flexing position. When the rotation reaches the maximum degree, the operator operates a narrow range, rapid pulling-rotation with his right hand. Meanwhile, his left thumb push-presses the affected spinous process of lumbar vertebrae with force left upwards and when the patient has a moving sensation in the spinous process or appears a crack, his right hand immediately helps the patient's upper body up into sitting-up position (Fig 2—38). The movements of left lateral rotation-pulling are the same as above but directions are the opposite.

3) Pulling of Waist with Backward Extension

① Pulling of lumbar vertebrae with backward extension of two-legs

The doctor with Hand A, holds the two knees of the patient who is in prone position and lifts them up slowly, and presses the operated part of the waist with the palm or palmar root of Hand

侧下肢，一手抵住其近术者侧的肩后部，另一手从受术者对侧的腋下伸入扳住肩前部，两手再同时朝相反方向用力，使其上身旋转以扳动腰椎（图2-37）。

（2）腰椎旋转复位法

受术者端坐于无靠背的方凳上。以向右侧旋扳为例：助手用双膝与双手将受术者左下肢固定，术者站在其右后侧方，用左手拇指按抵在其受术腰椎棘突的右旁，右手从受术者右侧腋下穿过，把握住其颈项。动作时，嘱受术者向前弯腰俯身至最大限度后，术者右手再用力将其上身扳向右侧，使其腰椎在前屈位时再向右侧旋转。旋转至最大限度时，术者右手再顺势用力做一小幅度的快速牵扳与旋转的动作；同时，左手拇指发力将受术腰椎的棘突向左上方推按，待手下的棘突有动感或出现"喀嗒"的响声后，右手立即将受术者上身扶正至端坐位（图2-38）。左侧旋扳法动作相同，方向相反。

（3）腰椎后伸扳法

①双腿腰椎后伸扳法

受术者俯卧位。术者甲手托住受术者两膝部，缓缓向上提起，

B. When the affected lumbar vertebrae are extended backwards to the maximum degree, Hand A operates an upward, narrow range, and rapid holding-up with force. At the same time, Hand B gives a forceful press downwards for an over-extension of the lumbar vertebrae and thus achieving the goal of pulling-extending the lumbar vertebrae (Fig. 2—39).

② Pulling of lumbar vertebrae with backward extension of one leg

The doctor stands to the left of the patient who is in prone position, holds the right knee of the patient with his right hand and presses the affected spinous process of the lumbar vertebrae with the left palmar root. The right hand of the doctor slowly raises the right lower limb of the patient, the left palmar root presses tight the affected lumbar vertebrae. When the affected lumbar vertebrae are extended backwards to the maximum degree, the right hand operates a rapid lifting-pulling. At the same time, the left hand push-presses downwards rapidly and powerfully for an over-extension of the lumbar vertebrae to end the manipulation (Fig. 2—40). An extension of lumbar vertebrae by raising the left lower limb may also be used. The operation is the same as that by raising the right lower limb.

4) Pulling of Shoulder Joints (Fig. 2—41)

(1) Shoulder-pulling in Abducting Manner

The doctor, squatting to the affected side of the patient who is sitting, puts the patient's forearm or elbow on his right shoulder; presses the upper end of the affected shoulder joints by two hands; rises slowly and, when the affected joint is gradually abducted to a maximum degree, stands up abruptly to cause a 90 degree abduction of the shoulder. Meanwhile, two hands press downwards with force to make the stress reach the operated joint and release articular adhesion for the recovery of its moving function.

(2) Shoulder-pulling of Forward-flexion and Backward

乙手以手掌或掌根处按压在腰部患处，当受术腰椎后伸到最大限度时，甲手用力向上做一个小幅度的快速托举动作；同时，乙手向下用力按压使受术腰椎过伸，从而达到扳动牵伸腰椎的目的(图2-39)。

②单腿腰椎后伸扳法

受术者俯卧位，术者站在其左侧，用右手把握住受术者的右膝部，左手掌根按压在受术腰椎的棘突上。术者右手将受术者的右下肢慢慢向上提起，左掌根紧压患椎，使受术腰椎后伸至最大限度时，右手再用力向上做一快速的提拉动作；同时，左手向下发力快速推压，使受术者腰椎过伸而完成手法(图2-40)。也可抬举左下肢使腰椎后伸，其动作与抬右下肢后伸腰椎法相同。

4) 肩关节扳法(图2-41)

(1) 外展扳肩法

受术者端坐，术者在其患侧，下蹲。将患肢的前臂部，或肘部放置于自己的右肩上，术者双手按压在受术肩关节的上端。术者慢慢起立，使受术关节渐渐外展至最大限度时，突然起立至使肩外展90°的水平；同时，双手向下用力按压，使应力传递至受术肩关节，以解除关节粘连，恢复其运动功能。

(2) 前屈、后伸扳肩法

Extension

The doctor holds the lower end or elbow of the affected fore-arm with Hand A and props the posterior of the shoulder with Hand B. He first slowly flexes the affected limb forwards or extends it backwards to the maximum degree. At this moment, Hand A suddenly pulls the operated shoulder in the direction of forward-flexion or backward-extension. Meanwhile, Hand B fixes this shoulder and gives a force opposite to that of Hand A to strengthen the stress that has reached the shoulder joint, thus achieving the goal of shoulder-pulling.

3) Shoulder-pulling in an Adducting Manner

The patient sits up straight and keeps his hands before the chest. The doctor who stands close to the patient's back supports the affected shoulder with Hand A and grasps the elbow of the affected side with Hand B. When the affected forearm is pulled inwards to the maximum degree, Hand B operates a rapid pulling-drawing in the adducted direction.

In addition, there are pullings of some other joints such as the elbow, wrist, finger, hip, knee, ankle, toe, etc. The principle of their operation is: giving a force in opposite directions to the lower and upper ends of a joint so that it may have over-extension, flexion, adduction, abduction, and rotation-pulling along its moving axis within the limit of physiological function.

To conclude it, pulling at the beginning should be steady and moderate, while at the moment of pulling, resolute and rapid, and firm force and coordination between the two hands are needed. The range of pulling should not be beyond the limit of normal physiological movements. As for the direction of pulling, only the direction of one moving axis can be chosen in the pulling, in the case of joints of multi-moving axes or a single moving axis. In addition, in the course of pulling, there is usually a crack in the operated joint, which means the stress by pulling has reached the required position and success of the reduction has succeeded. But clinically it is not necessary for

受术者端坐，术者甲手握住患肢前臂下端或肘部，乙手按扶住肩后部。先将患肢慢慢前屈，或后伸，至最大限度时，甲手突然用力向前屈，或后伸方向扳动受术肩关节，同时，乙手将该肩固定，并用力从相反方向与甲手扳肩的力量对抗，以加强传递到肩关节的应力，从而达到扳肩的目的。

（3）内收扳肩法

受术者端坐，将手置于胸前，术者站在其背后，并紧靠其身，用甲手扶住患肩，乙手握住其同侧肘部。乙手将患侧前臂向内收扳动至最大限度时，再用力向其内收方向做一快速的扳拉动作。

另外，还有肘、腕、指、髋、膝、踝、趾等关节的扳法。其施术原则是：在关节上、下端用一相互对抗的力量，使受术关节顺着其运动轴的方向，在生理功能允许的范围内，作过伸、屈曲、内收、外展方向及旋转扳动。

总之，扳法动作在起势时，要稳妥、缓和，而在扳动的瞬间，则必须动作果断而快速，且用力刚强，两手配合要协调。扳动的幅度不得超越正常的生理活动范围；扳动的方向，无论是多运动轴关节或单运动轴关节，在每一次扳动时，只能选择一个运动轴所限定的方向施术。另外，在施用扳法时，往往受术关节会发生弹响声，这表明扳动的应力传递到位，手法复位成功。但在临床上，不一定每个人每次都会有此反应，只要扳动的方向与幅度正确，

everyone to have such a crack in every pulling. The operating is effective so long as the direction and range are right. For this reason, there's no need for each pulling to have such a crack-standard, still less to concentrate on cracks by blindly enlarging the pulling range. Otherwise an over-pulling would result in injuries of joints and ligaments.

CLINICAL APPLICATION

This manipulation is applied to all the moving joints and amphiarthroses, especially joints of the neck, lumbar vertebrae and four limbs. It has the function of restituting articular disturbance and semiluxation, releasing adhesion, lubricating joints, correcting deformity and renewing articular-moving ability.

Before the clinical pulling, other manipulations are usually operated around the affected joints. This manipulation is applied to it only when spasmodic muscles are relaxed and contracted ligaments and tendons softened, and the pain remitted. In this way not only the success rate of pulling can be increased but that the doctor saves his efforts, the patient has less pain, and pulling injuries are avoided.

20. Traction and Counter-traction

The doctor operates a pulling-extending with much force in opposite directions on the upper and lower ends of joints along the longitudinal direction of limbs to enlarge joint spaces. This is called traction and counter-traction, or pulling or leading.

STRUCTURE OF OPERATION

1) Traction and Counter-Traction of Cervical Vertebrae.
(1) In Sitting Position

The doctor who stands behind the sitting patient props the patient's suboccipital bone by two thumbs, holds the lower part of the bilateral angles of mandible with his palmar root, and presses the two shoulders of the patient with both of his forearms. The doctor's two hands hold the patient's head up with force

就会有效。故不必每次都以出现声响为手法成功的标准，更不能盲目地以扩大扳动幅度来追求弹响声。否则，往往会因过度的牵拉而造成关节、韧带的损伤。

【临床应用】

本法适用于全身所有的运动关节与微动关节，特别适用于颈、腰椎及四肢关节，具有整复关节紊乱及半脱位、松解粘连、滑利关节、矫正畸形、恢复关节运动机能等功效。

临床在施用扳法时，往往先用其他手法在关节周围操作，待痉挛的肌肉放松、挛缩的韧带、筋腱软化以及痛势缓解后，再用本法整治罹病关节。这样不但可提高扳法的成功率，而且术者省力，受术者也可以少受痛苦，并避免手法造成的损伤。

20．拔伸法

术者在关节上、下端，沿肢体的纵轴方向，用力做相反方向的牵拉、引伸动作，从而使关节间隙增宽的手法，称为拔伸法，或牵引法、牵拉法。

【动作结构】

1）颈椎拔伸法

(1)坐位颈椎拔伸法

受术者端坐，术者站在其背后，用双手拇指顶在枕骨下方，掌根托住两侧下颌角的下方，并用两前臂压住受术者的两肩。两

and meanwhile his two arms press the patient's shoulders down with force (Fig. 2—42).

(2) In Lower Sitting Position

The patient sits up straight on a square stool and the doctor half-squats to one side of the patient. The doctor holds the patient's chin with the cubital fossa of his flexed left elbow, holds the patient's head tight in upper arms and fore arms, and supports the patient's occiput with his right palm. The doctor straightens his upper body with his two hands holding tight the patient's head to cause a general relaxation of the patient, then stands up erect, and lifts up the upper body of the patient to make him leave the square stool to finish the traction of the cervical vertebrae with the help of the patient's body weight (Fig. 2—43).

(3) In Supine Position

The patient lies in supine position without a pillow. The doctor sits to one side of the patient's head with a steady tread of two feet on the ground while the two knees are pushing against bed-legs, with upper body inclined forewards, waist and back straightened erect, left hand down holding the patient's occiput, and right hand up holding the patient's chin. The doctor's left and right hands grasp and fix the patient's occiput and chin with force respectively. His two upper limbs stretch straight. The force given by waist and back makes the patient's upper body incline backwards, which brings in a pulled-sliding of the patient's body on the bed by the doctor's two hands. In such a way traction of cervical vertebrae is operated with the help of the patient's body weight (Fig. 2—44).

2) Traction and Counter-Traction of the Lumbar Vertebrae

(1) In Prone Position

The doctor asks his assistant to fix the subaxillary regions of the patient who is in supine position or tells the patient to hold the bed edge, and grasps the lower ends of the patient's two shanks with two hands; then tells the patient to have a general re-

手用力向上将头部托起，同时，两臂向下用力压肩（图2-42）。

（2）低坐位颈椎拔伸法

受术者端坐在无靠背的矮凳子上，术者在其一侧，取马步势。术者左肘屈曲用肘窝将受术者的颏部托住，并用上臂与前臂将其头部抱紧，用右手掌支托住其枕部。术者上身挺直，两手环抱将受术者头部挟紧抱住，令其全身放松，然后从马步势站直，将受术者上身提起，使其离开矮凳，利用其自身的重量，完成对颈椎的牵引（图2-43）。

（3）仰卧位颈椎牵引法

受术者仰卧，不用枕头，术者在其头侧取坐位，两足分开踏稳，用双膝顶住两侧床腿，上身略向前倾，腰背挺直，左手在下，垫在受术者的枕部下并将其托住，右手在上，托握住受术者的下颏部。术者的左、右手分别将受术者的枕部与颏部用力握固，两上肢伸直，由腰背部发力，使上身向后仰伸，并带动两手将受术者的身体在床面上滑行拖动，利用其自身的重量完成对颈椎的牵引（图2-44）。

2）腰椎拔伸法

（1）卧位腰椎拔伸法

受术者俯卧，令助手固定其两腋下，或嘱受术者两手拉住床头边缘，术者用两手握紧受术者两小腿下端。令受术者全身放松，

laxation or a cough. At this moment, the doctor and his assistant give force in opposite directions for counter-traction of lumbar vertebrae (Fig. 2—45).

(2) In Backward-extension Position

This is also called back manipulation. Standing back against back with the patient, the doctor stretches his two upper limbs backwards, holds the patient's elbow knees with his two elbows; and puts his hip against the patient's lumbar vertebrae or lumbosacral portion. The patient is asked for a cough and the operator, taking this chance, bends his waist, flexes his knees and throws out his hip to pull the patient off the ground; then operates a rhythmical knee-flexion and hip-throwing-out. At this moment, the hip gives force to vibrate and shake the patient's waist to make the lumbar vertebrae pulled by the lower body weight of himself in backward extension position (Fig. 2—46).

3) Traction and Counter-Traction of Shoulder Joints

The doctor holds the lower end of the fore arm of the patient who is sitting and asks his assistant to fix the patient's body. Then they two slowly give force in opposite directions to tract and counter-tract the patient's shoulder joints (Fig. 2—47).

In addition, there are also traction and counter-traction of some other joints such as elbow, wrist, finger, hipbone, knee, ankle, toe, etc. Their operations are as follows: with one hand holding the proximal end of the operated joint, the other hand holding its distal end, the doctor gives force simultaneously by two hands and operates traction and counter-traction in opposite directions to enlarge joint spaces (Fig. 2—48).

In the course of this manipulation, the force given should be even, lasting, and slowly increased. Pulling with violence is forbidden. Direction of pulling force should be along the longitudinal axis of a joint. This manipulation must be applied with great care to articular deformity and rigidity.

CLINICAL APPLIATION

或令其咳嗽一声，此时术者与助手同时相对用力，拔伸腰椎（图2-45）。

(2) 背势腰椎牵引法

本法亦称背法。术者与受术者相背而立，两上肢后伸，用两肘套钩住受术者的肘弯部。术者用臀部抵住受术者的腰椎或腰骶部后，即令其咳嗽一声，术者趁其咳嗽的瞬间，弯腰、屈膝、挺臀将其双足离开地面，再做有节律的伸膝、挺臀动作，同时以臀部用力，颤动或摇动受术者的腰部，使其腰椎在后伸位受到下半身自身重量的牵引（图2-46）。

3) 肩关节拔伸法

受术者取坐位。术者用双手握住其前臂下端，令助手固定受术者身体。术者与助手缓缓地相对用力拔伸肩关节（图2-47）。

另外，还有肘、腕、指、髋、膝、踝、趾等关节的拔伸法。其操作方法是：术者用一手握住受术关节的近侧端，另一手握住其远侧端，用两手同时用力，作相反方向的对抗牵引的动作，牵引关节使其间隙增宽（图2-48）。

本法操作时，用力要均匀，持久，缓缓加大力量，切忌用暴力牵引；牵引力的方向要沿受术关节的纵轴进行。对畸形、僵直的关节，要慎用本法。

【临床应用】

This manipulation can be applied to joints of cervical vertebrae, lumbar vertebrae and extremities, with the function of restoring and treating injuried soft tissues, reducing dislocated joints, enlarging joint spaces, remitting nerve compression, and relaxing adhesion. It may be used to treat symptoms of cervical spondylopathy, prolapse of lumbar intervertebral disc, torsiversion malposition of tendon ligament, constriction of joint capsule, disturbance and semiluxation of joints.

Section 2

Methods and Measures of Manipulation Practices

Manipulation practices are a professional training in basic skills aiming at making students acquire skills of manipulation-practicing to master skillful techniques and possess a constant force in operating, a strict training of basic techniques is needed to establish a "conditioned reflex" according to standard movement structure, thus forming a correct "movement stereotype." Some manipulations, especially those with complicated structures and greater difficulty of their operating techniques, such as pushing with one-finger meditation, rolling, rubbing, vibrating, digital striking, etc. must be practised again and again to be handled skillfully for a better effectiveness. For this reason, Chinese Massage Science thinks highly of professional training of manipulation techniques and has summerized a set of effective training methods in practice.

Training measures of basic manipulation techniques may be divided into three periods: rice sack practice, practice of routine operation in parts of human body, and practice of routine operation of common diseases. The practising methods and requirements are as follows:

本法适用于颈椎、腰椎及四肢关节，有理筋、复位、增宽关节间隙、解除神经挤压、松解粘连等功效。可用于治疗颈椎病、腰椎间盘突出症、肌腱韧带扭错移位、关节囊缩窄、关节紊乱及半脱位等病证。

第 二 节

手法的练习方法与步骤

手法练习，是指旨在使学员获得规范手法操作技能而进行的一种专业基本功训练。要掌握熟练的技巧和具有持续手法操作的能力，必须通过严格的基本技能训练，按照规范的动作结构建立"条件反射"，形成正确的"运动定型"。特别是对一些动作结构复杂、操作技巧难度较大的手法，如一指禅推法、滚法、摩法、振法、击点法等，更须长期反复练习，才能在临床上运用自如，取得良好的疗效。所以，中国推拿学十分重视手法技能的专业训练，并在实践中总结出一套行之有效的训练方法。

手法的基本功训练步骤，可分为米袋练习、人体各部操作常规练习与常见病操作常规练习三个阶段。每个阶段的练习方法与要求如下：

1. Rice Sack Practice (Fig. 2–49)

Practicing basic skills of manipulation with a rice sack is the basic technique training a beginner must undertake first. Except for manipulations of passive movements of joints, all the other manipulations should be practised first with a rice sack. Standards and methods of the sack are: stitch a sack 25 cm long and 16 cm wide, 4/5 of which is filled with polished round-grained nonglutinous rice of good quality (or sands may be used instead) and then stitch the sack mouth. Coat the sack with a wearable clothing, one end of which has an opening with a thread, the other end is closed. At the beginning of practices, the sack may be tied tight and loosened gradually later.

In practices, the rice sack is put up straight on a table. This is the case of pushing with one-finger meditation, kneading, vibrating, etc; and now the doctor is in sitting position. The doctor stands when practising rolling manipulation. In the course of operation, movement structures of every manipulation, from preparing postures to movement essentials, must be observed, which include position of force-directing point, angle of every joint moving, swinging range and frequency, and the general coordinating links such as posture, breathing and one's will. And the standardized strict training is carried on under a correct guidance.

Firstly, at the beginning of practices, the main efforts should be concentrated on "whether the movement is correct". There is no hurry for greater force, for under the condition of incorrect movement, a blindly-increased force would cause a stiffness of operated muscles which would prevent the acquisition of correct postures and result in a possible sprain of joints and ligaments. After a period of time's serious training, manipulatings may be more skillful, movements more correct and standard. Consequently, as soon as manipulation movements start, they will reach the "best mechanical

1. 米袋练习（图2-49）

在米袋上进行手法基本动作练习，是初学者必须首先进行的基本功训练。除关节被动运动手法外，几乎所有手法都要先在米袋上进行练习。米袋的规格与制法是：先缝制一个长25厘米、宽16厘米的布袋，内装4/5的优质粳米（用洗净的黄沙代替亦可），然后将口袋缝合，外面再做一耐磨的布质外套，布套的一端留有带线绳的扎口，另一端缝合封口。开始练习时，米袋可扎得紧一些，以后逐渐放松。

练习时，先将米袋端放在桌上，如练一指禅推法、揉法、振法等手法时，应取坐位；练习擦法时，取站位。操作时，必须按照每种手法的动作结构，从预备姿势到动作要领，包括着力点的位置，各运动关节的角度、摆动幅度与频率，以及全身配合的姿势、呼吸、意念等各个环节，在教师正确指导下进行规范化的严格训练。

首先，在开始练习时，主要的精力应放在"动作是否正确"这一环节上，不要急于加力。因为在动作不正确的情况下，一味地加重手法的压力，会引起术手肌肉的僵硬而有碍于正确动作姿势的获得，而且有发生关节、韧带损伤的可能。通过一段时间的认真训练，使手法熟练并动作正确、规范，那末，手法动作一旦启动，就会"自动地"达到"最佳力学状态"，力量也就会自然地产

state", and produce force "automatically".

Secondly, the left and right hands should be practised alternatively to make them master the operating skills of every manipulation. After practising one-finger meditation by one hand, operating by two hands at the same time should be practiced.

In addition, in the beginning period of rice sack practices, operating ability of localized points of every manipulation is usually practised first, namely, skills of "localized force" and "attracting force" of manipulations. For this period, "localized force" of manipulation must be emphasised (skills of operating along a line may be practised in later period) because it is one of the primary quality criteria of manipulation and an important factor of clinical effectiveness. To practise it, move slowly along a straight line while operating repeatedly from above to below and from below to above. Practices of the two skills may lay a foundation for the operating skills of "pushing at points, moving along channels" in a human body.

With the development of modern technology, China has lunched the experimental teaching methodology of kinematic biomechanical gradually since 1982, which substitutes information determining instrument for a rice sack to carry on practices of manipulation skills in the first period. The student may practice the above-mentioned manipulations on the force-measuring arch platform of the instrument or by putting the rice sack on it. The students may practice imitatedly on the instrument following the teacher's wave curves of dynamic power and compare them with their own wave shapes which are directly watched on the oscilloscope to find and correct their mistakes and to avoid wrong movements (Fig. 2—50). Practice has proved that by adopting this scientific training method, blindness and dullness of practices can be decreased and interest increased. And the teacher is thus provided with realistic basis for aspects of teaching activities such as demons-

生。

其次，要注意左、右手交替练习，使双手都能熟练掌握各种手法的操作技能。一指禅推法在单手练习后，还要进行双手同时操作的训练。

另外，米袋练习的初始阶段，一般先练各种手法的定点操作能力，即所谓手法的"定力"与"吸定"功夫。因为手法的"定力"是手法质量的主要标准之一，是临床取得治疗效果的重要因素，所以，在此阶段练习时要特别予以重视。以后再练习走线操作的技能。练习时，应沿米袋的纵轴线，由上而下，由下而上，往返地边操作边缓慢地做直线移动。这两种技能的训练，可为以后在人体进行"推穴道、走经络"的操作技术打下基础。

随着现代技术的发展，我国自82年以来，逐步展开了手法运动生物力学实验教学法。该法用推拿手法力学信息测定器作为手法练习器，以代替米袋进行第一阶段的手法技能训练。学员可直接在测定器弧形测力平台上，也可将米袋放在平台上进行上述手法练习。此时，学员可以按照教师所示范的手法动态力波形曲线，在测定器上做模拟练习，并通过示波器直接观察自己所做手法的曲线形态与之比较，以及时发现并纠正其中的缺点，从而避免错误动作的产生(图2-50)。实践证明，采用这种科学的训练方法，可减少学员练习时的盲目性和枯燥感，提高其对手法训练的

tration teaching, training instructions, a timely understanding of students' training degree, and academic records.

The students may enter the second period——practice on human body after the first period's practices which focus on mastering standard movement structures of manipulation and acquisition of skillful operation techniques.

2. Practices of Routine Operating on Parts of the Human Body

After finishing aspects of manipulation practices in the first period, the students should carry out manipulation practices on the human body without delay so as to further acquire operating techniques and experiences of human body to lay a better basis for clinical applications. There are two kinds of practices. One is to practice the operating of points-localizing and moving along channels by one hand in every manipulation by choosing the regarding channel routes and points in their corresponding parts of the human body. The other is, according to the constructive features of formation of different human parts and distributing rule of channels and points, to choose various manipulations applicable to the operation of these parts and to form a group of routine skills of operation for comprehensive practices by a certain route and order.

3. Practices of Routine Operating of Common Diseases

Manipulation practices in this period focus on practicing basic routine operating of clinical common diseases one by one. And imitated practices of this clinical therapy can not only make the students skillfully grasp massage operating methods and measures of every common disease as well as the special manipulations which are not dealt with in the human body practice period and are especially used in treating each diseases, but also make them understand and preliminarily grasp the prescription

兴趣和效率；教师在手法的示范教学、指导训练与及时了解学员的训练程度与学习成绩等教学活动方面都有了客观的依据。

通过第一阶段的练习，在重点掌握主要手法的规范动作结构与习得娴熟的操作技巧后，即可进入第二阶段——人体练习。

2. 人体各部操作常规练习

为进一步获得在人体上进行手法操作的技能与体验，为临床实用打好基础，学员在完成了第一阶段手法训练的各项课目之后，要及时进行人体手法练习。其练习方法有二，一是将各种手法，在其所适用的人体部位上，选择有关的经络路线与穴位，进行单手的定点与循经操作练习；二是根据人体各部位的形态结构特点与经络、穴位的配布规律，选择适用于在该部操作的多种手法，按一定的路线与次序，编排组合成一组手法操作的常规套路，来进行综合练习。

3. 常见病操作常规练习

此阶段手法训练，主要是要求对临床各种常见病的基本操作常规逐一进行练习。通过这种临床治疗的模拟练习，不但能使学员比较熟练地掌握每种常见病的推拿操作方法与步骤，以及在一般人体练习阶段中没有涉及到的、治疗每种疾病时所专用的特

rules of differential points-selecting of clinical massage and manipulation-choosing for treatment. For this reason, this is a very important training step before the real beginning of clinical applications.

Section 3

Clinical Knowledge of Adult Massage

1. Requirement for the Consulting Room

The consulting room should be tidy, clean, commodious, bright and its size should be decided in accordance with the number of doctors. If conditions permit, it should be installed with an air-conditioner and the floor be covered with carpet. At least one of the walls should be fitted with mirror in order that both doctors and patients can correct their postures by themselves in training.

The consulting bed should be solid, 2m long, 80cm wide, 80 cm high and covered with foam-rubber cushion well wrappped with imitation leather. It should be placed away from the walls with a stool of which the height can be adjusted at one side of it so that the doctors can manipulate properly. The medium cupboard should be placed beside the consulting bed with various media in it.

2. Medium for Massage

Media should be used while massaging to increase the curative effect, moist and protect the skin. The use of media for massage has a long history in China. In ancient times, ointment made from various herbal medicines was used as a medium for massage and it was called ointment massage. For example, in the 4th volume of *General Collec-*

殊手法；而且，还可以使其了解并初步掌握推拿临床辨证取穴和选用手法的组方治疗规律。因此，这是正式进入临床应用之前的一个十分重要的训练过程。

第 三 节

成人推拿临床须知

1. 对诊疗室的要求

诊疗室应整洁、宽敞、明亮，大小可根据医生的多少而定。有条件的应装有空调设施，地面铺设地毯。在一面墙上装有落地镜子，以备医生、患者练功时能自我纠正练功时的姿势。

诊疗床应坚固，规格一般为长2米、宽80厘米、高80厘米，床面铺有薄海绵垫并用人造革面封好。诊疗床应放置在四周不靠墙壁的位置，一侧放有能调整高低的凳子，以便于医生操作。介质柜应放在诊疗床的一侧，内备各种介质。

2. 推拿介质

推拿时应用介质，能增强疗效，润滑和保护皮肤。推拿介质的应用，在我国已有悠久的历史。古代应用各种药物制成的膏作为推拿时的介质，称为膏摩。如《圣济总录·卷四》："若疗伤寒，以

tion for Holy Relief, it is mentioned that "When treating the case of febrile diseases, rubbing manipulation is used with ointment for a thousand times, then the ointment of herbal medicine will take its effect. It must be known that massage is ever used with drugs.". Sesame oil is also used as a medium. For instance, the 45th Volume of *Complete Works of Zhang Jingyue* says: "Illness of fever with lumbar pain can be cured by pressing and kneading with pot sesame oil at the painful portion." At present, media used in the clinical practice of massage are: talcum powder, Chinese holly ointment, massage cream, onion and ginger water, sesame oil, etc.

1) Talcum Powder

Talcum powder can be used all the year round, particularly in summer. In summer, people are likely to sweat and that will hurt the skin if manipulation is performed where there is sweat. But if talcum is used, both the doctors' and patients' skin can be protected.

2) Chinese Holly Ointment

The mixture of methyl salicylate and vaseline is called Chinese holly ointment and frequently used in spring, autumn and winter. When it is used with scrubbing and pressing-kneading manipulations, it can increase the diathermal effect of the manipulation. If a little dosage of musk (moschus) is added, it can achieve greater curative effect on promoting blood circulation and alleviating pain by removing blood stasis.

3) Massage Cream

It can be used all the year round. If it is used for scrubbing and pressing-kneading manipulations, it can improve the curative effect for promoting blood circulation by removing blood stasis and clearing and activating the channels and collaterals.

4) Sesame Oil

A little dosage of sesame oil with the scrubbing manipulation can increase the diathermal effect of the manipulation.

白膏摩体，手当千遍，药力乃行，则摩之用药，又不可不知也"。

也有用麻油作为介质的，如《景岳全书·卷四十五》："治发热便见腰痛者，以热麻油按痛处揉之可止"。目前，推拿临床治疗中常用的介质有：滑石粉、冬青膏、按摩乳、葱姜水、麻油等。

1）滑石粉 四季均可应用，但以夏季多用。夏季易出汗，在出汗部位运用手法时，容易造成皮肤破损，局部敷以滑石粉，可保护患者和医生的皮肤。

2）冬青膏 将冬青油（水杨酸甲脂）与凡士林混和称冬青膏。春、秋、冬季多用。用擦法或按揉法时用此膏可加强手法的透热效果。若加少量麝香，更能增强活血化瘀、止痛的疗效。

3）按摩乳 四季均可应用。擦法或按揉法时用此药，能增强活血化瘀、通经活络之功效。

4）麻油 擦法时涂上少许麻油，可加强手法的透热作用。

Other media such as turpentine oil, lotion for relaxing muscles and tendons to promote blood circulation, carthamin oil etc. can all be used. All the ordinary non-poisonous vegetable oils can be used according to the local conditions.

Appendix

1) The Ointment Prescription for Massage

Indications: Pain due to traumatic injuries.

Ingredients: 45 grams of castor seed (*Semen Ricini*) (ground after chaff is removed); 15 grams of kusnezoff monkshood root (*Radix Aconiti Kusnezoffii*) (crude drug powder); 3 grams of olibanum (*Resina Olibani*) (ground). It is seen in The 145th Volume in *General Collection for Holy Relief*.

2) The Green Ointment Prescription for Massage

Indications: Headache, stiffness of neck and pain in the extremities due to febrile diseases.

Ingredients: 90 grams of Chinese angelica root (*Radix Angelicae Sinensis*), 90 grams of chuanxiong rhizome (*Rhizoma Ligustici Chuanxiong*), 90 grams of peppertree pricklyash peel (*Pericarpium Zanthoxyli*), 90 grams of dahurian angelica root (*Radix Angelicae Dahuricae*), 90 grams of evodia fruit (*Fructus Evodiae*), 90 grams of mankshood root (*Radix Aconiti Praeparata*), 90 grams of Kusnezoff monkshood root (*Radix Aconiti Kusnezoffii*), 90 gram of *mangcao* (*Folium Illicii Lanceolati*). This prescription is seen in The 9th Volume of *Prescriptions Worth a Thousand Gold for Emergencies*.

3. Prevention of Accidental Injuries and Autolesion

1) Prevention of Accidental Injuries: Careful, overall and acurate diagnosis of the illness should be made. For patients with violent trauma, doctors should be able to know whether or not there is fracture, dislocation or bleeding inside. For the aged and weak patients, while using the passive movement manipulation, the doctor should operate lightly, softly and carefully,

其他如松节油、舒筋活络药水、红花油等均可应用。一般无毒性的植物油均可酌情选用。

【附】

1）摩膏方　治打扑内损疼痛。蓖麻子（去皮研）45克，草乌头（生为末）15克，乳香（研）3克（见《圣济总录·卷一百四十五》）。

2）青膏方　治伤寒头痛项强、四肢疼痛。当归、川芎、蜀椒、白芷、吴茱萸、附子、草乌头、莽草各三两（见《备急千金要方·卷九》）。

3. 防止误伤与自伤

1）防止误伤：医生在诊疗过程中，应仔细、全面、正确的诊断病情，对暴力外伤患者，应排除骨折、关节脱位，明确是否有内出血继续存在。对年老体弱者采用被动运动手法时，应轻柔谨

and exclude the other pathological fracture factors such as tuberculosis, phymatosis, etc. When the passive movement manipulations with quite big amplitude such as pulling, shaking-tracting and tracting manipulations are used, they should be well-coordinated, soft and must not be rough or harsh at all.

2) Prevention of Autolesion: A massage doctor should have quite strong constitution, qualified skills and should carry on self-training in ordinary times. In the course of clinical manipulation, it should be noted that he should always take proper postures, hold in the chest, pull up the back and contract the abdomen but not drop the shoulders or bend the back. He should have his hands move along with his mind and his body move along with his hands. It is not proper to move only the hands while the body remains still. While standing, the doctor should keep his feet in a "八" posture thus they can step forward or backward freely, turn nimbly and keep every part of the body in proper coordination in the process of manipulation. The above mentioned is a basic skill of the massage doctors. Only in this way can the self-strain be reduced or avoided so as to increase the curative effect. A good command of the manipulation principles can also prevent autolesion and reduce self-strain. For example, lowering the shoulders, dropping the elbows, suspending the wrists and bending or stretching the interphalangeal joints of the thumbs by the swaying force of the wrists are the principles in the pushing manipulation of one-finger meditation. Only by doing so, can the muscles of the upper limbr remain in the best state of alternate relaxation.

In addition, massage doctors should do what they are capable of. When the patient is stout and beyond your strength, some of the manipulations such as back-packing may be left out. When the passive movement manipulation with big amplitude is necessary and the patient is stout, he should be told to co-operate properly and ingenious skills should be used.

慎，并应除外病理骨折因素如结核、肿瘤等。做幅度较大的被动运动手法如扳、抖拉、牵引等，应协调柔和，切忌粗暴生硬。

2) 防止自伤：推拿医生应具备较强健的身体素质，应有一定的功力，平时应注意自我练功。临床操作过程中，应注意正确的身体姿势。要含胸拔背收腹，不要挺胸凸肚，亦不要塌肩屈背。要意到手到，身体相应移动，不要只是手移动而身体不动。站立时两足成丁八步，这样可使身体进退自如，转侧灵活，保持操作过程中身体各部动作协调一致。以上是推拿医生的一项基本功。只有这样才能减少或避免自我劳损，提高疗效。掌握每一手法的操作要领，也能防止自伤，减少劳损。如一指禅推法中的沉肩、垂肘、悬腕，靠腕关节的摆动带动拇指指间关节的屈伸，只有这样，在操作时上肢的肌肉才处于交替放松的最佳状态。

另外，推拿医生应当量力而行。对形体高大的患者施术时，若自觉力量相差悬殊，则有些手法可不必做，如背法。若做较大幅度的被动手法且患者形体又较大时，应当让患者配合好，采用巧力。

4. Prevention and Treatment of Adverse Reaction

In clinical massage, sometimes the patients may have adverse reaction such as syncopy, exacerbation of pain, etc.

1) Syncopy: For the patients who are weakly constituted, nervous, over sensitive to pain, and hungry, heavy manipulations can easily cause transitory syncopy. Therefore, for the weak patients, manipulations should be light and soft. According to the patients' conditions, doctors should try to reduce the amplitude and use less strength so as to avoid syncopy when passive movement manipulation is adopted. Generally speaking, it is not advisable to offer massage treatment for the patient while he or she is hungry. If it is highly necessary, manipulations should be soft and light or patients should drink some sugar water before the treatment. For the over-nervous patients, they should be urged to get rid of the tension before treatment to ensure a good cooperation and avoid syncopy. In the treatment, if the patient feels dizzy, dim-sighted, and palpitant, etc., doctors should stop the manipulation at once, let the patients have a bed rest and knead softly their Neiguan (P 6) with the thumbs. If it is necessary, 20 ml intravenous injection of 50% glucose can be given.

2) Exacerbration of Pain: Patients with lumbocrural pain, shoulder ache and backache may feel the pain worsened if the manipulation is heavier or they are not used to the first massage treatment. This pain will, generally speaking, disappear within 1—3 days. Drugs of activating the blood and resolving the stasis can be used in coordination. Manipulations should be as light and soft as the patients can bear.

5. Indications and Contraindications

1) Indications: Massage indications have gradually got increased with the rapid development of massage speciality.

4 不良反应的预防与处理方法

在推拿临床中，有时可遇到个别患者出现某些不良反应，如晕厥、疼痛加重等。

1）晕厥 体质虚弱，疼痛过于敏感，或过于饥饿或过度紧张的患者，若推拿治疗时手法过重，易引起一时性晕厥。因此，对体质虚弱的患者，治疗时手法宜轻柔，被动活动手法应视患者忍受情况，幅度尽量减小，用力稍轻，避免晕厥的发生。饥饿状态的患者，一般不宜做推拿治疗，必要时手法应轻柔或先让患者喝些糖水。精神过度紧张的患者，治疗前应做好思想工作，消除紧张心理，积极做好配合，避免晕厥的发生。在治疗过程中，若患者出现头晕、眼花、心慌等感觉时，应立即停止操作，让患者卧床休息，可以拇指轻揉内关穴。必要时可静脉推注50％葡萄糖20毫升。

2）疼痛加重 对腰腿、肩背疼痛患者，若手法过重或第一次推拿治疗患者不适应，有时出现疼痛加重，一般1～3天后多能自行消除，亦可配合活血化瘀药物。在手法操作时应尽量轻柔和缓，以患者能忍受为度。

5 适应症与禁忌症

1）适应症 随着推拿学科的迅速发展，推拿的适应症也逐

There are massage indications in all the departments of traumatology, internal medicine, surgery, gynechology, pediatrics and the five sense organs. The chief indications may be referred to the related contents in the therapeutic chapter of this book.

2) Contraindications: So far as contraindications are concerned, they are not absolute in massage therapy. For some diseases, massage can be used as an auxiliary measure to increase the curative effect and eliminate the symptoms. In the clinical practice, attention should be paid to the following points:

① Massage can't be used to treat motion organ disease due to tuberculin and pus organism.

② Generally speaking, it is not suitable for the patient with cancer to be treated by massotherapy.

③ Massage is not used for dermatosis with pathologic changes and injuries, bruise and scald.

④ It's not proper to massage at the part which is bleeding.

⑤ Dislocations should be treated chiefly with taxis.

⑥ Massage can't be applied to the abdomen and lumbosacral portions of women who are pregnant or with menses.

⑦ Attention should be paid to avoiding syncopy in the massage treatment for patients who are hungry and just after strenuous exercise.

6. Other Warnings

1) Male doctors should be accompanied by nurses when they treat female patients for the disease of breast, coxa, groin, and the inside of the thighs in order to avoid unnecessary disputes.

2) So far as the treatment courses are concerned, manipulations with strong stimulations should be given every other day for the purpose of the recovery of the pathologic portion while light and soft manipulations with less stimulations given once a day. For acute diseases or syndromes, 3 to 5 days may be regarded as one course of treatment; for chronic ones 10 to 15 days as one course.

渐扩大。在伤科、内、外、妇、儿、五官等各科疾病，都有推拿的适应症。主要适应症见本书治疗篇的有关内容。

2）禁忌症　关于推拿的禁忌症，亦并非绝对的。有些疾病在治疗中，推拿可做为辅助治疗，能够提高疗效，消除症状。在推拿临床中下列情况应注意：

①由结核菌、化脓菌所引起的运动器官病症不宜进行推拿。

②癌症一般不宜推拿治疗。

③皮肤病病变损害处，皮开肉绽及烫伤处一般不宜推拿。

④正在出血的部位不宜推拿。

⑤脱位处以整复手法为主。

⑥妇女在怀孕期和月经期，腹部和腰骶部不宜使用推拿方法。

⑦患者饥饿时及剧烈运动后，推拿时应防止晕厥。

6. 其他注意事项

1）男医生在诊治女性患者的某些疾病如乳房疾患、髋部疾患、腹股沟及大腿内侧疾患等，应由护士陪伴，以免引起不必要的医疗纠纷。

2）关于疗程，对治疗操作时手法刺激量较大的，一般采取隔日治疗，以便于病变处自我恢复；而操作手法轻柔，刺激量较小者，多采用每日治疗。急性病症以3～5次为1疗程；慢性病症以10～15次为1疗程。

Section 4

Treatment of Common Diseases

Stiff Neck

This disease is, generally speaking, caused by long-time over strain of the muscle group in the neck and the nuchal region (usually one side only) due to improper height of pillow or improper posture during sleep, or caused by myospasm or myofibrositis due to exposure to wind-coldness, or caused by synovial incarceration of the cervical vertebra joints, due to muscular sprain or sudden turn of the head. In TCM, it is also called "*lao zhen*" (stiff neck).

CLINICAL MANIFESTATIONS

The main symptoms are spasm, rigidity and pain of sternocleidomastoid muscle and trapezius muscle, one side only, which are manifested as oblique head to the diseased side, lower jaw turning to the normal side, obvious limitation of neck movement, possible involvement of the head, upper back and shoulder in severe cases and marked tenderness at the diseased area. The mild cases may recover all by themselves within 2—3 days, while the severe cases, with unbearable pain and minimum freedom of neck movement, may last several weeks.

TREATMENT

Massage therapy gives satisfactory curative effect. Usually, the case may get cured after 1 or 2 times of treatment. The shorter the course of disease is, the better the therapeutic effectiveness will be.

1. Manipulation: Pushing with one-finger meditation, pressing, kneading, rotating, pulling, grasping, etc.

2. Location of Points: Ashi, Fengchi (GB 20),

第 四 节

常见病的治疗

落 枕

本病多因睡眠时枕头高低不适或姿势不良，使一侧颈项部肌群在较长时间内处于过度紧张状态；或睡卧时颈肩部当风受凉，该部肌肉发生痉挛、肌纤维炎所致。亦有因扭伤肌肉，或颈部突然扭转不当，造成颈椎后关节滑膜嵌顿所致者。中医亦称之为"落枕"。

【临床表现】

患者颈项部以单侧胸锁乳突肌或斜方肌痉挛、僵硬、疼痛为主要表现。头向患侧倾斜，下颌转向健侧，颈部活动明显受限，疼痛重者可涉及头部、上背部及肩部。患处有明显压痛。轻者2～3天可自愈；重者疼痛难忍，颈部运动功能严重受限，可延至数周不愈。

【治疗】

推拿治疗落枕，有良好疗效，一般1～2次可愈。病程越短，疗效越好。

1. 手法：一指禅推、按、揉、摇、扳、拿等。

2. 取穴：阿是、风池、天柱、风府、肩井、曲垣、天宗穴

Tianzhu (UB 10), Fengfu (DU 16), Jianjing (GB 21), Quyuan (SI 13), Tianzong (SI 11), etc.

3. Operation: The patient sits naturally and the doctor stands behind the patient at the affected side. The doctor, with gentle one-finger pushing manipulation, pushes the points of Fengchi (GB 20), Ashi, Tianzhu (UB 10), Jianjing (GB 21) and Quyuan (SI 13) on the affected side of the neck with one hand. At the same time, he holds the patient's lower jaw with the other hand, and shakes the head slowly and gently. When the cervical muscles are relaxed and the neck can move to some extent, he tells the patient to bend the head forward at about 30 degrees and he himself pushes the patient's lower jaw to the affected side to make his neck turn within the extent of tolerance. With the thumb pressing the corresponding cervical vertebral process, the two hands pushing the neck at the same time in opposite directions so that the extent of neckturning can increase by 5 degrees or so. This method may help the spasmatic cervical muscles get released or the incarcerated synovium return to normal, which may then alleviate the pain and cure the disease. The two hands, while in operation, should be coordinative, light, gentle, precise and nimble. The last part of the treatment includes grasping of Fengchi (GB 20) point and the posterior muscles of the neck, pressing and kneading of Tianzong (SI 11), even pushing of the shoulder and back (till heat sensation is felt locally), and lifting-up and grasping of Jianjing (GB 21) point.

4. Course of Treatment: It is performed once daily. Generally the patient can recover after 1—3 times of treatment.

Cervical Spondylopathy

Cervical spondylopathy, also called cervical spondylotic syndrome, is a syndrome caused by atrophy of the cervical intervertebral discs, narrowing of cervical intervertebral space, or inflammation due to servical hyperplasia that compresses cer-

等。

3.操作：患者坐位，医者站其患侧后方，先用一手以轻柔的一指推法在患侧颈项及肩部风池、阿是、天柱、肩井、曲垣等穴施术，同时另一手托患者下颌部，轻轻摇动，手法宜轻柔和缓，边推边摇。待颈椎活动幅度渐大、肌肉放松后，即令其颈部微向前屈约30°，并将下颌扳向患侧，使颈椎旋转至能耐受的最大幅度。此时，另一手拇指按在相应颈椎棘突，再双手同时向相反方向用巧力扳动颈椎，使之在上述位置再扩大5°左右即可。本法可使痉挛的颈肌伸展平复，或使被嵌顿的滑膜退出而解除患者的病痛。操作时两手应协调一致，轻巧灵活。最后，拿风池及项后大筋，按揉天宗，平推肩背部至局部发热，提拿肩井穴。

4.疗程：每日1次，一般1～3次即愈。

颈 椎 病

颈椎病又称颈椎综合征，是由于颈椎间盘萎缩、椎间隙变窄，或颈椎增生后引起的炎症、刺激、压迫颈神经根、颈部脊

vical nerve root, spinal cord of the cervical region, vertebral artery or sympathetic nerve, all resulting in this syndrome. This syndrome is common in the old and middle-age, and belongs to "*bi zheng*" (arthralgia-syndrome), "*tou tong*" (headache) or "*xuan yun*" (vertigo) in traditional Chinese medicine.

CLINICAL MANIFESTATIONS

1. Cervical Spondylopathy of the Nerve Root Type

It is caused by retroplasia of the intervertebral joints or unci-vertebral joints which stimulates or compresses the nerve root, manifested as cervical-shoulder pain, cervical-occiput pain, sensory disturbance of the occiput, or stiffness and limited movement of the neck, radiated pain in the neck or shoulder or arm (one side or both sides), accompanied by numbness of the fingers, flaccidity of the upper arms, weekness in holding objects, etc. Other symptoms include unsymmetrical limitation of cervical movement and agravated pain upon extending backward or turning to the affected side. Compressing vertex test, traction test, traction and pulling test of brachial plexus, test of finger-compression on spinous process and raising head backward, as well as test of forced head-turning, may all be positive. Reflex pain and secondary tender points may be found at the inner edge of the scapula in the scapular region or in the shoulder.

2. Cervical Spondylopathy of the Spinal Cord Type

It is caused by the hyperplasia of posterior edge of the vertebral body or the invasion of the vertebral canal by the intervertebral disc, the posterior longitudinal ligament or the thick yellow ligament, which further compresses the spinal cord and the nerve roots in the canal. Symptoms of this type include numbness and flaccidity of extremities (upper or lower, unilateral or bilateral), quivering or trembling of the neck and shoulder, or even incomplete spasmatic paralysis which is manifested as limited movement of the extremities, staggering gait, confinement in bed due to inability to walk, and even dyspnea, hypermyotonia, tendon hyperreflexia, weakening or loss

髓、椎动脉或交感神经而引起的综合征候群。多发于中老年人。本病属中医"痹证"、"头痛"、"眩晕"等范畴。

【临床表现】

1. 神经根型

此型是由于退变增生的椎间小关节或钩椎关节刺激或压迫神经根出现颈肩痛或颈枕痛及枕部感觉障碍等，或见颈部僵硬、活动受限，一侧或两侧颈、肩、臂放射痛，并伴有手指麻木、肢冷、上肢发沉无力、持物坠落等症状。颈部活动呈不对称性限制，后伸或向患侧旋转时疼痛加剧。压顶试验、牵引试验、臂丛牵拉试验、棘突指压头后仰试验及转头加力试验均可为阳性。患者肩胛内缘、肩胛区或肩部可有反射性疼痛和继发性压痛点。

2. 脊髓型

此型是由于椎体后缘增生，膨出的椎间盘和后纵韧带或肥厚的黄韧带突入椎管，压迫脊髓和神经根椎管内部分所致。可见上肢或下肢、一侧或两侧麻木、疲软无力，颈颤臂抖，甚者可表现为不同程度的不全痉挛性瘫痪，如活动不便，步态笨拙，走路不稳，以至卧床不起，甚至出现呼吸困难，四肢肌张力高，腱反射

of superficial reflex as well as clonus of the patella and the ankle and positive Babinski's sign. Usually there is no neck pain and dyskinesia. Dynamic test of cerebrospinal fluid commonly reveals incomplete obstruction.

3. Cervical Spondylopathy of the Vertebral Artery Type

This type, also called ischemic cervical spondylopathy, is caused by poor blood supply of the vertebral artery due to degeneration and hyperplasia of the cervical vertebrae which make the vertebral artery wrenched, spasmodic or compressed. Because of blood deficiency of the inner ear and the brain, the patient may have cervical and shoulder pain, cervical and occiput pain, dizziness, vomiting, nausea, positional vertigo, sudden falling to the ground, dysfunction in holding object, tinnitus, deafness, blurring of vision, etc. The above-mentioned symptoms are induced or deteriorated by the movement of the head and neck or their bending laterally to certain extent.

4. Cervical Spondylopathy of the Sympathetic Nerve Type

This type is caused by stimulation of the sympathetic nerves. The symptoms include occipital pain, heaviness in the head, dizziness or migraine, palpitation, chest distress, coldness of the extremities, low skin temperature, feverish sensation in the palms and soles, soreness and swelling sensation in the extremities. Generally, there is no radiation pain or numbness in the upper arms. Postbulbar pain, blurring of vision, photophobia, lacrimation, rhinorrhea, sensation of foreign body in the throat, pain in the anterior pectorial region and facial sweating may be noticed in a few patients.

5. Cervical Spondylopathy of Mixed Type

It refers to cervical spondylopathy having the symptoms of the two or more types mentioned above. Cervical x-ray film reveals such abnormal changes as disappearance of physiological lordosis, lateral curvature of the cervical vertebrae, narrowing of the intervertebral space, sclerosis of the edges of the intervertebral facet joints, hamate vertebral articulations and the vertebral

亢进，浅反射减弱或消失以及髌、踝阵挛，巴氏征阳性。多无颈部疼痛和运动障碍。脑脊液动力试验常为不完全梗阻。

3. 椎动脉型

椎动脉型又称缺血型，是由于颈椎退变增生，使椎动脉扭曲、痉挛或受压，引起椎动脉供血不足所致。患者因内耳和脑部缺血，表现为颈肩痛或颈枕痛、头晕、恶心、呕吐、位置性眩晕、猝倒、持物落地、耳鸣、耳聋、视物不清等。上述症状常因头颈转动或侧屈到某一位置而诱发或加重。

4. 交感神经型

此型是由于交感神经受刺激而出现枕部痛、头沉、头晕或偏头痛、心慌、胸闷、肢凉、皮肤温度低或手足发热、四肢酸胀等症状，一般无上肢放射痛或麻木感，个别病人也可出现眼球后痛、视物不清、畏光、流泪、流涕、咽部异物感、胸前区痛、面部出汗等。

5. 混合型

混合型为同时表现出上述两型及两型以上的症状。

颈部X线片示颈椎生理前凸消失或反向，颈椎侧弯，椎间隙变窄，椎间小关节、钩椎关节和椎体边缘硬化，椎间小关节间隙

body, stricture of the intervertebral facet joint space, and backward and downward sliding excursion of the inferior articular process. Abnormal sliding excursion of the intervertebral space in the affected region can also be shown by roentgenograms of the anterflexion and retroflexion of the neck. Vertebral arteriography is helpful to the diagnosis of cervical spondylopathy of the vertebral artery type. Complete or incomplete obstruction may be seen in the diseased space of the subarachnoid cavity of the cases with cervical spondylopathy of the spinal cord type.

TREATMENT

Massage therapy has certain therapeutic effect on cervical spondylopathy, except that caused by direct osseous compression. It is more efficacious in the treatment of cervical spondylopathy of nerve root type, vertebral artery type and the sympathetic nerve type. However, it is not advisable to apply the replacement manipulation by turning the cervical vertebrae to patients with cervical spondylopathy of spinal cord type and with hypertension and arteriosclerosis, and attention must be paid to the manipulation, which should be light and gentle in the treamtnet of cervical spondylopathy of all the other types.

1. Manipulations: Pushing with one-finger, pressing, kneading, grasping, tracting-countertracting, tracting-counter-tracting-turning, foulage, flat-pushing, rotating, shaking, etc.

2. Location of Point: Fengchi (GB 20), Tianzhu (UB 10), Dazhui (Du 14), Dazhu (UB 11), Jianjing (GB 21), Tianzong (SI 11), Quchi (LI 11), Waiguan (SJ 5), etc.

3. Operation

1) With the patient sitting erect, the doctor stands behind him, and pushes from Fengchi (GB 20) along the sides of the spinous processes of cervical vertebrae down to Dazhu (UB 11) with one-finger pushing manipulation (to and fro) for 5—7 times. The two sides of the spinous processes of cervical vertebrae should be pushed alternatively.

2) Pinch-grasp the dorsocervical area with the tender

变窄，下关节突向后下滑移等异常征象。颈前屈、后伸位X线片可显示病变处椎体间的异常滑移。椎动脉造影对诊断椎动脉型有帮助。脊髓型患者蛛网膜下腔可见病变间隙有不全或完全梗阻影像。

【治疗】

推拿治疗本病，除骨性直接压迫者外，均有一定效果。其中，对神经根型、椎动脉型、交感神经型效果尤为显著。但对脊髓型和伴有高血压及严重动脉硬化的病人，不宜使用颈椎旋转复位法。其他类型使用本法时手法亦应轻柔，切忌暴力。

1. 手法：一指推、按、揉、拿、拔伸、拔伸旋转、搓、平推、摇、抖等。

2. 取穴：风池、天柱、大椎、大杼、肩井、天宗、曲池、外关等。

3. 操作

1) 患者正坐，医者站其背后，先以一指推法从风池穴向下沿颈椎棘突旁推至大杼穴。往返5～7遍，两侧交替。

2) 以捏拿法，捏拿颈项部，重点在压痛点处，同时轻轻旋转

points as the main sites to exert strength. At the same time, rotate the head and neck gently for 2—3 minutes.

3) Intervally press-knead the points of Tianzong (SI 11), Bingfeng (SI 12), Quepen (St 12) and Jianwaishu (SI 14) with the tip of the thumb or tips of the index and middle finger, followed by pinching and grasping Jianjing (GB 21) with both hands. Then flick-pluck the area of the upper 1/3 of the medial side of the upper arm with the index, middle, and ring fingers. Press-knead Quchi (LI 11), Shousanli (LI 10) and Waiguan (SJ 5) with the thumb. Rotate the shoulder joint, and shake the upper extremities.

4) The tracting-countertracting of the neck includes the following three methods:

(1) The patient assumes supine position with his legs stretched straight and the arms put along the sides of the bodys, while the doctor sits at the patient's head with the knees against the bed side. Then, the doctor holds the patient's lower jaw with one hand and holds the occipital tuberosity with the other, leans the upper part of the body backward to exert a pulling force on the patient's neck, to pull and shake the cervical vertebrae gently and slowly for 2—3 minutes. While pulling and shaking, gently turn the patient's head to the right or left side. Often a sound of "crack" may be heard.

(2) The patient sits while the doctor stands behind him. The doctor places his two ulnar sides of the forearms against the patient's bilateral shoulders and exerts force downward, places the two thumbs respectively against the regions above the two Fengchi (GB 20) points, while gets the rest fingers and the palms holding up the lower jaw, and exerts force upward. The upward and downward force of the forearms and hands naturally enlarge the cervical vertebral spaces to some extent. While pulling, bend the head and neck of the patient forward and backward and turn it right and left.

(3) The patient sits on a low stool while the doctor stands

头颈 2～3 分钟。

3）继以拇或食、中指端按揉天宗、秉风、缺盆、肩外俞等穴，后以双手捏拿肩井穴。再以食、中、无名指弹拨上臂内侧上 1/3 处，以拇指按揉曲池、手三里、外关等穴，环转摇动肩关节，抖上肢。

4）颈部拔伸常用以下三种拔伸法

（1）患者仰卧，下肢伸直，上肢平放于体侧。医者坐于患者头侧，以双膝顶住床腿，一手放于患者下颌部，另手托住枕骨粗隆处，以腰及上身后仰拔伸，边拔伸边轻柔摇动颈椎 2～3 分钟。在拔伸摇动的同时，可以柔和之力向左或右旋转摇动。可听到"咔嚓"响声。

（2）患者正坐，医者站在患者背后，两前臂尺侧放于患者两肩部向下用力，双手大拇指顶在风池穴上方，其余四指及手掌托起下颌部，并向上用力，前臂和手同时向相反方向用力，把颈椎间隙拉宽，边牵边使头颈部前屈后伸及左右旋转。

（3）患者坐于低凳上，医者站于患者患侧，肘关节屈曲并托

at the patient's affected side. The doctor bends one arm to hold the patient's lower jaw with the bent elbow and places the hand against the patient's temporo-occipital area of the healthy side. Then, he pulls slowly upward and turns the head and neck right and left. At the same time, with the thumb of another hand placed on the corresponding side of the vertebral process of the affected part, he presses and kneads the tender points with the thumb while the patient's neck is moved.

For patients with headache and dizziness, in addition to the manipulations mentioned above, the following manipulation should be performed: rubbing the forehead from the middle part to the two sides, rubbing the two superciliary arches from the inner parts to the outer, pecking Jingming (UB 1), wiping-rubbing Yingxiang (LI 20), Renzhong (Du 26) and Chengjiang (Ren 24), sweeping-rubbing the temporal areas and pressing and sliding from the temporal and occipital area to the back of the neck.

5) While receiving massage therapy, the patient may practise the following exercises themselves:

(1) Bending the neck forward and backward: Sit or stand with the hands placed naturally on the thighs in sitting position or falling at the two sides in standing position. Relax generally, bend the head and neck slowly forward and backward to the utmost extent for 20—30 times.

(2) Bending from side to side: Sit or stand, slowly bend the head and neck to the normal side, then to the affected side to the utmost extent for 20—30 times.

(3) Rotating: Sit or stand, slowly rotate the head and neck to the normal side, then backward, then to the affected side, then back to the original position. Repeat the rotation 20—30 times. Then rotate in an opposite direction for another 20—30 times.

(4) Self traction: A self-made traction support may be

住患者下颌部，手扶健侧颞枕部，向上缓缓用力拔伸，并做颈部左右旋转活动；另一手拇指置于患处相应棘突旁，随颈部的活动在压痛点上施以按揉法。

对伴有头痛、头晕等症者，除用上述手法外，可加分抹前额、眉弓，点睛明，分迎香、人中、承浆，扫散二侧颞部，从颞枕至项部。

5）本病在推拿治疗的同时，应配合以下颈部功能锻炼方法：

（1）前屈后伸法　坐位或站立，两手自然下垂（坐位时两手轻放于两大腿上），全身放松，头颈缓缓前屈至最大限度，再缓缓后伸至最大限度，如此反复20～30次。

（2）左右侧屈法　坐位或站立，头颈先缓缓向健侧侧屈至最大限度，再缓缓向患侧侧屈至最大限度，反复20～30次。

（3）左右环转法　坐位或站立，头颈先缓缓由正中位向健侧、后方至患侧复原位，如此环转20～30周，再向相反方向环转20～30周。

（4）自我牵引法　可用自制牵引托（托住下颌及枕部），坐于

used to hold the lower jaw and the occipital part to tract the neck while the patient is seated on a chair. The head and neck should remain erect, without bending forward, backward or to the left or to the right. The traction weight is usually 3—5 kg, and each traction lasts 30 minutes, 1—2 times each day.

6) Course of Treatment: One course consists of 15 times, once every other day. The interval between every two courses is 5—7 days.

Acute Lumbar Sprain

It refers to the sudden sprain of muscles, fasciae, ligaments and other soft tissues in the lumbar region, and is usaully caused by forward or backward over-flexion (beyond the normal range of movement), carrying over-weighted object in improper posture, or direct knock on the waist due to accident. Traditional Chinese medicine regards this disease as *"niu cuo shang"* (sprain / contusion) in its classification.

CLINICAL MANIFESTATIONS

Patients with acute lumbar sprain have, in general, obvious history of sprain. Severe lumbar pain, limitation and difficulty in movements, e.g., sitting, lying and walking, and deteriorated pain while coughing, sneezing or breathing deeply usually occur immediately after the sprain in severe cases. The patients of mild cases feel no obvious lumbar pain immediately after the sprain but they begin to experience progressive pain or limited lumbar movement several hours or 1—2 days later. Examination reveals obvious local tenderness in the sprain area and marked muscular tense and spasm, with no tenderness and percussion pain radiated to the lower extremities. Compensatory lateral curvature of the lumbar vertebrae may be seen in severe cases.

TREATMENT

Massage therapy has a marked efficacy in the treatment of

方凳上牵引，头勿前屈、后伸及左右侧屈，宜保持正中位。牵引重量为3～5公斤，每次牵引半小时，每日1～2次。

6)疗程：隔日1次，15次为1疗程。各疗程之间间隔5～7天。

急性腰扭伤

本病多因腰部过度后伸与前屈、扭转弯曲，超过了正常活动范围，或搬运重物时负重过大，加之姿势不正；或跌仆或暴力直接撞击腰部。以上均可使腰部的肌肉、筋膜、韧带等软组织受到剧烈的扭转、牵拉而卒然发病。该病属中医"扭挫伤"范畴。

【临床表现】

多有明确的扭伤史，重者伤后随即出现腰部剧痛，活动受限，坐、卧、行走均困难，咳嗽、打喷嚏及深呼吸时疼痛加重。轻者扭伤当时腰部疼痛不明显，数小时或1～2天后，腰痛渐重，以至腰部不能活动。检查可见：伤处明显的局限性压痛，无下肢放射性压痛及叩击痛，肌肉明显紧张、痉挛。重者腰椎可见代偿性侧弯。

【治疗】

推拿治疗急性腰扭伤疗效显著。治疗期间应卧床休息，防止

acute lumbar sprain. Bed rest is advised to avoid further sprain during treatment. Hot compress may be applied to the case of severe pain. Comfortable position is usually assumed during treatment.

1. Manipulations: Kneading, rolling, scrubbing, and digital-pressing and pressing.

2. Location of Points: Ashi points, Shenshu (UB 23), Dachangshu (UB 25), Yaoyangguan (Du 3), Weizhong (UB 40), Chengshan (UB 57), etc.

3. Operation

1) With the patient in a prone position, the doctor stands at the affected side of the patient and lightly and gently knead the bilateral lumbar muscles and the surrounding area of the tender points with finger-kneading and thenar-kneading manipulations for 2—3 minutes.

2) While gradually increasing the strength, finger-knead the tender points and then rub the lumbar muscles around the sprain to and fro for 3—5 times with scrubbing manipulation. At the same time, lift one lower limb in coordination with the back ward flexion of the lumbar vertebrae of the patient. The extent of lifting and backward flexion should be increased slowly.

3) Press and digitally hit the points of Shenshu (UB 23), Dachangshu (UB 25), Yaoyangguan (Du 3), Ashi Points, Weizhong (UB 40) and Chengshan (UB 57), and press and knead the bilateral lumbar muscles.

4) Apply some Chinese holly leaf ointment or massage cream on the surrounding area of the tender point, then rub this area till it becomes warm.

5) The patient lies on his back with the knees and hips bent. The operator holds and slowly rotates the patient's knees, which leads to a movement of the waist and hips, to end the manipulations.

4. Course of Treatment: Once every day, usually 2—3 times may get the illness cured.

再度扭伤。疼痛剧烈者，可配合热敷。治疗时应选择患者自觉舒适的体位进行操作。

1. 手法：揉、㨰、擦、点、按等。

2. 取穴：阿是、肾俞、大肠俞、腰阳关、委中、承山等。

3. 操作

1）患者俯卧位，医者站其患侧，先以柔和的指揉法或掌根揉法在双侧腰肌与痛点周围轻轻操作2～3分钟。

2）再在痛点用指揉法，用力由轻渐重，然后用擦法在伤处上下的腰肌上往返操作3～5遍；同时，用另一手扳动同侧或对侧下肢，配合做腰椎后伸活动，幅度从小渐大，用力渐加。

3）再按、点肾俞、大肠俞、腰阳关、阿是穴及委中、承山穴，按揉双侧腰肌。

4）在伤处周围涂以冬青油或按摩乳等介质，用擦法将局部皮肤擦热。

5）患者仰卧位，屈膝屈髋，双手扶患者双膝部，轻轻转动腰髋部，结束手法。

4. 疗程：每日1次，一般2～3次可愈。

Semi-dislocation of Sacro-iliac Joint

It is commonly caused by carrying overweighted objects or improper posture for carrying, which leads to torsiversion malposition of sacrum and ilium and abnormal arrangement and improper interlock of the articular surfaces, and consequently the widened joint space, or even worse, incarcerated articular synovium in the articular cavity due to its vacuum suction. It can also be caused by an inadvertent stretch, flexion and turning when the muscles and ligaments arround the sacro-iliac joint are flaccid, or by local exposure to cold. Semi-dislocation of sacro-iliac joint includes two kinds: the anterior and the posterior, classified on the basis of the malposition of the sacrum and the ilium. Traditional Chinese medicine regards this disease as "*gujie cuofeng*" (belonging to the joint semi-dislocation).

CLINICAL MANIFESTATIONS

Patients with semi-dislocation of sacro-iliac joint feel severe pain at the affected buttock with difficulty in standing, walking, and bending the waist. When lying, they feel more severe pain; when sitting, the affected side can not bear the body weight. The severe cases often have radiated pains in the groin and heel. If there is a marked tenderness of the sacro-iliac joint of the affected side, and the posterior superior iliac spine is below the level of the normal side, it is a case of posterior semi-dislocation of sacro-iliac joint; otherwise, it is one of the anterior. "4" test, bedside test, knee / hip-bending test and lower extremity-stretching test all give positive results. Lateral lumbosacral curvature is often seen in severe or protracted cases.

TREATMENT

Massage therapy has marked efficacy in the treatment of the disease. If the case receives timely treatment of this kind, the therapeutical result is better. Bed rest for 2—3 hours is necessary after massage therapy to facilitate the stabilization of the joint and the self-adjustment of the muscles and ligaments.

骶髂关节半脱位

本病多由弯腰负重或搬重物时姿势不当等，使骶骨与髂骨扭错，关节面排列紊乱，失去正常的凹凸相嵌的关系，导致关节间隙相应加宽，甚至关节滑膜在关节腔负压的作用下吸入关节间隙，发生嵌顿，或在骶髂关节附近肌肉韧带松弛的情况下，无意的伸屈、扭转以及局部受寒冷侵袭等原因引起本病。根据骶骨与髂骨相对位置的不同，有向前和向后半脱位两种情况。本病属中医"骨节错缝"范畴。

【临床表现】

骶髂关节错位后，患侧臀部疼痛剧烈，下肢不能站立负重，尤其不能弯腰，行走、抬腿困难，平卧后疼痛加剧，坐时需用健侧负重。严重者疼痛不仅局限于臀部，且向腹股沟及足跟放射。患侧骶髂关节压痛明显，其髂后上棘在健侧髂后上棘水平线下者，为骶髂关节向后半脱位；反之，为向前半脱位。"4"字试验、床边试验、屈膝屈髋试验及下肢后伸试验均呈阳性。病情严重或发病时间较久者，可见腰骶部脊柱侧弯。

【治疗】

推拿治疗本病疗效显著，发病后及时推拿治疗，疗效更佳。手法治疗后宜平卧休息2～3小时，以利关节稳定和肌肉、韧带的自我调整。

1. Manipulations: one-finger pushing, pressing-kneading, tracting and pulling obliquely.

2. Location of Points: Ashi, Baliao (UB 31–34), Huantiao (GB 30), Dachangshu (UB 25), etc.

3. Operation

1) The patient assumes a prone position, while the doctor stands at the affected side, press and push to and fro the sacro-iliac joint and its surrounding area of the affected side with one-finger pushing manipulation for 5 minutes, then press intervally with the thumb of one hand the points of Baliao (UB 31–43), Huantiao (GB 30), Dachangshu (UB 25), etc. while holding with the other hand the knee of the affected side to make the hip practise hyperextension.

2) The patient assumes a supine position while the doctor stands on the affected side (supposing the right side), holds the patient's right big toe (hallux) in the right hand and the heel in the left hand, tells the patient to bend his knee and hip and then stretch the leg with strength, while he himself still holds the toe and heel, and pulls along with the patient's movement for 3 times.

3) If it is a case of anterior semi-dislocation of sacro-iliac joint, tell the patient to lie on his healthy side with the lower extremity of the healthy side stretched and that of the affected side bent. The doctor puts one of his elbows against the patient's anterior part of the shoulder and the other against the hip of the affected side. Then he pushes the shoulder backward while pulling the hip forward with the two elbows. The patient lies on his back, while the doctor stands at the affected side, holds the posterior part of the shank of the affected side with one hand and presses the hip of the same side with another. The doctor bends the knee and the hip to the utmost extent, then stretches the leg quickly, and tracts the disordered leg to end the operation.

1. 手法：一指推、按揉、牵引、斜扳等。

2. 取穴：阿是、八髎、环跳、大肠俞等。

3. 操作

1）患者俯卧，医者站其患侧，以一指推法在患侧骶髂关节及其周围往返推拿约5分钟，然后以一手拇指点按八髎、环跳、大肠俞等穴，同时以另一手扳住膝部使骶髂关节做过伸活动。

2）患者仰卧，医者站其患侧（以右侧为例），右手握住患者右踇趾，左手托住足跟部，嘱患者屈膝屈髋后用力蹬腿，医者同时顺牵，反复3次。

3）若骶髂关节向前半脱位，病人侧卧位，健肢在下，伸直，患肢在上，屈曲，医者将屈曲的肘分别放于肩前部和臀部，使肩部向背侧，臀部向腹侧相反用力行扳法；然后患者取仰卧位，医者站于患侧，一手托住患肢小腿后侧，另一手扶住患侧髋部，使髋膝强力屈曲至最大限度，继之做快速伸膝动作，最后拔伸患肢。

4) If it is a case of posterior semi-dislocation of sacro-iliac joint, tell the patient to lie on his healthy side with the normal lower extremity straightened and the affected one flexed at 90 degrees. The doctor stands at the patient's back, holds the sacro-iliac joint of the affected side with the rear part of one palm, and the ankle of the affected side with the other hand to pull it to the utmost extent. Then the two hands push and pull in the opposite directions.

5) The patient assumes a prone position. The doctor applies some Chinese holly leaf ointment on the sacro-iliac joint, then press-rubs the joint and its surrounding area with evenly-pushing manipulation, till this area becomes hot in depth.

Posterior Articular Disturbance Syndrome of the Lumbar Vertebrae

It is commonly caused by malposition of the small joints of the lumbar vertebrae or incarceration of the synovium due to knock of external force or improper waist movement. Its main symptoms are severe lumbar pain and difficulty in lying supine and turning the waist. Traditional Chinese medicine regards this disease as "*shanyao chaqi*" (sudden sprain in the lumbar region).

CLINICAL MANIFESTATIONS

Most patients have a history of acute sprain or unremarked injury of the waist. They usually feel a sudden lumbar pain when bending or turning the waist, which is then followed by difficulty in movement and increased pain in coughing and sneezing. Generally, there is no radiated pain in the lower extremities. It is not rare that coughing or sneezing causes this disease. There is usually a marked fixed tenderness point in the projection area of the posterior vertebrae and obvious waist movement limitation, especially limitation of the active or passive backward flexion of the lumbar vertebrae. Muscular tension and spasm at the waist on the affected side and local pain on percussion are usually experienced, but no

4）若骶髂关节向后半脱位，病人健侧卧位，健侧下肢伸直，患肢屈膝至90°。医者站其背侧，一手掌根部抵住患侧骶髂关节部，另一手握住患肢踝部向后扳至最大限度时，两手做相反方向推拉。

5）患者俯卧，在骶髂关节处涂以冬青膏，用平推法，擦推骶髂关节及其周围，以热深透为宜。

腰椎后关节紊乱症

本病多因外力或腰部活动不当，导致腰椎小关节的错位或滑膜嵌顿所致。主要表现为腰部疼痛，不能仰俯及转侧。中医称之为"闪腰岔气"。

【临床表现】

大多数患者腰部有急性扭伤史，亦有无明显外伤史者。多于弯腰或腰部左右侧屈或旋转时突感腰部疼痛，随即不能活动，咳嗽、打喷嚏时疼痛加重，无下肢放射性疼痛。亦有因咳嗽、打喷嚏而致发病者。在发病的后关节投影处有明显固定的压痛点，腰部活动明显受限，尤以腰椎主、被动后仰动作受限为甚。痛侧腰肌紧

marked radiated tenderness and movement limitation in the lower limbs are noticed. Roentgenogram reveals no abnormal changes of the bones or the inter vertebral space.

TREATMENT

Massage therapy can ensure a complete cure of this disease. If the patient receives such treatment immediately after the injury, one time is enough.

1. Manipulations: Pressing, kneading, pulling obliquely and tracting-countertracting.

2. Location of Points: Ashi Point, Shenshu (UB 2), Yaoyan (Extra), Dachangshu (UB 25), Weizhong (UB 40) and Chengshan (UB 57).

3. Operation

1) The patient lies prone while the doctor sits or stands on the affected side. Gently the latter kneads with a thumb the tender point and the points of Shenshu (UB 23), Yaoyan (Extra) and Dachangshu (UB 25) to relax the muscles; at the same time, presses and kneads with another thumb the points of Chengshan (UB 57) and Weizhong (UB 40) of the affected side to relieve spasm and pain and promote circulation of *qi* and blood.

2) The patient lies supine and the manipulation of pulling obliquely the lumbar vertebrae is used; lateral recumbent position is also applicable for the pulling. The disordered side should be manipulated first. Then the patient is told to stretch his leg quickly. Along with the stretching, the doctor holds the patients ankle and tracts his leg 3 times. Being treated like this, the patient may feel that the lumbar area is relaxed and the pain has disappeared. The final step is to knead gently the original tender point and the lumbar points previously kneaded for 2— 3 minutes.

Chronic Lumbar Muscle Strain

It is caused by long-term and repeated lumbar strains, or

张痉挛，局部叩击痛，无明显下肢放射性压痛，双下肢活动不受限。X 线腰椎片无骨质及椎间隙异常改变。

【治疗】

推拿治疗腰椎小关节紊乱症，有手到病除之效。若发病后立即治疗，1 次可愈。

1. 手法：按、揉、斜扳、拔伸等。

2. 取穴：阿是、肾俞、腰眼、大肠俞、委中、承山等。

3. 操作

1) 患者俯卧，医者站或坐其痛侧，先以一手拇指轻揉痛点、肾俞、腰眼、大肠俞等穴，使其肌肉放松；同时以另一手拇指按揉痛侧承山或委中穴，以解痉镇痛，行气活血。

2) 患者仰卧位，行仰卧位腰椎斜扳法，亦可取侧卧位腰椎斜扳法，均先扳患侧后扳健侧。然后，嘱患者用力蹬腿，顺患者下蹬之力牵引足踝部，蹬拉 3 次即可。此时患者感到腰部轻松，疼痛消失，再轻揉原痛点与腰部诸穴 2～3 分钟。

慢性腰肌劳损

本症是由于长期反复地腰部劳损，或因腰部肌肉急性损伤未

delayed or mal-treated acute lumbar muscular injury, by re-peated lumbar injuries, or by chronic inflammation of the lumbar muscle fibers due to cold-dampness. This disease is clas-sified in the category of *"yao tong"* (lumbar pain) and *"bi zheng"* (arthralgia) in TCM.

CLINICAL MANIFESTATIONS

Patients with chronic lumbar muscular strain have a history of long-term lumbar pain, which is usually marked by an aching one, occurs repeatedly and becomes paroxysmal or deteriorates af-ter overfatigue. Lumbar pain appears when bending the waist or sitting or standing for some time. The tender area is compara-tively large and no fixed tenderness point can be found but tender mass may be felt in long-term and severe cases. There is usually no marked disturbance in waist and leg move-ment. Upon acute attack, the above-mentioned symptoms be-come more serious, muscular spasm and lateral vertebral curva-ture can be seen and pain is felt when stretching the lower extremities.

TREATMENT

1. Manipulations: Rolling, pushing with one-finger medi-tation, kneading, digital-pressing, scrubbing, and patting-hitting.

2. Lication of Points: Shenshu (UB 23), Mingmen (Du 4), Dachangshu (UB 25) and Weizhong (UB 40).

3. Operation

1) With the patient lying prone, the doctor sits or stands on either side of the patient and practises rolling and pushing with one-finger meditation on the lumbar muscles of the two sides for 5 minutes, then presses and kneads with one thumb or the root of a palm the sacrospinal muscles of the two sides from top to bottom for 5—10 times, laying stress on the points of Shenshu (UB 23), Dachangshu (UB 25) and Zhibian (UB 54). At the same time, he presses the points of Wei-zhong (UB 40) and Chengshan (UB 57) with another thumb.

2) Apply some of ointment of Chinese holly leaf or

予及时治疗或治疗不当，或因反复损伤，或因腰部受寒湿造成腰部肌纤维慢性炎症所致。慢性腰肌劳损属中医"腰痛"、"痹症"等范畴。

【临床表现】

有长期反复发作的腰痛史，多呈酸痛，每因劳累发作或加重，弯腰及久坐、久立时腰部疼痛。腰部压痛较广泛，多无固定压痛点，痛久病重者可触及痛性硬结，腰腿活动多无明显障碍。急性发作时各种症状均显著加重，并可有肌痉挛、腰脊椎侧弯、下肢牵掣作痛等症状。

【治疗】

1. 手法：𢵈、一指禅推法、揉、点按、擦、拍击等。

2. 取穴：肾俞、命门、大肠俞、委中等。

3. 操作

1）患者俯卧，医者站或坐其一侧，先以𢵈法、一指禅推法施于两侧腰肌约 5 分钟，继以拇指或掌根自上而下按揉两侧骶棘肌 5～10 遍，重点按揉肾俞、大肠俞、秩边等穴，同时以另手拇指点按委中、承山穴。

2）在腰椎两侧涂以冬青膏或按摩乳，行擦法，以热深透为

massage cream on the two sides of lumbar vertebrae and rub these areas till a sensation of heat runs deep.

3) To end the treatment with patting and hitting the sacrospinal muscles of the lumbar vertebrae region.

4. Course of Treatment: One course includes 7 times, once every other day. The interval between courses is of 5—7 days.

Retrograde Osteoarthropathy of Lumbar Vertebrae

It is a chronic retrograde affection commonly seen in the middle and old-aged, which usually involves those lumbar joints that bear heavy weight and move in large extent. This illness is classified into the category of *"yao tong"*, (waist pain) and *"gu bi"* (arthralgia syndrome) in traditional Chinese medicine.

CLINICAL MANIFESTATIONS

Most of the patients are over 40 years of age, and the male are more often affected than the female. At the early stage, the patient may have stuffiness in the waist which is more severe in the morning and will be relieved after movements. However, aching pain appears and becomes deteriorated after fatigue. Symptoms of compression of spinal cord or nerve roots may be found in a small number of patients. Examination shows that the physiological curve of the lumbar vertebrae becomes flat or reversed, waist movement is limited, pain is felt on the two sides of the lumbar vertebrae upon deep pressing, and hypermyotonia in the lumbar region is noticeable. Backward stretching test of the lower extremities is positive in most cases. Limit is mostly felt in straight-lifting. Roentgenogram shows spur formation and flatten physiological curve of the lumbar vertebrae.

TREATMENT

Massage therapy is efficacious in the treatment of this disease, but the course is longer (about 2 months). Besides, some

度。

3) 以拍击腰脊部两侧骶棘肌结束手法。

4. 疗程：隔日1次，7次为1疗程。各疗程之间间隔5～7天。

腰椎退行性骨关节病

腰椎退行性骨关节病是中老年人常患的一种慢性退行性病变，常累及负重和活动范围较大的关节。本病属中医"腰痛"，"骨痹"等范畴。

【临床表现】

患者多在40岁以上，男多于女。早期患者自觉腰部有僵硬感，以晨起为重，活动后稍减，但劳累后酸痛加重，少数病人可出现骨髓或神经根受压症状。检查时可见腰椎生理曲线变平或倒置，腰部活动受阻，腰椎两侧深压痛，腰部肌肉张力增高。下肢后伸试验多为阳性。直腿抬高多不受限。X线片可见骨刺形成，脊柱正常的生理弧度消失，变平。

【治疗】

推拿治疗本病疗效可靠，但疗程较长，一般需2个月左右。

waist exercises are needed during the treatment.

1. Manipulations: Pushing, digital-pressing, patting, pulling and flat-pushing.

2. Location of Points: Huatuojiaji (Extra), Shenshu (UB 23), Mingmen (Du 4), Weizhong (UB 40) and Baliao (UB 31–34).

3. Operation

1) The patient lies prone with the whole back exposed, while the doctor stands on the patient's side. Apply some ointment of Chinese holly leaf on the lumbar region and the back, and push flatly with the palm the two sides of the lumbar vertebrae from top to bottom for 30—50 times, then push flatly the lumbosacral portion from side to side.

2) The doctor bends his own arms and press-pushes the two sides of the vertebrae from the lower thoracic vertebral area down to the sacral area with the elbow, then pushes obliquely to the point of Huantiao (GB 30) and presses it with the tip of the elbow. This step is repeated 3—5 times.

3) Pat the lumbo-sacral area with the bent palms 3—5 times.

4) Stretching-pulling backwards the thighs so as to help the lumbosacral region bend backwards.

5) The patient assumes lateral position. The doctor pulls obliquely backward the upper thigh. Then the patient lies on the other side to receive the manipulation of the other thigh.

6) The patient lies supine with his knees and hips bent. The doctor holds the knees with his two hands and rotates and shakes the lumbosacral part.

Rupture Syndrome of the Fibrous Rings of the Lumbar Intervertebral Disc

This illness, also called "protrusion of nucleus pulposus of the lumbar intervertebral disc", is due to acute sprain, chronic strain or exposure to cold. These factors cause partial

在推拿治疗的同时，须适当配合腰脊部活动锻炼。

1. 手法：推、点按、拍、扳、平推等。

2. 取穴：华佗夹脊、肾俞、命门、委中、八髎等。

3. 操作

1）患者俯卧位，医者站其腰部一侧，充分暴露腰背部皮肤，在腰背部皮肤涂以冬青膏，以手掌平推法在腰背部分别沿脊柱两侧做自上而下的平推 30～50 次，然后在腰骶部行横向平推。

2）医者屈曲肘部，以肘部分别沿脊柱两侧自下胸部至骶部压推，推至骶部后，再斜推向环跳穴，点按该穴，如此推动 3～5 遍。

3）以空掌拍 3～5 下。

4）做腰骶部后伸扳法。

5）患者侧卧位，做腰椎斜扳法，左右各 1 次。

6）患者仰卧位，屈膝屈髋，医者双手扶患者双膝部，行腰髋部旋转摇动。

腰椎间盘纤维环破裂症

本症又名"腰椎间盘髓核脱出症"，是由于急性扭伤、慢性劳损或受凉等原因，促使已发生退行性改变的腰椎间盘纤维环部分

or total damage of the degenerated fibrous rings of the lumbar intervertebral disc which will protrude together with the nucleus pulposus and compress the nerve roots or the spinal cord. The disease occurs most commonly in labourers of 20—40 years old, and clinically common is the protrusion of the disc from the 4th to 5th vertebrae and that from the 5th vertebra to the 1st sacrum. Traditional Chinese medicine regards this disease as "*bi zheng*" (arthralgia-syndrome), "*yao tui tong*" (lumbocrural pain) or "*shanyao chaqi*" (sudden sprain of the lumbar region).

CLINICAL MANIFESTATIONS

1. Symptoms

1) Pain in the Waist and Lower Extremities: Patients with the disease have a history of long term and repeated lumbago. In some patients, the pain is gradually felt radiating to one of the lower extremities (rarely radiating to both extremities), and the radiating pain becomes worse when the abdominal pressure is increased during coughing or sneezing, while in some other patients, pain or numbness is felt first in the lateral or posterior part of one leg, then lumbago appears. Generally, the patient likes to lie on the normal side, and the affected lower limb is often bent.

2) Disturbance of Waist Movement: Limit in waist movement in every direction is obvious in the acute stage, and the scope of waist movement can gradually be enlarged with the alleviation of the disease.

3) Numbness: Numbness is common in the patients with longer course of illness and is limited in the lateral aspect of the leg, the dorsum of the foot, the heel or the great toe. Protrusion of the nucleus pulposus of the central type may lead to numbness in the sella area.

4) Coldness of the Affected Limb: Most of the patients feel lower body temperature and intolerance to cold in the

或全部破坏,连同髓核一并向外膨出,压迫神经根或脊髓所致。多发于 20 ～ 40 岁的中青年体力劳动者。临床以腰 4 ～ 5 或腰 5 ～骶 1 椎间盘脱出为多见。该症属中医"痹证"、"腰腿痛"、"闪腰岔气"等范畴。

【临床表现】

1. 症状

1) 腰腿疼痛:大多数患者有长期反复发作的腰痛病史。逐渐感觉疼痛向一侧下肢放射(双侧者少见),咳嗽、喷嚏等腹压增大性动作使放射性疼痛加重;亦有开始先表现为一侧小腿外侧或后侧疼痛或麻木,而后渐感腰部疼痛者。患者常取健侧卧位,患侧下肢屈曲。

2) 腰部活动障碍:急性期腰部各方向活动均明显受限,随着病情的缓解,腰部活动幅度渐大。

3) 麻木感:病程较久者,常有麻木感,多局限于小腿外侧、足背、足跟或足踇趾。中央型髓核突出可发生鞍区麻痹。

4) 患肢发凉:大部分患者自觉患肢怕冷,皮温较健侧低。

affected limb.

2. Physical Signs

1) Lateral curvature of the lumbar vertebral column, decrease or disappearance or even reverse of the physiological curve of the lumbar vertebrae.

2) Tenderness and percussion pain in the waist which radiate to the sole through the lower extremity of the affected side and marked tenderness in the distributing areas of the sciatic nerve of the affected side.

3) Positive results of straight-leg lifting test and dorsi-flexion test.

4) Decreased myodynamia of dorsi-flexion of the great toe or metatarsal flexion.

5) Positive result of supine-position-abdomen-straightening test and neck flexion test.

6) Positive result of lower-limb-extension test.

7) Decreased Achilles tendon or knee reflex, and hypoesthesia of the dorsum of the foot and the posterior and lateral parts of the leg.

8) Narrowing of the intervertebral spaces, with no other vertebral and joint lesions, on x-ray examination.

9) Protrusion to one or all directions of the intervertebral disc on CT examination.

TREATMENT

Massage therapy is only second to surgical operation concerning the effectiveness in the treatment of the protrusion of lumbar intervertebral disc. Patients should be confined to bed rest (in a wooden bed, not soft bed) and the waist kept warm during the attack and treatment. When the symptoms are relieved, they are asked to practise some functional exercises of the lumbar region.

1. Manipulations: Rolling, pressing, digital-pressing, kneading, tracting-pulling-countertracting and pulling obliquely.

2. Location of Points: Ashi Point, Shenshu (UB 23),

2．体征

1）腰脊柱侧弯，腰椎生理前凸减小或消失，甚至后凸。

2）腰部有压痛、叩击痛，并向患侧下肢放射至足底，沿患侧坐骨神经分布区有明显压痛。

3）直腿抬高试验及背屈加强试验阳性。

4）踇趾背屈或跖屈肌力减弱。

5）仰卧挺腹试验或屈颈试验阳性。

6）下肢后伸试验阳性。

7）膝或跟腱反射减弱，小腿后外侧及足背皮肤感觉减退。

8）X线检查多表现为椎间隙变窄，并除外其他椎骨及关节病变。

9）CT检查示椎间盘向不同方向脱出或向四周膨出。

【治疗】

在腰椎间盘突出症的非手术疗法中,目前仍以推拿最为有效。发病及治疗期间，病人应卧板床休息，并注意腰部保暖。症状缓解后，应做适当的腰部功能锻炼。

1．手法：撩、按、点、揉、牵引拔伸、斜扳等。

2．取穴：阿是穴、肾俞、大肠俞、腰阳关、秩边、环跳、

Dachangshu (UB 25), Yaoyangguan (Du 3), Zhibian (UB 54), Huantiao (GB 30), Yinmen (UB 37), Weizhong (UB 40), Chengshan (UB 57), Yanglingquan (GB 34) and Jiexi (St 40).

3. Operation

1) The patient lies prone, while the doctor stands on the patient's affected side. Alternately apply the manipulations of finger-kneading, palm-pressing, palm-kneading and rolling to the two sides of the lumbar vertebrae, the hip muscles and the points of Shenshu (UB 23), Yaoyangguan (Du 3), Dachangshu (UB 25), Zhibian (UB 54) and Huantiao (GB 30). The strength of manipulations should be light at first and gradually become moderate.

2) Alternately apply the manipulations of rolling, palm-kneading and digital pressing to the points of Chengfu (UB 36), Yinmen (UB 37), Weizhong (UB 40), Chengshan (UB 57), Yanglingquan (GB 34), Feiyang (UB 58) and Juegu (GB 39) in the affected limb for 2 or 3 times.

3) Apply the manipulations of pressing-kneading or thumb-kneading (one on top of the other) to the point of Ashi on the sides of the lumbar vertebrae for 2—3 minutes, the manipulation strength should be light and shallow first, and then gradually be deep and heavy.

4) Four lumbar vertebral pulling manipulations are often applied: stretching-pulling backward, lateral recumbent or dorsal position oblique pulling and sitting rotational replacement. In treatment, the first manipulation is compulsory and any one of the other three can be used selectively depending on the situation.

5) Lumbar vertebral traction can be applied depending on conditions and facilities. Manual tracting-pressing reposition or instantaneous intermittent or continued lumbar vertebral tracting with a mechanical traction bed can be selected.

殷门、委中、承山、阳陵泉、解溪等。

3. 操作

1）患者俯卧，医者站其患侧。在腰两侧、臀部肌肉及肾俞、腰阳关、大肠俞、秩边、环跳穴处，交替使用指揉、掌按、掌揉及擦法，反复2～3遍，用力始轻而渐至中等强度。

2）再沿患肢的承扶、殷门、委中、承山、阳陵泉、飞扬、绝骨一线，交替使用滚、掌揉及按点法，往返操作2～3遍。

3）用指按揉法或双手拇指叠揉法，在椎旁阿是穴处操作2～3分钟，用力由轻浅至深重。

4）腰椎扳法可选用腰椎后伸扳法、侧卧位腰椎斜扳法或仰卧位腰椎斜扳法等，亦可取坐位做腰椎旋转复位法。以上四种扳法在应用时，除第一种为必选手法外，后三种可根据情况任选一种。

5）腰椎牵引法根据需要与条件，可选用人工拉压复位法，或用机械牵引床做瞬间断续腰椎牵引或持续腰椎牵引。

6) With the patient lying supine, bend, stretch and rotate his knee(s) and hip(s) to help move the lumbar vertebrae 3—5 times.

4. Course of Treatment: The patient recieves treatment once every other day, ten times of treatment make one course. The interval between every two courses is 3—5 days.

Injury of Superior Cluneal Nerves

Injury of superior cluneal nerves, also called "superior cluneal neuralgia", refers to a pain syndrome caused by injury of the superior cluneal nerves. Big-range lateral flexion and rotation of the waist or forced traction of the lumbo-cluneal muscles may lead to the injury of the superior cluneal nerves which gives rise to hyperemia, edema or bleeding. Chronic injury may also lead to degeneration of the neural axon process and myelin sheath, i.e. fusiform thickening of the nerve-tract, which then gives rise to the symptoms of neuralgia. This disease is classified into the categories of "*shang jin*" (injury of the muscle and tendon), "*jin chu cao*" (displacement of muscle and tendon after trauma) or "*bi zheng*" (arthralgia-syndrome) in traditional Chinese medicine.

CLINICAL MANIFESTATIONS

Most of the patients have a history of lumbo-cluneal sprain, contusion and other injuries, and have experienced an aching pain or a splitting pain in the lumbo-cluneal spinous process of one side. The pain in the acute stage is severe, accompanied with tracting pain in the thigh. Patients usually have difficulty in lumbar flexion and in the movement from sitting to standing or vice versa. Physical examination reveals tension or prominence of the lumbo-cluneal muscles, cluneal bending towards the affected side, limitation in forward flexion of the waist, marked tenderness and painful hard and fusiform cord at the medial aspect 2—3 cm from the top of the iliac crest of the affected side.

6）仰卧位，做单、双腿屈膝屈髋动作，并摆动腰椎 3～5 次。

4．疗程：隔日 1 次，10次为 1 疗程。各疗程之间间隔 3～5 天。

臀上皮神经损伤

本症为臀上皮神经损伤所致的一种疼痛综合征，故又称"臀上皮神经痛"。当人体做较大幅度的侧屈、旋转或腰臀部肌肉强力收缩时，易伤及臀上皮神经而引起神经充血、水肿以至出血；慢性损伤亦可导致神经轴突和髓鞘发生变性反应，即神经束呈梭状增粗，出现神经痛症状。该症属中医"伤筋"、"筋出槽"、"痹症"等范畴。

【临床表现】

多数患者有腰臀部扭伤、闪挫或劳损史。自觉一侧腰臀部棘突酸痛或撕裂样疼痛。急性期疼痛较剧，并可伴有下肢牵扯性痛。但一般不超过膝盖。弯腰困难，坐位起立或站位下坐时均感困难。检查时可见腰臀部肌肉紧张或高起，臀部歪向患侧，腰部前屈受限，痛侧髂嵴最高点内侧 2～3 厘米处明显压痛，并可触及痛性梭形硬质条索。

TREATMENT

Massage therapy has a better curative effect. Bed rest for 1—2 days and avoidance of big-range movement after treatment are advisable to prevent another injury.

1. Manipulations: Flicking-poking, rolling, digital-pressing and kneading.

2. Location of Points: Shenshu (UB 23), Dachangshu (UB 25), Zhibian (UB 54), Huantiao (GB 30), Weizhong (UB 40), Yanglingquan (UB 34) and Ashi point.

3. Operation

1) The patient lies prone and the doctor stands on the patient's affected side. The doctor presses intervally with a thumb the points of Zhibian (UB 54), Yanglingquan (GB 34) Chengshan (UB 57), Kunlun (UB 60) one minute for each. The manipulation is light initially and heavy thereafter.

2) Press-knead with the rear part of the palm the cluneal area of the affected side till the muscles become slightly heated, then let the muscles relax for 3—5 minutes.

3) Overlap the two thumbs (the left above the right) and press with them the pain point (i.e., 2—3 cm medial to the hight of the iliac crest) with the strength exerted from light to heavy and from shallow to deep, for one minute, followed by flicking-poking towards the medial front for 30—50 times. The hard cord may be felt softened at this time. When these manipulations are performed, the patient should be asked to breathe deeply and relax all over. The pressing should be heavy during expiration and light during inspiration.

4) Apply rolling manipulation to the affected side of the waist and buttocks for 2—3 minutes.

5) Spread some ointment of Chinese holly leaf on the affected buttock and scrub with the hypothenar. The scrubbing should be deep and penetrating and should give the patient a warm sensation.

【治疗】

推拿治疗本病疗效较好。治疗后宜卧床休息1～2天，避免活动幅度过大，以防止重复损伤。

1．手法：弹拨、㨰、点按、揉等。

2．取穴：肾俞、大肠俞、秩边、环跳、委中、阳陵泉、阿是穴等。

3．操作

1）患者俯卧位，医者站其患侧，先以拇指点按患者秩边、阳陵泉、承山、昆仑等穴各1分钟，用力由轻而重。

2）以掌根部按揉患侧臀部，由轻渐重，至臀部肌肉微热，放松约3～5分钟。

3）以两拇指重叠（右拇指在下），点按痛点（即髂嵴最高点内侧2～3厘米处），由轻渐重、由浅至深地持续按压1分钟后，再向内上方向弹拨30～50次。此时可觉指下硬索变软。按压、弹拨时嘱患者深呼吸，全身放松，呼气时用力按压，吸气时稍放松。

4）在患侧腰及臀部用㨰法，反复2～3分钟。

5）在患侧臀部涂以冬青膏，以小鱼际行擦法，以热深透为度。

3. Course of Treatment: One course is composed of 10 times, one time daily. The interval between courses is 3—5 days.

Syndrome of the Third Lumbar Vertebral Transverse Process

The 3rd lumbar vertebra is located at the apex of the physiological anterior process of the lumbar vertebra. It is the centre of lumbar vertebral movement. Its transverse process is longer than all of the others. The stress it receives during lumbar vertebral movement is the strongest and the pulling force the lumbar muscles give it is the biggest. This can easily cause strain of the attaching point of the lumbar muscular faciae, resulting in lumbago. The syndrome is a kind of common clinical lumbago, belonging to "pain in loins" in traditional Chinese medicine.

CLINICAL MANIFESTATIONS

The patient usually has a history of sprain or strain of the waist of different extent. The pain is often in one side of the waist and buttock and radiates from the thigh downwards to the knee, which may be worsened with bending and rotating of the waist. Clinical examination may reveal obvious tenderness at the ends of the transverse process of the 3rd lumbar vertebra. A hard, cordlike mass can be felt on palpation. Mild lumbar muscle atrophy may be found at the late stage.

TREATMENT

Massage treatment usually yields satisfactory effect. The manipulation should be gentle at the first stage of treatment lest it cause new injury. Bending, Stretching and rotating movements of the waist should be avoided or reduced during treatment.

1. Manipulations: Pushing with one-finger meditation, scrubbing, flicking-poking, and pressing-kneading.

2. Location of Points: Ashi point, Chengshan (UB

3. 疗程：每日 1 次，10次为 1 疗程。各疗程之间间隔 3 ～ 5 天。

第三腰椎横突综合征

第三腰椎位于腰椎生理前凹的顶点，是腰椎活动的中心，其横突最长，在腰椎运动中所受应力最大，所受腰肌牵拉亦最多，极易致腰肌筋膜附着点发生劳损而引起腰痛。本症是临床常见的一种腰痛病症，属中医"腰痛"范畴。

【临床表现】

多有不同程度的腰部扭伤史或劳损史。病人一侧腰臀部疼痛，并沿大腿向下放射到膝平面以上，弯腰及旋转腰部则疼痛加重。检查时第三腰椎横突尖端有明显压痛，并可触及粗硬的条索样硬块。晚期可见轻度腰肌萎缩。

【治疗】

本病以推拿治疗效果较满意。初期手法宜轻柔，否则会引起新的损伤。治疗期间，要避免或减少腰部的伸屈及旋转活动。

1. 手法：一指禅推、擦、弹拨、按揉等。

2. 取穴：阿是、承山、阳陵泉等。

57) and Yanglingquan (GB 34).

3. Operation

1) With the patient lying supine, the doctor stands at the affected side of the patient and press-kneads with the thumb Chengshan (UB 57) and Yanglingquan (GB 34) to dredge the channels and collaterals and relieve spasm and pain. Then he pushes gently with one-finger meditation on the 3rd lumbar transverse process as well as its periphery for 3—5 minutes.

2) Flick-poke the cord-like mass vertically. The force should be exerted from light to heavy, just right for the patient to stand.

3) Apply some ointment of Chinese holly leaf or other lubricant and scrub until a sensation of hotness runs deep.

4) As a last procedure, perform the backward extensional pulling manipulation and the manipulation of oblique pulling of the normal side. Hot compress on the waist can be applied after the above treatment.

4. Course of Treatment: One course includes 3 times, one time a day.

Scapulohumeral Periarthritis

The disease is mainly related to chronic shoulder strain, acute traumatic injury, retrograde affection, invasion by cold, infection and reduced amount of movement. Other important causes may include dystrophy of the shoulder nerves caused by cervical spondylopathy. It is called in TCM *"dong jie jian"* (frozen shoulder), *jian ning zheng* (congealed shoulder) and *"lou jian feng"* (omalgia). It is also named "omalgia at 50" for it often occurs in people around the age of fifty.

CLINICAL MANIFESTATIONS

The disease often affects one shoulder, usually the right. The main symptoms are pain and rigidity in the shoulder. The pain is felt gradually with no special cause. Sometimes it occurs suddenly after traumatic injury or invasion by cold. At the initial stage of the disease, the main symptom is

3．操作：

1）患者俯卧，医者站其患侧，先以拇指按揉患肢承山、阳陵泉穴，以疏通经络，解痉镇痛。继以轻柔的一指禅推法在患侧第三腰椎横突及其周围推3～5分钟。

2）以弹拨法垂直弹拨条索状硬块。用力由轻渐重，以患者能忍受为度。

3）在局部涂以冬青膏或其他润滑介质，行擦法，以热深透为度。

4）最后行后扳伸法及健侧斜扳法。术后可配合腰部热敷。

4．疗程：每日1次，3次为1疗程。

肩关节周围炎

肩关节周围炎的发生主要与肩部的慢性劳损、急性外伤、退行性变、受凉、感染以及活动减少等因素有关。此外，颈椎病所致的肩部神经营养性障碍也可能是一较重要的发病因素。中医多称之为"冻结肩"、"肩凝症"、"漏肩风"。又因其多发生于50岁左右的中年人，故又有"五十肩"之称。

【临床表现】

本病好发于单侧，以右侧受累居多。其主要症状为肩部疼痛与僵硬。疼痛常无特殊原因而缓慢开始，但也可在外伤或受凉后而急性发病。一般初发时以疼痛为主，多为酸痛，遍及肩关节周

pain, usually aching-pain, which may be felt all round the shoulder joint. However it often around the anterior side of the shoulder and radiates towards the forearm. The patient can not lie on the affected side. The patient usually has to keep a fixed posture. The pain can be caused by a sudden touch on the shoulder or by shoulder joint movement. At the advanced stage, the pain may become relieved gradually but movement disturbance becomes increasingly obvious. It is especially difficult for the patient to abduct, rotate outwardly and raise the arm, not to mention the difficulty in drawing in and forward inclining of the shoulder. When abducting the arm there may be typical "shoulder-pole-carrying posture". Combing the hair and dressing or undressing become hard for the patient. In severe cases, the function of the elbow joint may be affected. The hand can not reach the shoulder even if the patient bends his elbow and try to do it. Long course of the disease may result in atrophy of the triangular muscle of different extent.

TREATMENT

At the initial stage as the pain is severe, gentle manipulations may be performed locally and repeatedly to dredge the channels and collaterals, promote blood circulation, alleviate pain and improve the function of the local muscls and tendons. At the late stage of the disease, heavy manipulations such as holding-pulling / pushing, pulling-stretching and rotating may be performed in combination with other kind of shoulder movements to relieve adhesion, lubricate the joints and promote recovery of the function of the joints.

1. Manipulation: Pushing with one-finger meditation, digital-pressing, pressing, grasping, pulling, tracting-countertracting, rotating and shaking.

2. Location of Points: Jianqian, Jianyu (LI 15), Jianliao (SJ 14), Jianzhen (SI 9), Tianzong (SI 11), Jianjing (GB 21), Quchi (LI 11), Hegu (LI 4).

3. Operation

围，但常以肩关节前面为著，有时可向前臂放射。不能患侧卧位。患者经常保持着固定位置，突然碰及肩部或活动肩关节可引起肩部剧烈疼痛。至后期，疼痛往往逐渐减轻，肩部活动障碍却日趋严重。特别是外展、外旋及上举动作最为困难，内收和前屈动作也有障碍。外展时出现典型的"扛肩"现象，梳头、穿脱衣服等动作难以完成。严重时肘关节功能亦受限，屈肘时手不能摸肩。日久，三角肌等可有不同程度的萎缩。

【治疗】

初期，病人因疼痛较甚，可用较轻柔的手法在局部反复治疗，以疏通经络，活血止痛，加强局部肌肉及韧带的功能；晚期，可用较重手法，如扳、拔伸、摇法以及配合肩关节的其他活动，以松解粘连，滑利关节，促使关节功能逐渐恢复。

1. 手法：一指禅推、点、按、拿、扳、拔伸、摇、抖等。

2. 取穴：肩前、肩髃、肩髎、肩贞、天宗、肩井、曲池、合谷等。

3. 操作

1) The patient lies supine or sits, the doctor stands or sits at the affected side of the patient. Push with one-finger meditation the anterior aspect of the shoulder and the medial aspect of the arm to and fro for 3—5 minutes cooperated by the passive abduction, adduction, up-lifting and outward rotation of the arm of the disordered side.

2) The patient lies on the healthy side. The doctor holds the elbow of the disordered side with one hand and performs, with another hand, pushing with one-finger meditation, kneading or rolling manipulations on the lateral aspect of the shoulder and the posterior part of the armpit in combination with the passive movements of raising and adducting of the disordered arm.

3) With the patient sitting the doctor carries out grasping-nipping on Jianjing (GB 21) and digital-kneading on Tianzong (SI 11), Jianzhen (SI 9) Jianyu (LI 15), Jianliao (SJ 14), Jian-qian, Quchi (LI 11) and Hegu (LI 4).

4) The doctor stands in front of the affected side holding the disordered shoulder of the patient in one hand and the wrist or the elbow in another to carry out rotating movement with the shoulder joint as the axis with the movement extent from small to large. Then the doctor holds up the patient's forearm to get the elbow of the disordered side flexed and adducted and places the hand on the healthy shoulder, and then have the hand of the patient go over the head and fall on the affected shoulder. Repeat this for 5—10 times. The doctor should nip-grasp the disordered shoulder with another hand at the same time.

5) The doctor stands in front of the affected side of the patient, holding the wrist of the affected side of the patient and pushing against the anterior aspect of the disordered shoulder with his own chest. With his hand holding the wrist of the patient, the doctor pushes the disordered arm of the patient towards the back and gradually sets it stretched backwards. Do it for 3—5 times.

6) The doctor stands at the back of the healthy side of the

1）患者仰卧或坐位，医者站（或坐）其患侧，用一指推法推患侧肩前部及上臂内侧，往返3～5分钟，同时配合患肢的被动外展、内收、上举、外旋等活动。

2）健侧卧位，医者一手握住患肢的肘部，另一手在肩外侧和腋后部用一指推、揉或㨰法，同时配合患肢上举、内收等被动活动。

3）患者坐位，拿捏肩井，点揉天宗、肩贞、肩髎、肩髃、肩前、曲池、合谷等穴。

4）医者站在患者的患肢稍前方，一手扶住患肩，一手握住腕部或托住肘部，以肩关节为轴心做环转运动，幅度由小到大。然后医者一手托起前臂，使患肢屈肘内收，手搭健肩，再由健肩绕过头顶到患肩，反复环绕5～10次，同时用另一手捏拿患肩。

5）医者站在患者患侧稍前方，一手握住患侧腕部，并以胸部顶住患肩前部。握腕之手将患臂由前方扳向背后，逐渐用力，使之后伸，重复3～5次。

6）医者站在患者健侧稍后方，用一手扶健肩，另一手握住

patient. Supporting the healthy shoulder with one hand, he holds the wrist of the affected side of the patient with another and pulls the disordered arm via the back towards the healthy side. The doctor should exert strength and increase the extent of movement gradually within the patient's bearing.

7) The doctor stands lateral to the disordered shoulder and holds with both hands the part slightly above the wrist of the disordered side. While lifting up the disordered arm, he shakes it and pulls it up obliquely. The patient should, cooperatively, relax the shoulder and drop the elbow before pulling. The manipulations should be gentle and slow.

8) The doctor rotates the disordered shoulder of the patient clockwise and counterclockwise for 3 rounds respectively and then with the two palms facing each other rub-kneads from the shoulder to the forearm for 3—5 times, and lastly shakes the disordered arm to end the treatment.

4. Course of Treatment: One course includes 10 times, once every other day. The interval between courses is 5—7 days.

In treatment of the disease, better effect may be obtained if some functional exercises of the shoulder are carried out in cooperation. The exercises should be carried out orderly, step by step and perseveringly. The following exercises may be selected according to the severity of illness.

1) Raising the Shoulder: Bend forward with the two arms falling and the two hands grasping each other. Swing the arms forward with the extent increased gradually.

2) Abducting the Shoulder: Bend forward with the two arms falling. Swing the arms left and right naturally with the extent increased gradually.

3) Streching the Shoulder Backward: Get the feet apart at shoulder-width and the hands grasped each other behind the body with the pamls facing outside. With the healthy arm in lead of the affected one, stretch the arms backward as far as possible with the body kept straight.

患侧腕部，从背后将患肢向健侧牵拉，逐渐用力，加大活动范围，以患者能忍受为度。

7）医者站在患肩外侧，用双手握住患肢腕部稍上方，将患肢提起，边提边抖，向斜上牵拉。牵拉时要求患者先沉肩、曲肘，且手法宜轻柔缓和。

8）前、后分别环转摇动患肩，各3周，然后两掌相对，从肩部搓揉至前臂反复3～5遍，抖患肢结束治疗。

4. 疗程：隔日1次，10次为1疗程。各疗程之间间隔5～7天。

本病治疗时，须配合适当的肩部功能锻炼，方能收到较好疗效。锻炼应循序渐进，持之以恒，根据具体病情可选下面诸法：

1）抬肩：弯腰，两上肢下垂，两手相握，两上肢向前摆动，幅度逐渐增大。

2）肩外展：弯腰，两上肢下垂，向左右自然摆动，幅度逐渐增大。

3）肩后伸：两足分开与肩同宽，两手在体后相握，掌心向外，用健手带动患手，尽力做后伸动作，身体不能前屈。

4) Rotating the Shoulder: Set the feet apart as wide as the shoulder with the two arms stretched straight. Rotate the arms with the rotating extent being increased gradually.

5) Climbing the Wall with the Hands: Face the wall. With the two hands climbing the wall, raise the arms as high as possible and then resume the original posture. Carry out the procedure repeatedly.

6) Adduction and Abduction Drawing: Cross the hands at the back of the neck and draw in and stretch out the shoulders repeatedly.

Sub-acromial Bursitis

Sub-acromial bursa is also named "subdeltoid bursa". It is located inferior to the acromion and the deltoid and covered by the rotator cuff. Its main function is to reduce friction of the upper end of the humerus when it is at motion below the acromion. The disease of sub-acromial bursitis may be caused by collision injury or by injury due to frequent friction and pressure of the bursa between the upper end of the humerus and the acromion induced when the shoulder exerts strength repeatedly.

CLINICAL MANIFESTATIONS

There is pain in the lateral side of the shoulder which often radiates to the upper end of the deltoid and may be aggravated by the abduction and extorsion movements of the upper arm. There is apparent tenderness in the lateral and anterior aspects of sub-acromial region. At the acute stage the anterior border of the deltoid looks round swollen because of the inflation of the bursa. Initially, there may be mild restriction of the shoulder movement, which may become activity impediment later when adhesion with the tendinous cuff occurs. Muscular atrophy appears firstly in suprospinous and infrospinous muscles, and at the late stage, deltoid mucular atrophy may be seen.

4）肩环绕：两足分开与肩等宽，两臂伸直，做前、后环绕动作，幅度逐渐增大。

5）双手爬墙：面对墙壁，双手沿墙壁缓慢向上爬动，使上肢尽量高举，然后再回原处，反复数次。

6）内收外展：双手在颈后交叉，肩关节尽量内收及外展，反复数次。

肩峰下滑囊炎

肩峰下滑囊又名"三角肌下滑囊"，位于肩峰与三角肌之下，覆盖着肩袖。其主要功能是使肱骨上端在肩峰下活动时减轻摩擦。当肩部遭受外力的直接撞伤，或肩部反复用力，使滑囊在肱骨头与肩峰之间经常受到磨擦与嵌挟等损伤时，即可致成本病。

【临床表现】

肩外侧疼痛，常引向三角肌上端，上臂外展、外旋运动时疼痛加剧。肩峰外下及前下压痛明显。急性期因滑囊膨胀，三角肌前缘呈圆形肿胀。初期肩部活动受限较轻，日久与肩袖粘连，而使肩部活动障碍。肌肉萎缩以冈上肌和冈下肌出现较早，晚期可出现三角肌萎缩。

TREATMENT

Manipulations for treatment at the acute stage should be gentle. Force pressing on the affected region should be avoided lest the bursa be injured further. Heavier manipulations may be performed at the chronic stage. The patient should not restrict the shoulder too much; he can conduct some gentle movement at the acute stage and do some functional exercises at the chronic stage. The affected part should be kept warm.

1. Manipulation: Pushing with one-finger meditation, rolling, kneading, foulaging, flat-pushing, shaking and rotating.

2. Location of Points: Jianyu (LI 15), Binao (LI 14), Jianqian, Tianzong (SI 11) and Quchi (LI 11).

3. Operation

1) The patient takes a sitting posture. The doctor stands at the affected side of the patient and carries out the manipulation as mentioned below. Firstly, carry out pushing with one-finger meditation and then rolling on the deltoid region 3—5 minutes.

2) Apply some ointment of Chinese holly leaf or some safflower oil on the lateral, anterior and posterior aspects of the upper arm, and push flatly till the region is very warm and the manipulation penetrates deeply. Then, with the two palms facing each other, foulage-knead the upper arm and the forearm up and down 3—5 times.

3) Press-knead with the tip of the thumb or the middle finger the points Tianzong (SI 11), Jianyu (LI 15), Quchi (LI 11), Shousanli (LI 10) and Hegu (LI 4) until the patient feels soreness and distension.

4) Finally, rotate and shake the affected arm gently and then shake-pull it to end the treatment.

Hot compress may be applied as a cooperative therapy after the above-mentioned treatment so as to promote the subsiding of the inflammation.

4. Course of Treatment: One course includes 7 days, once daily. The interval between courses is 3—5 days.

【治疗】

急性期治疗手法宜轻柔，切勿用力按压患部，以免加重滑囊损伤；慢性期手法可适当加重。患者不要过分制动，急性期可做适当的轻度活动，慢性期则应进行适当的功能锻炼。患部宜保暖。

1．手法：一指禅推、㨰、揉、搓、平推、抖、摇等。

2．取穴：肩髃、臂臑、肩前、天宗、曲池等。

3．操作

1）患者坐位，医者站其患侧，先以一指禅推法，后用㨰法，施于三角肌部位约3～5分钟。

2）继在上臂外侧及前后侧涂以冬青膏或红花油，以平推法推至热深透为度。再以两掌相对搓揉上臂及前臂，上下往返3～5次。

3）以拇指或中指端按揉天宗、肩髃、曲池、手三里、合谷等穴，以酸胀为度。

4）最后，轻轻旋转摇动患肢，并以轻抖拉患肢结束治疗。

治疗后可配合局部热敷，以促进炎症物的吸收。

4．疗程：每日1次，7次为1疗程。各疗程之间间隔3～5天。

Tendinitis of Supraspinatus Muscle

The disease is a kind of acute or chronic aseptic inflammation due to traction, abrading, sprain or strain of the supraspinatus tendon caused by large-extent strenuous movement or repeated abducting of the shoulder joint.

CLINICAL MANIFESTATIONS

The main symptoms of the disease are pain, movement restriction and tenderness. The pain may be localized at the lateral aspect of the shoulder and may spread to the attaching point of the deltoid. It may sometimes radiate upwards to the neck and downwards to the elbow, the forearm and the fingers. There is obvious tenderness in the greater tubercle at the extremity of the supraspinatus tendon. There may be little restriction of the shoulder movement, but there will be severe pain which may even hinder the movement of the shoulder when it is abducted at 60—120 degrees. Prolonged illness may result in adhesion of the shoulder joint and local muscular atrophy. Calcification of the muscle tendon may be seen by X-ray examination of the shoulder.

TREATMENT

Massage yields satisfactory results. At the acute stage, manipulations should be performed slowly and gently, with the shoulder joint being restricted in movement appropriately. At the chronic stage, the manipulation should be carried out deeply and in combination with certain functional exercises done by the patient. The affected region should be kept warm; cold irritation should be avoided.

1. Manipulation: Pushing with one-finger meditation, pressing, kneading, grasping, flat-pushing, rotating and shaking.

2. Location of Points: Jianjing (GB 21), Bingfeng (SI 12), Quyuan (SI 13), Tianzong (SI 11), Jianliao (SJ 14), Jianzhen (SI 9), Binao (LI 14) and Quchi (LI 11).

冈上肌肌腱炎

本病是由于肩关节大幅度强力运动或反复外展，使冈上肌肌腱受到应力的牵拉、磨损、扭伤或劳损所致的急、慢性无菌性炎症。

【临床表现】

本病的主要症状为疼痛、活动受限和压痛。表现为肩外侧疼痛，并扩散到三角肌附丽点附近。有时疼痛可向上放射到颈部，向下放射到肘部、前臂及手指。在冈上肌肌腱抵止点大结节处有明显压痛。肩关节活动一般不受限制，但在肩部外展 60°～120° 范围时疼痛剧烈，甚则影响肩部活动。日久可致肩关节粘连和局部肌肉萎缩。肩部 X 线片可见肌腱钙化。

【治疗】

推拿治疗本病，疗效较好。急性期手法宜轻柔和缓，肩关节要适当制动；慢性期手法宜深沉，同时应配合适当的功能锻炼。局部宜保暖，避免寒冷刺激。

1. 手法：一指禅推、按、揉、拿、平推、摇、抖等。

2. 取穴：肩井、秉风、曲垣、天宗、肩髎、肩贞、臂臑、曲池等。

3. Operation

1) The patient assumes a sitting posture. The doctor stands at the affected side. The disordered arm is abducted at 30 degrees to get the muscles relaxed. The doctor, with one hand holding the elbow of the affected arm, carries out pushing with one-finger meditation by the thumb of the other hand on the sub-acromial greater tuberosity of humerus to and fro along the suprospinous muscle for 3—5 minutes.

2) Perform thumb-flicking-poking and pressing-kneading alternatively on the affected part for 3—5 minutes.

3) Apply some ointment of Chinese holly leaf or some other massage media on the superior fossa of the spina scapulae and then push flatly with the palm rear or the hypothenar and meanwhile, press with the tip of the middle or index finger on the points of Bingfeng (SI 12), Quyuan (SI 13), Jianliao (SJ 14) and Quchi (LI 11). The pressing should be deep, penetrating and give the patient a sensation of hotness, soreness and distension.

4) Nip and grasp Jianjing (GB 21) and the deltoid muscle, rock the shoulder joint, and foulage and shake-pull the affected arm to end the treatment. Local hot compress may be applied in combination with the manipulation.

4. Course of Treatment: The course is composed of 7 days, once daily.

External Humeral Epicondylitis

Also named "syndrome of external epicondyle of humerus", "tennis elbow" or "humeroradial bursitis", the disease is a kind of syndrome manifested mainly as pain in the lateral aspect of the elbow joint. The pathogenesis of the disease remains unknown. It is seen most frequently in workers who often rotate the forearm and stretch the wrist strenuously. It belongs to the syndrome "shang jin" (injury of the tissues) in traditional Chinese medicine.

3．操作

1）患者坐位，医者站其患侧，患肢被动外展30°，使肌肉放松。医者一手托住患肢肘部，另一手拇指在肩峰下肱骨大结节顶部，以一指禅推法沿冈上肌行走方向往返操作3～5分钟。

2）以拇指弹拨法与按揉法在患部交替操作3～5分钟。

3）然后在肩胛骨冈上窝处涂以冬青膏或其他推拿介质，以手掌根部或小鱼际行平推法。同时，以中指或食指端点按秉风、曲垣、肩髎、曲池等穴，以热感深透、点按酸胀为度。

4）捏拿肩井、三角肌，摇动肩关节，以搓、抖拉患肢结束治疗。可配合局部热敷。

4．疗程：每日1次，7次为1疗程。

肱骨外上髁炎

本病又称"肱骨外上髁综合征"、"网球肘"或"肱桡滑囊炎"，是以肘关节外侧疼痛为主要表现的综合征。其发病原因尚未完全了解，多见于经常反复旋转前臂和用力伸腕的作业人员。该病属中医"伤筋"范畴。

CLINICAL MANIFESTATIONS

The patient has soreness and pain in the posterior and lateral aspects of the elbow, which may become severe on movements such as rotating, stretching backward, lifting, pulling, holding levelly and pushing. The pain radiates downwards along the extensor muscle of the wrist. There may be slight swelling locally; it is difficult for the patient to rotate the forearm and hold things. There is obvious tenderness in the external humeral epicondyle or in the fissures of humeroradial articulation. Both the extensor muscle tension test and the tennis elbow test give positive results.

TREATMENT

Massage yields satisfactory effect especially in patients with short course of illness. Surgical operation may be performed for those who have a longer course of illness and fail to recover by conservative treatment.

1. Manipulation: Pushing with one-finger meditation, kneading, flicking-poking and scrubbing.

2. Location of Points: Quchi (LI 11), Ashi, Shousanli (LI 10), Waiguan (SJ 5) and Hegu (LI 4)

3. Operation

1) The patient assumes a sitting posture while the doctor sits by his affected side, firstly carries out pushing with one-finger meditation to and fro from the external humeral epicondyle to the forearm for 3—5 minutes, and then flick-pokes the local site 5—10 times.

2) Take the right elbow of the body as an example. ·Hold the wrist of the patient with the right hand and get his right forearm turned back. Press heavily the anterior region of the external humeral epicondyle with the tip of the bent thumb and rest the other four fingers on the medial aspect of the elbow joint. Bend the elbow joint of the patient slowly with the right hand until the elbow can not be bent any further and press heavily with the left thumb the anterior region of the external humeral

【临床表现】

患者肘后外侧酸痛，尤其在旋转、背伸、提、拉、端、推等动作时疼痛更为剧烈。同时，沿伸腕肌向下放射，局部可微呈肿胀，前臂旋转及握物无力，肱骨外上髁或肱桡关节间隙有明显压痛，伸肌紧张试验和网球肘试验阳性。

【治疗】

推拿治疗本病有较好效果，对病程短者疗效更佳。病程较长而保守治疗无效者，可行手术治疗。

1．手法：一指禅推、揉、弹拨、擦等。

2．取穴：曲池、阿是、手三里、外关、合谷等。

3．操作

1）患者坐位，医者坐其患侧。先以一指禅推法沿肱骨外上髁向前臂往返推3～5分钟，再在局部弹拨5～10次。

2）以推右侧为例，以右手持腕部，使患者右前臂旋后位，左手用屈曲的拇指端压于肱骨外上髁前方，其他四指放于肘关节内侧，医者以右手逐渐屈曲患者肘关节至最大限度，左手拇指用力按压患者肱骨外上髁的前方，继之伸直其肘关节，同时医者左

epicondyle. Then get the elbow joint of the patient straightened and at the same time push the left thumb to the anterior and upper region of the head of radius and flick-poke the starting point of the wrist extensor backwards along the anterior lateral border of the head of radius.

3) Finally, apply some ointment of Chinese holly leaf or safflower oil on the lateral aspect of the elbow and scrub with the major thenar eminence on the external humeral epicondyle at the lateral aspect of the elbow as well as on the extensor group of the forearm until a sensation of hotness runs deep. Hold the far end of the humerus with the left hand and the four fingers of the patient with the right and shake-pull the forearm and the elbow joint to end the treatment.

4. Course of Treatment: Seven days is required in one course, with one session of treatment everyday. The interval between two courses is 2—3 days.

Tenosynovitis Stenosans

Styloid process of radius is a kind of longitudinal bony groove. Covered by dorsal carpal ligament, it forms a bony fibrous tube through which the tendons of short extensor muslce and long abductor muscle of thumb and their common tendon sheath pass. The tube is narrow and its bottom is hard and rough. So when the thumb is drawn in and the wrist is bent frequently, there will be repeated friction between the muscle tendon and tendon sheath and the fibrous wall of the tube, resulting in aseptic inflammation, edema and thickening of the tendon sheath as well as narrowing of the tube's diameter. Then the muscle tendon may become thinner because of the extra pressure on it, and its motion may be hindered, thus resulting in tenosynovitis stenosans. In traditional Chinese medicine the disease belongs to "*shang jin*" (injury of the tissues).

CLINICAL MANIFESTATIONS

The onset of the disease is slow. There is often a history of persistent, repeated strain of the wrist and fingers,

手拇指推至患肢桡骨头之前上面，沿桡骨头前外缘向后弹拨伸腕肌起点。

3) 最后，在肘外侧涂以冬青膏或红花油，以大鱼际擦肘外侧肱骨外上髁及前臂伸肌群，以热深透为度。左手握肱骨远端，右手握患者四指，以抖拉前臂及肘关节结束手法治疗。

4. 疗程：每日1次，7次为1疗程。各疗程之间间隔2～3天。

桡骨茎突部狭窄性腱鞘炎

桡骨茎突是一骨性纵沟，上覆有腕背韧带，形成一骨性纤维管，拇短伸肌和拇长展肌肌腱及其共同的腱鞘在此经过。由于管径狭窄，管底质硬而粗糙不平，故当经常做拇指内收和腕关节尺屈动作时，肌腱、腱鞘与此骨纤维管壁之间所产生的反复磨擦会造成腱鞘无菌性炎症、水肿、增厚及腔径狭窄；肌腱则因之受压而变细及活动受阻等，从而引起本病。该病属中医"伤筋"范畴。

【临床表现】

本病多起病缓慢，常有腕指长期、反复的劳损史，亦有因短

Overstrain of the wrist and fingers for even a short time may give sudden rise to the disease. At the early stage, the patient may only feel soreness and pain and mild tenderness in the region around the styloid process of radius, and asthenia of the thumb. The pain turns severe gradually and may radiate downward to the thumb, upward to the forearm and even to the upper arm. As the times goes by, atrophy of the major thenar eminence may occur because of the disuse of it and a soybean-sized soft bone-like mass may be felt at the styloid process of radius. Friction sound can be heard when the thumb is moved and a sensation of friction can be felt. There may be local swelling. Fist-making test is positive.

TREATMENT

Massage yields good result at the early stage of the disease. In patients with longer course of illness, a longer course of massage treatment is needed and there is often relapse. When treatment is carried out, the movement amount of the wrist and fingers should be reduced. Washing of the affected part with hot herbal decoction should be conducted in cooperation with the massage in order to promote the absorption of the inflammatory exudate.

1. Manipulation: Pushing with one-finger meditation, rolling, pressing-kneading, flicking-poking, tracting-countertracting, and scrubbing.

2. Location of Points: Shousanli (LI 10), Pianli (LI 6), Yangxi (LI 5), Lieque (Lu 7), Hegu (LI 4) and Ashi point.

3. Operation

1) The patient assumes a sitting posture. The doctor sits opposite to him. Carry out rolling manipulation and pressing-kneading with the thumb on Quchi (LI 11), Shousanli (LI 10), Waiguan (SJ 5) and Hegu (LI 4) alternatively for 2—3minutes.

2) Push with one-finger meditation around the disordered styloid process of radius for 3—5 minutes.

3) Conduct pressing-heavily and flicking-poking with the

期用力过度而突发者。早期仅觉桡骨茎突部酸痛、轻压痛、拇指乏力,渐渐疼痛加重,疼痛可向下放射至拇指,上达前臂,甚者至上臂。久之,可因废用而出现大鱼际肌萎缩,在桡骨茎突处可触及一黄豆大小的软骨样硬块。拇指活动时可有摩擦音,触之有摩擦感觉,局部可有肿胀。握拳试验阳性。

【治疗】

本病早期采用推拿治疗疗效较好。病程长者,推拿治疗疗程较长,且易反复。治疗期间应减少腕指部活动,配合中药烫洗,以促进炎性渗出物的吸收。

1. 手法:一指禅推、揉、按揉、弹拨、拔伸、擦等。

2. 取穴:手三里、偏历、阳溪、列缺、合谷、阿是穴等。

3. 操作

1)患者坐位,医者坐其对面患侧,先以揉法与拇指按揉法在曲池、手三里、外关、合谷穴交替操作2～3分钟。

2)医者以一指禅推法在患侧桡骨茎突周围推动约3～5分钟。

3)以拇指沿前臂外展拇长肌和伸拇短肌到第一掌骨背侧,

thumb to and fro from the long abductor muscle and the short extensor muscle of thumb to the dorsal aspect of the 1st metacarpal bone for 3—5 times.

4) Tracting-counter-tracting the Thumb: Hold the wrist of the patient with one hand and grip the thumb of the patient near the thumb joint with the index and middle fingers of the other hand. Tract the thumb of the patient hard in the opposite direction. At the same time press-knead Hegu (LI 4) with the thumb of the hand which is holding the patient's wrist and abduct and adduct the thumb of the patient with the other hand.

5) Scrub the Wrist: Apply some ointment of Chinese holly leaf or some safflower oil on the patient's wrist and scrub from the dorsal side of the 1st metacarpal bone to the forearm. The scrubbing should be done deeply and penetratingly and should give the patient a local sensation of hotness. Then foulage, knead and shake-pull the upper arm and the wrist to end the treatment.

4. Course of Treatment: One course consists of 15 times, once daily. There is a 7 days' interval between each two courses.

Sprain of the Wrist Joint

The sprain of the wrist joint is resulted when the wrist receives an abrupt hitting or has a rotation, flexion, stretching and lateral bending beyond the range and of excessive load; or when the wrist works too long and is fatigued repeatedly. This causes a partial laceration of the ligament and tendon around the wrist or synovitis of the tendon. In TCM this is called "wanbu shangjin". (injury of the muscle and tendon of the wrist).

CLINICAL MANIFESTATIONS

Injury of the wrist mostly has an obvious history of acute injury or chronic strain.

An acute injury may cause swelling and pain in the wrist

行按压、弹拨，上下往返 3～5 遍。

4）拔伸拇指。医者一手握住患者腕部，另一手食、中两指夹持拇指近指关节处，向相反方向用力拔伸。拔伸的同时，握腕之手拇指按揉阳谷穴，夹持拇指的手做拇指的外展、内收被动活动。

5）擦腕。在腕部涂以冬青膏或红花油，从第一掌骨背侧至前臂行擦法，以热深透为度，然后再以搓、揉、抖拉上臂和腕部结束治疗。

4．疗程：每日 1 次，15 次为 1 疗程。各疗程之间间隔 7 天。

腕关节扭伤

腕关节扭伤是腕部遇受外力的突然撞击，或超负荷大幅度旋转、屈伸、侧屈，或长期反复劳作而引起的腕关节周围韧带、肌腱的部分撕裂伤或肌腱滑膜炎。中医称之为"腕部伤筋"。

【临床表现】

腕关节损伤大多有明确的急性外伤或慢性劳损史。

急性损伤，可有腕部肿胀疼痛，功能活动受限，活动时疼痛

and limit the functional activities. When the wrist moves the pain will become severe and tenderness may appear; as for the chronic strain there is no distinct pain and swelling. There may be pain in the wrist when it moves beyond range, with a sensation of weakness and limitation in movement. In examination if there is pain on the back when the wrist joint is given a palmar flexion it thus means an injury of the ligamentum carpi dorsale and the extensor digitorum; otherwise it means an injury of the ligamentum carpi volare or the flexion tendon. If the wrist has an ulnar flexion and the radial feels a pain, it thus means injury of the radial collateral ligament; otherwise it is injury of the collateral ulnar ligament. If there is pain when the wrist moves in any direction and its activities are appearently limitted, mostly it is a compound injury of the ligament and tendon.

TREATMENT

The anatomic structure of the wrist is complex and there are a lot of traumatic diseases, thus in clinical practice it must be distinguished from the fracture of the distal end of the radius and ulna, the fracture of scaphoid, the fracture or dislocation of the lunate bone, the avulsion fracture of the dorsum of the triangular bone, and the aseptic necrosis of the navicular and lunate bone. When one of the above-manifestations is the case, orthopedic restitutionor operative treatment should be adopted. Massage therapy may achieve good results.

1. Manipulation: Pushing with one-finger meditation, digital-pressing, kneading, rotating, grasping, scrubbing and pulling-extension.

2. Location of Points: Shaohai (H 3), Tongli (H 5), Shenmen (H 7), Chize (Lu 5), Lieque (Lu 7), Taiyuan (Lu 9), Hegu (LI 4), Yangxi (LI 5), Quchi (LI 11).

3. Operation

1) When acute injury is the case, the pain and swelling are comparatively distinct. Soft and slow manipulations

加剧，局部有明显压痛；慢性劳损，腕关节疼痛不甚，无明显肿胀，做较大幅度活动时伤处可有疼痛，腕部有乏力和不灵活感。

检查时，若将腕关节用力掌屈，在背侧发生疼痛，则为腕背侧韧带与伸指肌腱损伤；反之，则为腕掌侧韧带或屈指肌腱损伤。如果将腕关节向尺侧屈曲而疼痛在桡侧，则为桡侧副韧带损伤；反之，则为尺侧副韧带损伤。如果向各个方向运动均发生疼痛，且活动明显受限，则多为韧带和肌腱等的复合损伤。

【治疗】

腕部解剖结构复杂，损伤疾病繁多，临床上须注意与桡、尺骨远端骨折、舟状骨骨折、月骨骨折或脱位、三角骨背侧撕脱骨折及舟月骨无菌性坏死等相鉴别。若属上述情况之一者，则应采取骨科整复或手术治疗。推拿治疗腕关节扭伤，可收到良好效果。

1．手法：一指禅推、点、揉、摇、拿、擦、拔伸。

2．取穴：少海、通里、神门、尺泽、列缺、太渊、合谷、阳溪、曲池。

3．操作

1）急性损伤，往往疼痛和肿胀较为明显，手法操作宜轻柔和

are needed. And appropriate points on the corresponding channels should be selected first near the injury. For example, on the palmar surface of the ulna, the Shaohai (H 3), Tongli (H 5) and Shenmen (H 7) of the Heart Channel of Hand-*Shaoyin* may be chosen; on the radial palmar surface, the Chize (Lu 5), Lieque (Lu 7) and Taiyuan (Lu 9) of the Lung Channel of Hand-*Taiyin* may be chosen; on the dorsal surface of the ulna, the Hegu (LI 4), Yangxi (LI 5) and Quchi (LI 11) of the Large Intestine Channel of Hand-*Yangming* may be chosen. Then press and knead the above-mentioned points with the thumb tip to produce *qi*, that is, an sensation of soreness and distension, which will last about one minute for promoting the flow of *qi* and blood in the channel.

2) Then push with one-finger meditation upwards, downwards, to the left and to the right, around the injury for about 3 to 5 minutes to dissipate blood stasis and improve blood circulation around the injury, meanwhile, grasping and muscle-plucking should be used together with this for relieving spasm.

3) Then, pulling-extension is done to make the wrist do activities of passive circling, dorsiflexion, palmar flexion and hemilateral bending in order to restitute its normal function of activity.

4) Daub the wrist region with the safflower oil and scrub it till a sensation of heat runs deep. If the swelling is distinct, topical application of herbal medicines may be applied after operation.

In the case of chronic sprain and in the later stage of acute injury, there are only slight pain and swelling so that the above-mentioned manipulation should be done with appropriately increased strength and the range of movement should be enlarged gradually to relieve spasm, prevent or relieve adhesion and improve the function of activity of the wrist.

4. Course of Treatment: Once a day, five times for one course, with an interval of 2 to 3 days between two courses.

缓。应先在伤处附近选取相应经络上的适当穴位，如尺侧掌面，可选少阴心经的少海、通里、神门等穴；桡侧面掌，可选手太阴肺经的尺泽、列缺、太渊等穴；桡侧背面，可选手阳明大肠经的合谷、阳溪、曲池等穴。用拇指点按揉上述穴位，使之得气，即有较强的酸胀感，持续约1分钟，以疏通经气，促使经络气血畅通。

2）在伤处的周围向上、下、左、右用一指禅推法，施术约3～5分钟，以散瘀活血，改善伤处周围的血液循环。同时配合拿法、弹筋，以缓解痉挛。

3）然后用摇腕手法，在拔伸的情况下，使腕被动地做绕环、背伸、掌屈、侧屈等动作，以恢复其正常的活动功能。

4）最后，在腕部涂以红花油，以擦法擦之，以透热为度。对肿胀明显者，可在治疗后用中药外敷。

急性损伤后期和慢性劳损，由于疼痛与肿胀较轻，选用以上手法时，要相应加重，活动幅度逐渐加大，以解除痉挛，防止或松解粘连，改善关节活动功能。

4. 疗程：每日1次，5次为1疗程。各疗程之间间隔2～3天。

Sciatica

Sciatica is a clinical syndrome caused by many factors manifested as a pain along the route of sciatic nerve and in its spreading area which is due to primary and secondary injuries of the sciatic nerve. It falls into the category of *"bi zheng"* (arthralgia-syndrome).

CLINICAL MANIFESTATIONS

At the beginning of the disease, there is usually a lateral pain in the waist and with the development of the disease the pain radiates suddenly or gradually along the buttock of the affected side, the posterior aspect of the thigh and the posterolateral side of the leg and the dorsum of the foot or the lateral margin of foot. And a burning, lancinating or electric-shock like pain may appear along the spreading area of the sciatic nerve. At the beginning, the pain is mostly paroxysmal, increases after tiredness, disappears after rest, and becomes severe and continuous gradually afterwards. Usually there is septal repeated attack which may last several weeks, several months or even several years. In examination, the physiological curvature of the lumbar vertebrae can be seen as flat and straight, or the lateral curvature and the lumbar muscle may look tense. And near the spinous process of the affected side of the lumbar vertebrae there is a distinct tenderness point which radiates towards the lower limbs of the affected side. The test of straight leg-raising is positive. Neck flexion and neck pressure test are also positive. In a long-standing case, there may be hypoesthesia or anesthesia or muscular atrophy of the affected limb.

TREATMENT

A massage therapy of this disease may produce obvious curative effect in most cases. A secondary case should be treated comprehensively by integrating with the manipulation of massage for the primary case. In addition, a careful differenti-

坐骨神经痛

坐骨神经痛是由多种原因引起的原发性或继发性坐骨神经损害所产生的一种沿坐骨神经通路及其分布区域疼痛的 临 床 综 合征。本症属中医"痹证"范畴。

【临床表现】

发病初期常为一侧腰痛，随着病情进展，可突然或逐渐向患侧的臀部、大腿后侧、小腿后外侧以至足背或足外缘放射，沿坐骨神经分布区域发生烧灼样、刀割样或触电样疼痛。开始多为阵发性，于活动劳累后加重，休息后消失，以后逐渐加重，并呈持续性，常有间歇性反复发作，可历时数周、数月甚至数年。检查时，往往可见腰椎生理弯曲平直，或侧弯，腰肌紧张，在腰椎的患侧棘突旁有明显压痛点，且向该侧下肢放射。直腿抬高试验阳性，屈颈、压颈试验通常亦为阳性。久病者可有患肢感觉减退或缺失，乃至肌肉萎缩。

【治疗】

推拿治疗本症多有明显疗效。对继发性者，要注意结合运用治疗原发病症的推拿手法，综合施治。另外，要仔细进行鉴别诊

al diagnosis is needed and the massage therapy is forbidden in sciatica caused by tumor, metastatic carcinoma, tuberculosis, etc.

1. Manipulation: Digital-pressing, pressing, kneading, rolling and traction.

2. Points Selection: Dachangshu (UB 25), Zhibian (UB 54), Huantiao (GB 30), Chengfu (UB 36), Yinmen (UB 37), Liangqiu (St 34), Yanglingquan (GB 34), Chengshan (UB 57), Jiexi (St 41), Kunlun (UB 60).

3. Operation

1) The doctor stands at the affected side of the patient who is in prone position and then applies rolling manipulation for 3 to 5 times to the lumbar muscle of the affected side of the lower lumbar vertebrae and along the posterior aspect of the affected thigh and the posterolateral part of the leg softly at first and then hard and deeply.

2) Then the doctor, with the thumbs overlapped press-kneads Ashi on the waist and the buttock for 1 to 2 minutes repeatedly with a bit more strength.

3) Using his elbow, the doctor presses the points of Dachangshu (UB 25) and Huantiao (GB 30) and the Ashi point of the waist and buttock.

4) The doctor digit-presses the points of Chengfu (UB 36), Yinmen (UB 37), Weizhong (UB 40), Chengshan (UB 57), Kunlun (UB 60), etc.

5) The doctor holds the lumbus and pulls it backwards, once for the right and once for the left.

6) Repeat "Operation 1)" for 2 to 3 times.

7) The patient is in prone position, while the doctor, digit-presses to stimulate the points of Futu (St 32), Liangqiu (St 34), Zusanli (St 36), Yanglingquan (GB 34), Juegu (GB 39) and Jiexi (St 41). Then the doctor rolls from the upper part to the lower part and repeats the operation 2 or 3 times.

8) Ask the patient to flex his knee and hip bone. Then

断，对肿瘤、转移癌、结核等所致本症者，则禁用推拿。

1．手法：点、按、揉、擦、牵引。

2．取穴：大肠俞、秩边、环跳、承扶、殷门、梁丘、阳陵泉、承山、解溪、昆仑。

3．操作

1）患者俯卧位，医者站其患侧，先用擦法在下腰椎患侧腰肌，并沿患肢后侧及小腿后外侧，反复往返操作3～5遍，用力先轻柔后重深。

2）再用双拇指重叠按揉法，按揉腰、臀部阿是穴，各1～2分钟，用力稍重。

3）用肘压法，按点大肠俞、环跳及腰臀部阿是穴。

4）用指点承扶、殷门、委中、承山、昆仑等穴。

5）做腰椎后扳法，左右各1次。

6）再重复1)项操作2～3次。

7）患者仰卧位，医者用按点法，刺激伏兔、梁丘、足三里、阳陵泉、绝骨、解溪等穴；再用擦法自上而下，反复操作2～3遍。

8）令患者屈膝屈髋，然后医者一手握患者足掌，一手扶住患

the doctor, with one hand grasping the foot sole, the other supporting the affected knee, makes the patient do compulsory flexion of the hip bone, stretch the knee and extend the ankle, for 2 to 3 times. Be sure that the stretching angle of the lower limb should be within the limits of the patient's movement.

9) Let the patient's lower limb stretch straight and end the operation with the manipulation of foulaging and shaking of the lower limb.

4. Course of Treatment: Once a day, 10 days for one course with an interval of 5—7 days between two courses.

Injury of the Lateral Collateral Ligament of the Knee Joint

When the knee joint has slight flexion and the heel is fixed on the ground, the medial and lateral collateral ligaments become relaxed and the steadiness of the knee is poor; and at this juncture if there is stress from the lateral side that makes the knee joint turn outwards, there will be injury of the medial collateral ligament of the knee joint; the other way round, injury of the lateral collateral ligament of knee joint will occur. Clinically the former case is more common. This is called "*shang jin*" (injury of the tissues) in TCM.

CLINICAL MANIFESTATIONS

Generally speaking, a patient with an injury or partial laceration has a distinct traumatic history. There is pain or tenderness in the medial aspect of the knee joint of the patient and the pain increases when the leg has a passive abduction, and there is local swelling in the medial aspect of the knee. Ecchymosis and hemarthrosis appear within 2 or 3 days. When the medial collateral ligament is completely broken, space between the two sections of the broken ligaments may be felt by touching. Test of the lateral knee joint is positive. And the outward-turning activity of the superjoint of the knee can be seen. From the X-ray orthophoric roentgenogram

膝，做强制性屈髋伸膝，踝背伸动作2～3次。要注意，伸下肢的角度要掌握在患者能忍受的范围内。

9）令下肢伸直，用搓抖下肢法结束治疗。

4. 疗程：每日1次，10次为1疗程。各疗程之间间隔5～7天。

膝关节侧副韧带损伤

当膝关节轻度屈曲，并足跟着地固定时，膝内、外侧副韧带松弛，膝关节稳定性较差。此时，如果在外侧受到使膝关节外翻的应力，则会造成膝内侧副韧带损伤；反之，则引起膝外侧副韧带损伤。临床以前者为多见。本症属中医"伤筋"范畴。

【临床表现】

内侧副韧带损伤或部分撕裂的患者，一般有明确的外伤史，患者膝关节内侧疼痛、压痛，小腿被动外展时疼痛加剧，膝内侧有局限性肿胀，2～3天可出现皮下瘀斑，膝关节内积血。内侧副韧带完全断裂时，可摸到断裂韧带的间隙。膝关节侧向试验阳性，并可见到膝关节的超关节外翻活动。膝关节X线正位片可见

we can see that the medial space (compared with the healthy side) is obviously widened. In the case of avulsion at the end of ligament, avulsion of little sclerite can be seen. In case of avulsion of the combined cruciate ligament, drawer-test is possitive.

TREATMENT

Massage therapy is generally used for the patient who has a sprain and partial laceration of ligament. If the ligament is completely broken, operative suture or neoplasty must be given as soon as possible.

1. Manipulation: Digital-pressing, pressing, pushing with one-finger meditation, kneading, palm-rubbing and flat-pushing.

2. Location of Points: Ashi point, Xuehai (Sp 10), Sanyinjiao (Sp 6), Yinlingquan (Sp 9), Xiguan (Liv 7) and Ququan (Liv 8).

3. Operation

1) The patient is in prone position with the injuried limb stretched straight and rotated outwards. The doctor digit-presses the points of Xuehai (Sp 10), Yinlingquan (Sp 9) and Sanyinjiao (Sp 6) to dredge the channel, promote the circulation of *qi* and blood, and relieve pain.

2) The doctor kneads the localized part with the palm or the major thenar eminance for 3—5 minutes, then pushes with one-finger meditation along the medial collateral ligament for 3—5 minutes, and afterwards, coat the locality with the ointment of Chinese holly leaf or safflower oil which is to be flat pushed till a sensation of heat runs deep.

In case of fresh injury with obvious swelling and pain, manipulation should be soft; in the case of an old injury, more strength should be used, and the manipulation should be integrated with the flexion and extension of the knee joint to prevent adhesion in the joint.

Clinically, there is seldom an injury of lateral collateral ligament, whose clinical manifestations are similar to those

内侧间隙明显加宽（与健侧对比）。若为韧带止点撕脱者，可见有小骨片撕脱；若合并十字韧带撕脱者，抽屉试验阳性。

【治疗】

推拿治疗一般仅用于韧带拉伤及部分撕裂伤者。韧带完全撕裂者，须尽早手术缝合或修补。

1. 手法：点、按、一指禅推、揉、摩、平推。

2. 取穴：阿是、血海、三阴交、阴陵泉、膝关、曲泉。

3. 操作

1）患者仰卧，伤肢伸直并旋外，医者先点按血海、阴陵泉、三阴交等穴，以疏通经络气血，缓解疼痛。

2）以掌或大鱼际轻揉局部3～5分钟，再以一指禅推法沿内侧副韧带做由轻渐重的上下推动3～5分钟，然后在局部涂以冬青膏或红花油，行平推法，以热深透为度。

新鲜损伤肿痛明显者，手法宜轻柔；陈旧损伤者，手法相对较重，并适当配合膝关节屈伸运动，以防止关节内粘连。

外侧副韧带损伤临床少见，其临床表现及推拿治疗方法与内

of the injury of the medial collateral ligament, and the manipulations to be used are just the same.

Sprain of the Ankle Joint

When a person jumps, goes down stairs or takes an inform step on uneven ground, his weight will fall on his flexed metatarsus due to the imbalance of his or her body. At this moment, the ankle is in a unsteady state and if it is suddenly given a stress it will turn inwards or outwards excessively, which will produce excesive leading-pulling or partial laceration of lateral or medial ligament of the foot, leading to sprain of the ankle joint. Clinically, cases of strain of lateral ligament are common. It falls into the category of *"shang jin"* (injury of the tissues) in TCM.

CLINICAL MANIFESTATIONS

The patient has a history of acute strain and distinct swelling and pain in the ankle which can't touch the ground. There is tenderness in the front-lower part of the lateral and medial ankles and the skin of the ankle is dark. In the case of a strain of the lateral ankle, pain increases when the ankle turns inwards. In the case of strain of joint capsule and anterior fibula ligament, the swelling is primarily located in the lateral side of the joint and in the front-lower part of the lateral ankle. A serious strain of medial ankle may cause fracture of lateral ankle. Consequently there is swelling and pain in both of the lateral and medial ankles.

TREATMENT

Massage therapy is effective for pure strain of ligament or partial fiber-breaking-up. To treat a complicated fracture or dislocation, a timely orthopedic operation or manual reduction is needed.

1. Manipulation: Digital-pressing, pressing, pushing with one-finger meditation, kneading, pulling-extension, shaking, etc.

2. Location of Points: Ashi point, Zusanli (St 36), Yanglingquan (GB 34), Taixi (K 3), Kunlun (UB 60), Qiuxu

侧副韧带相似。

踝关节扭伤

在跳跃、下楼或地面不平踩空时，人体因重心失衡而踝关节跖屈着地。此时，处于不稳定状态的踝关节突然遭受使其过度内翻或外翻的应力，致使足外侧或内侧副韧带受到过度牵拉或部分撕裂，从而造成踝关节扭伤。临床以外侧副韧带扭伤为多见。本症属中医"伤筋"范畴。

【临床表现】

有急性扭伤病史，踝部出现明显的肿胀疼痛，不能着地，内、外踝前下方均有压痛，皮肤呈紫色。外踝扭伤者，踝关节内翻则外踝部疼痛加剧。外侧关节囊及腓前韧带损伤时，肿胀主要在关节外侧和外踝前下方。内踝扭伤严重者可伴有外踝骨折。因此，内、外踝均肿胀疼痛。

【治疗】

推拿对治疗单纯的韧带扭伤或韧带部分纤维断裂者疗效较好。合并骨折或脱位者，应尽早行骨科手术或配合手法复位。

1. 手法：点、按、一指禅推、揉、拔伸、摇等。

2. 取穴：阿是、足三里、阳陵泉、太溪、昆仑、丘墟、绝

(GB 40), Juegu (GB 39), Jiexi (St 41), and Taichong (Liv 3).

3. Operation

1) The patient being in prone position, the doctor digit-presses the points of Zusanli (St 36), Taixi (K 3), Kunlun (UB 60), Qiuxu (GB 40), Juegu (GB 39), Jiexi (St 41), Taichong (Liv 3) to dredge the channel and relieve the pain.

2) Then the doctor kneads the local part with thenar eminance for 3 to 5 minutes, then pushes near the leg and ankle with thumb from above to below in order to promote blood circulation, remove blood stasis, relieve swelling, and alleviate pain.

3) The patient is in supine position. The doctor, taking the right side for example, grasp the right great toe of the patient with the right hand, and tracts upwards. First turns outwards to enlarge the medial space of the ankle joint and at the same time presses into the space with the left fore-finger; then, still tracting, turns the foot inwards to enlarge the lateral space of the ankle joint and presses into the space of the joint with the thumb. Holding the ankle joint with the thumb and fore-finger, the right hand rocks the affected foot right and left under traction and turns it inwards once or twice. After that, while making the ankle part do dorsiflexion and plantar flexion, the doctor pushes the two ankles downwards and upwards: downwards for dorsiflexion and upwards for plantar flexion.

4) In the case of ankle strain accompanied by muscular spasm and joint adhesion, based on the manipulation mentioned above, the doctor, with one hand holding the Achilles tendon, the other holding the great toe, asks the patient to relax the ankle. First, the pulling-stressing and plantar flexion are applied, followed by sudden flexions of the back, and then by turning the dorsum of the foot outwards and inwards to release the muscular spasm. Finally the doctor gives local manipulation of soft-rubbing, kneading and flat pushing till a sensation of heat runs deep.

In the acute stage of strain (within 24—48 hours), the

骨、解溪、太冲等。

3. 操作

1）患者仰卧，医者用点按法点按足三里、太溪、昆仑、丘墟、绝骨、解溪、太冲等穴，以疏通经络，缓解疼痛。

2）再以鱼际揉法揉局部3～5分钟，继以拇指推法由上而下在小腿及踝关节周围施术，以活血祛瘀，消肿止痛。

3）患者仰卧，医者以右手（以右侧为例）紧握患者右踇趾，并向上牵引，先外翻以扩大踝关节内侧间隙，同时以左手食指压入间隙内，然后仍在牵引下内翻足部，扩大踝关节外侧间隙，以拇指压入关节间隙内。使拇、食指夹持踝关节，右手在牵引下将患足左右轻轻摇摆，内翻1～2次，然后背屈、跖屈，同时夹持踝关节的食、拇趾下推上提两踝，背屈时下推，跖屈时上提。

4）对伴有肌肉痉挛、关节粘连的患者，在上述手法的基础上，医者可以一手握跟腱，一手握住踇趾，并嘱患者放松踝部，先行拔伸、跖屈，然后做突然的背屈动作（手法需适宜，不要用力太猛），最后外翻或内翻足背以解除肌肉痉挛。再于局部行轻摩法、揉法及平推法，以热深透为度。

在损伤的急性期（24～48小时内），手法要轻柔，以远端取穴

manipulation should be light and soft. The distal points should be selected to avoid bleeding of the ruptured vessel. In the stage of recovery, a manipulation with a corresponding strength is needed. In case of organization of hematoma, formative adhesion and malfunction of the ankle joint, the adhesion should be stripped with a manipulation of more strength to restore the function of the joint. The manipulation of tracting-rocking, shaking and flexing-extending are frequently used for ankle joint in passive activities.

4. Course of Treatment: Once a day, five times for one course, with an interval of 2 or 3 days between two courses.

Facial Paralysis

Facial paralysis is mostly caused by acute non-suppurative inflammation of the facial nerve in the stylomastoid foramen. Attack of wind-cold on the face is a frequent inducing factor. It may also be resulted by a complication of otitis media, mastoiditis and parotitis. Most of the patients are in their adolescence and adulthood. It is called "*kou yan wai xie*" or "*diaoxianfeng*" (deviation of the eye and mouth) in TCM.

CLINICAL MANIFESTATIONS

In the incipient stage, there is retroauricular or subaural pain which will disappear in a few days. Mostly, when the patient gets up in the morning, there is deviation of the eye and mouth, salivation of labial angle, widening of palpebral fissure, disappearance of nasolabial sulcus, and ptosis of labial angle to the healthy side. And the patient can't have the activities of forehead-wrinkling, brow-knitting, cheek-blowing, eyes-shutting, and whistle-blowing.

TREATMENT

There will be gradual recovery in 1 or 2 weeks after its onset. Manipulation of massage may help the recovery of facial nerves and muscular function and reduce sequelae. During

治疗为主，以免加重损伤处血管破裂出血；恢复期手法宜相应加重，对血肿机化、形成粘连、踝关节功能受损的患者，应以较重手法剥离粘连，以恢复关节功能，牵引摇摆、摇晃、屈伸等法是常用的被动活动踝关节的手法。

4. 疗程：每日1次，5次为1疗程。各疗程之间间隔2～3天。

面神经麻痹

本病多因茎乳孔内的面神经发生急性非化脓性炎症所致；局部受风寒，常为诱因。亦可并发于中耳炎、乳突炎及腮腺炎。患者多为青壮年。中医称之为"口眼歪斜"、"吊线风"等。

【临床表现】

初发时，耳后或耳下疼痛，数日即消失。多于晨起时发现口眼歪斜，口角流涎，眼裂扩大，鼻唇沟消失，口角下垂，牵向健侧。患者不能做皱额、皱眉、鼓腮、闭眼、吹哨等动作。

【治疗】

本病于发病1～2周后开始逐渐恢复，推拿手法可促进神经、

the treatment, stimulus of cold to the face and head should be avoided and the patient should knead the face frequently for enhancing the effectiveness.

1. Manipulation: Pushing with one-finger meditation, digital-pressing, pressing, grasping and kneading.

2. Location of Points: Hegu (LI 4), Quchi (LI 11), Xiaguan (St 7), Jiache (St 6), Yifeng (SJ 17), Taiyang (Extra 2), Jingming (UB 1), Sibai (St 2), Yingxiang (LI 20), Renzhong (Du 26) and Dicang (St 4).

3. Operation

1) The doctor stands in front and to the side of the sitting patient and holds the postero-lateral part of the head with one hand. Using one-finger meditation pushing or thumb-pressing-kneading, the doctor pushes with the other hand repeatedly from the Yintang (Extra 1) along the superciliary of the affected side to the Taiyang (Extra 2) for 2 or 3 times first; then pushes repeatedly from Yintang (Extra 1) upwards by way of Shenting (Du 24) to Baihui (Du 20) also for 2 or 3 times; finally, pushes repeatedly from the middle of the forehead via Yangbai (GB 14) of the affected part to Taiyang (Extra 2) for 2 or 3 times.

2) After that, in the above-mentioned way, the doctor pushes downwards repeatedly from Yintang (Extra 1) by way of Jingming (UB 1) of the affected side, along the side of the nose up to Yingxiang (LI 20) for 2 or 3 times. Then the doctor pushes from Yingxiang (LI 20), along the point of Sibai (St 2), Quanliao (SI 18), Xiaguan (St 7) and Jiache (St 6) passing the face, to the Dicang (St 4) at the labial angle.

3) Still in the same way mentioned above, the operator pushes from Dicang (St 4) to Renzhong (Du 26) circling the lips, by way of Chengjiang (Ren 24), and returns to the starting-point. Then the operator pushes along the mandible to Jiache (St 6). Finally he rubs and scrubs softly the affected side of the face with the palm till local warmth and heat are produced.

肌肉恢复功能，减少后遗症。治疗期间宜避免头面部受寒冷刺激，患者可多按揉面部，以提高疗效。

1. 手法：一指禅推、点、按、拿、揉等。

2. 取穴：合谷、曲池、下关、颊车、翳风、太阳、睛明、四白、迎香、人中、地仓等。

3. 操作

1）患者坐位，医者站于其侧前方。医者以一手扶住其头部之侧后方；另一手用一指禅推法或拇指按揉法，先自印堂穴沿患侧眉弓推向太阳穴，反复2～3遍；再自印堂向上，经神庭穴推至百会穴，反复2～3遍；再返回额中，并自额中推向患侧阳白直至太阳穴，反复2～3遍。

2）再用上法自印堂向下推，经患侧睛明穴，并沿鼻旁至迎香，反复2～3遍，继之，自迎香穴沿四白、颧髎、下关、颊车一线，并经过面部直推至口角旁之地仓穴。

3）仍用上法，自地仓穴至人中，环绕口唇一周经承浆穴返回，再沿下颌大迎穴推至颊车穴。再用手掌轻轻摩擦患侧面部，以局部产生温热为度。

In the above-mentioned operations, the movement of the hand should pass at every point with a bit more strength exerted and some heavy stimulating manipulations such as digit-pressing used in combination.

4) The doctor stands to the side of the patient and, with one hand holding his forehead, grasps the Fengchi (GB 20) and the tendons of the back nape up and down repeatedly for 3—5 times, finally pushes the Qiaogong point for 30 times.

5) The doctor, standing behind the patient, grasps Jianjing (GB 21) with two hands and in a orderly way presses and kneads Quchi (LI 11) and Hegu (LI 4).

4. Course of Treatment: Once a day, six days for one course with an interval of 3 days between two courses.

Neurosism

Neurosism is mainly caused by imbalance between excitation and inhibition of the cerebral cortex which result from excessive strain of mental activity. Its main clinical characteristics are excitability and fatigability, often accompanied with different kinds of malaise and somnipathy. In TCM it belongs to the categories of *"shi mian"* (insomnia), *"duo meng"* (dreamful sleep), *"xuan yun"* (dizziness), *"yang wei"* (impotence), *"yijing"* (spermatorrhea), etc.

CLINICAL MANIFESTATIONS

This disease has complicated symptoms, which are usually divided into the following five types:

1) Deficiency of the Liver-*yin* and Kidney-*yin*: Fullness and dizziness in the head, tinnitus, amnesia, irritability and excitability, lumbago, dry throat and mouth, red tongue with thin and yellow fur, wiry and rapid pulse.

2) Insufficiency of both the Spleen and Kidney: Pale face, listlessness, pain in waist and debility of legs, anorexia, light-coloured urine, chilliness and cold limbs, insomnia and unsound slumber, impotence, premature ejaculation,

以上操作，凡经穴位处稍驻，且用力稍加重，并配合按点等重刺激手法。

4）医者站于患者侧方，一手扶住其前额，另一手拿风池及项后大筋，上下反复3～5遍；再推桥弓穴30次。

5）医者站于患者后方，用双手拿肩井，再依次按揉曲池、合谷等穴。

4. 疗程：每日1次，6次为1疗程。各疗程之间间隔3天。

神经衰弱

神经衰弱多由患者精神活动长期过度紧张，引起大脑皮层兴奋与抑制失调所致。其主要临床特点是易于兴奋和迅速疲劳，常有各种躯体不适感和睡眠障碍。本病属中医"失眠"、"多梦"、"眩晕"、"阳痿"、"遗精"等范畴。

【临床表现】

本病症状繁杂，中医常归纳为以下几个类型。

1）肝肾阴虚型　头胀头晕，耳鸣，健忘，烦躁易怒，腰酸背痛，咽干口燥。舌质红，苔薄黄，脉弦数。

2）脾肾阳虚型　面色㿠白，精神萎靡，腰痛腿软，饮食减少，小便清长，形寒肢冷，少寐易醒，阳痿，早泄，遗精。舌质淡，

spermatorrhea, pale tongue, and deep, thready and feeble pulse, etc.

3) Breakdown of the Normal Physiological Coordination between the Heart and Kidney: Palpitation and dysphoria, insomnia and amnesia, spermatorrhea, tinnitus, lassitude in loins and legs, dry mouth, dysphoria with feverish sensation in the chest, palms and soles, red tongue tip and thready rapid pulse.

4) Deficiency of Qi and Blood in the Heart and Spleen: Excessive dreaming and unsound slumber, palpitation and amnesia, fatigue and weakness, poor appetite, pale complexion, pale tongue with whitish coating and thready weak pulse.

5) Stagnation of the Liver-qi: Mental depression, stuffiness in the chest, hypochondriac pain, abdominal distention and eructation, poor appetite, vomiting, nausea, abdominal distention and pain, sensation of impediment in the pharynx, white fur and taut pulse.

TREATMENT

Massotherapy for this disease proves effective. During treatment, the patient should have a good rest and be free from worries and cares.

1. Manipulation: Pushing with one-finger meditation, kneading, flat-pushing, wiping, sweeping, grasping and rubbing.

2. Location of Points: Yintang (Extra 1), Shenting (Du 24), Jingming (UB 1), Zanzhu (UB 2), Taiyang (Extra 2), Jiaosun (SJ 20), Fengchi (GB 20), Jianjing (GB 21), Zhongwan (Ren 12), Qihai (Ren 6), Guanyuan (Ren 4) and the Stream Points on the back.

3. Operation

1) The patient is in a sitting position. The doctor stands posterolateral to the patient, holding the patient's forehead with the palmar sides of the thumb, fore finger and middle finger of one hand, with the thumb and the two fingers grasping Fengchi (GB 20) and the tendon of back nape from above to

脉沉细无力。

3）心肾不交型　心悸心烦，失眠健忘，遗精，耳鸣，腰酸膝软，口干，五心烦热。舌尖红，脉细数。

4）心脾两虚型　多梦易醒，心悸健忘，神疲乏力，饮食无味，面色少华。舌质淡，苔白，脉细弱。

5）肝气郁结型　精神抑郁，胸闷胁痛，腹胀嗳气，不思饮食，或呕恶，腹胀痛，喉中如梗。舌苔白，脉弦。

【治疗】

推拿对治疗本病疗效较好。治疗期间病人应适当休息，尽量保持心情舒畅。

1．手法：一指禅推、揉、平推、抹、扫散、拿、摩等。

2．取穴：印堂、神庭、睛明、攒竹、太阳、角孙、风池、肩井、中脘、气海、关元、背部俞穴等。

3．操作

1）患者坐位，医者站其后外侧，以一手拇、食、中三指指腹扶持其前额，另一手用三指拿风池及项后大筋，自上而下往返10余

below for a dozen time, and pushing the left and right Qiaogong for 20—30 times respectively.

2) The doctor, standing in front of the sitting patient, separately wipes the forehead and digital presses Jingming (UB 1), separately wipes the Yingxiang (LI 20), Renzhong (Du 26) and Chengjiang (Ren 24) for 3—5 times [respectively, which is to be repeated 3 times, and then, with the tips of the thumb and fingers, from Shuaigu (GB 8) to Naokong (GB 19), sweep-dispers the temple for 20—30 times, and joins from the temporo-occipital to the neck; after that, grasps with the palmar sides of the fingers along Shaoyang, Taiyang and Du channels in succession for 3—5 times.

3) The doctor stands on one side behind the patient and flat-pushes the chest and back, the hypochondriac region, the upper abdomen and the lumbosacral portion for 30—50 times.

4) The doctor lifts and grasps two Jianjing (GB 21) points, upper arms and forearm for 3—5 times; flat-pushes upper arms and forearms for 5—10 times; restores the thumbs and four fingers and splits the cracks between fingers for one time respectively; sets the shoulders back and forth for 3 circuits respectively; foulaging arms to-and-fro for 3 times; shakes the shoulders and arms 3—5 times; pinch-grasps Hegu (LI 4) till there is a sensation of aching and distention.

5) Repeat Operation 2.

6) The doctor vibrates fontanel with the center of the palm; and Dazhui (Du 14) and the Baliao points (UB 31—34) with fist back for 3 times respectively.

4. Modification of Manipulation according to Different Sydromes

1) Type of Deficiency of the Liver-*yin* and Kidney-*yin*: In addition, knead Ganshu (UB 18), Shenshu (UB 23) and Sanyinjiao (Sp 6).

2) Type of Insufficiency of both the Spleen and Kidney: In addition, knead Xinshu (UB 15), Shenshu (UB 23) and

次，推左、右桥弓穴，每侧各20～30次。

2）患者坐位，医者站其前面，分抹前额，点睛明，分抹眉弓、迎香、人中、承浆各3～5次，反复3遍。以五指端自率谷向脑空扫散颞部20～30次，合颞枕至项部，然后以五指指腹沿少阳、太阳、督脉自前向后拿3～5遍。

3）医者站于患者身后一侧，平推胸背，两胁肋、上腹部、腰骶部各30～50次。

4）推拿两肩井穴、上臂、前臂3～5次，平推上臂、前臂5～10次，理五指、劈指缝各1次；运膀子前后各3周；搓手臂，往返3次，抖肩臂3～5下；捏拿合谷以明显酸胀为度。

5）重复第2）项操作。

6）以掌心震囟门，拳背震大椎、八髎各3下。

4．随证加减

1）肝肾阴虚型　加揉肝俞、肾俞、三阴交。

2）脾肾阳虚型　加揉心俞、肾俞、命门。

Mingmen (Du 4).

3) Type of Breakdown of Normal Physiological Coordination between the Heart and the Kidney: In addition, knead Xinshu (UB 15) and Shenshu (UB 23), and scrub Yongquan (K 1).

4) Type of Deficiency of *Qi* and Blood in the Heart and Spleen: In addition, knead Xinshu (UB 15), Pishu (UB 20), Weishu (UB 21), Zhongwan (Ren 12) and Zusanli (St 36).

5) Type of Stagnation of the Liver-*qi*: In addition, knead Ganshu (UB 18), Danshu (UB 19), Qimen (Liv 14) and Yanglingquan (GB 34).

5. Course of Treatment: Once a day, 10 times as one course with an interval of 5—7 days between two courses.

Gastric and Duodenal Ulcer

These are chronic ulcer occuring in the stomach and duodenum. They are also called peptic ulcer because of the participation of digestive function of gastric acid and pepsase in the formation of ulcer. Clinically, the characteristics are chronic and periodic attack and a rhythmic pain in the upper abdomen. In TCM it belongs to the categories of "*weiwan tong*" (stomachache) and "*xinkou tong*" (epigastric pain).

CLINICAL MANIFESTATION

The special symptoms of both gastric ulcer and duodenal ulcer are that the pains are located in the upper abdomen. But the pains are different in nature, which may include vague pain, dull pain, distending pain, suffocating pain, burning pain, hunger pain or even stabbing pain and gripping pain, etc. These pains are rhythmic: in the case of gastric ulcer, the pain appears about half an hour after food-entry, lasting about 1 to 2 hours, and remits gradually; in the case of duodenal ulcer, the pain mostly appears before food-entry, taking the form of hunger pain, and remits after food-entry. As for the location of pains, the pain of gastric ulcer is located in the cen-

3）心肾不交型　加揉心俞、肾俞，擦涌泉。

4）心脾两虚型　加揉心俞、脾俞、胃俞、中脘、足三里。

5）肝气郁结型　加揉肝俞、胆俞、期门、阳陵泉。

5．疗程：每日1次，10次为1疗程。各疗程之间间隔5～7

天。

胃及十二指肠溃疡

本病是指发生在胃和十二指肠的慢性溃疡，因溃疡的形成均

有胃酸和胃蛋白酶的消化作用参与，故又称消化性溃疡。临床上

以慢性周期性发作并有节律的上腹部疼痛为特点，属中医"胃脘

痛"、"心口痛"等范畴。

【临床表现】

胃与十二指肠溃疡均以上腹部疼痛为突出症状，但痛的性质

不一，有隐痛、钝痛、胀闷而痛、灼热样痛、饥饿样痛，甚则刺

痛、绞痛难忍等。疼痛有节律性，胃溃疡多在进食后半小时左右

发生疼痛，持续1～2小时后逐渐缓解；十二指肠溃疡多在饭前疼

痛，呈空腹痛或饥饿样疼痛，进食后疼痛缓解。疼痛的部位，胃

ter of the upper abdomen or slightly to the left; the pain of the duodenal ulcer, slightly to the right. In addition, there are eructation, acid regurgitation, etc. An X-ray barium meal examination of gastro-intestinal tract and gastroscopy are helpful to confirming diagnosis.

TREATMENT

Massotherapy has a curative effect on treating gastric and duodenal ulcer, especially a peculiar effect on an incipient mild ulcer, and a distinct analgesic effect. Massage should be avoided in the bleeding period of ulcer and in the case of perforation. During of treatment, a good rest is needed and the diet is to be observed. Excessive hunger and full meal are forbidden.

1. Manipulation: Pushing with one-finger meditation, rubbing, pressing, kneading, vibrating, pulling-obliquely, etc.

2. Location of Points: Shangwan (Ren 13), Zhongwan (Ren 12), Qihai (Ren 6), Pishu (UB 20), Weishu (UB 21), Yanglingquan (GB 34) and Zusanli (St 36).

3. Operation

1) The patient is in lying position with the limbs stretched and the whole body relaxed. The doctor, standing to the right of the patient and with the soft and light pushing with one-finger meditation, pushes to and fro from Zhongwan (Ren 12) upwards to Shangwan (Ren 13) and to below xiphoid process for 5—10 minutes.

2) The patient lies, the doctor rubs with his palm, centering on Zhongwan (Ren 12), clockwise and counterclockwise for 200—300 times respectively; then vibrates the upper abdomen with his palm for 3—5 minutes.

3) Press and knead Zusanli (St 36) for 3—5 minutes.

4) Push or press-knead for 2 to 3 minutes respectively with onefinger-meditation-pushing inhaled over Pishu (UB 20), Weishu (UB 21) or Ashi points on the back of the patient who is in supine position.

溃疡多在上腹正中或稍偏左;十二指肠溃疡多在上腹偏右。另外,还常兼有嗳气、吞酸等症。X线胃肠道钡餐透视或胃镜检查可帮助确诊。

【治疗】

推拿对治疗胃、十二指肠溃疡有较好的疗效,尤其对早期溃疡较轻者疗效显著,并有明显的止痛效果。溃疡病出血期或出现穿孔者不宜推拿治疗。治疗期间应适当休息,并注意饮食,勿过饥过饱。

1. 手法:一指禅推、摩、按、揉、振、斜扳等。

2. 取穴:上脘、中脘、气海、脾俞、胃俞、阳陵泉、足三里等。

3. 操作

1)患者卧位,四肢伸开,全身放松。医者坐其右侧,以轻柔的一指禅推法自中脘穴向上脘穴推至剑突下,往返推5～10分钟。

2)体位姿势同上,医者用掌摩法以中脘为中心按顺、逆时针各摩200～300次。然后以掌振法振上腹部3～5分钟。

3)按揉右足三里穴3～5分钟。

4)患者俯卧位,以一指推法吸定于脾俞、胃俞或背部阿是穴,各推动或按揉2～3分钟。

4. Modification of Manipulation according to Different Syndromes

1) In the case of abdominal pain and turgor involving the costal regions, accompanied by eructation and acid regurgitation, which is the hyperactive liver-*qi* attacking the stomach, press-knead additional points of Ganshu (UB 18), Danshu (UB 19), Qimen (Liv 14) and Yanglingquan (GB 34).

2) In the case of upper abdominal pain which can be relieved by pressing, spitting clear water, joy for warmth and aversion to cold and lassitude, This is called insufficiency of the spleen-*yang*, press and knead Zhangmen (Liv 13), Neiguan (P 6) and Dachangshu (UB 25) in addition.

3) In the case of an acute attack of stomachache, first press-knead and digital press with much force to constantly stimulate for 2—5 minutes Ashi point on the back, Pishu (UB 20) and Weishu (UB 21); when the pain is distinctly relaxed, other treatment is to be taken.

5. Course of Treatment: once a day, 15 times as one course; at an interval of 5—7 days between two courses.

Chronic Gastritis

Chronic gastritis is a chronic gastropathy, with nonspecific inflamation of gastric muscosa as the main pathological change. The main clinical feature is long-standing repeated attacks of upper abdominal pain or distending and oppressing sensation. It falls into the category of "*weitong*" (stomachache) or "*pizheng*" (distention or fullness in the abdomen) in TCM.

CLINICAL MANIFESTATIONS

This disease develops slowly and has repeated attacks. Superficial gastritis is manifested as an uncomfortable [sensation in upper abdomen after meal, sensation of fullness and opression, self-sensed comfort after eructation, and sometimes nausea, vomitus and transient stomachache; astrophic gastri-

4. 随证加减

1）上腹部疼痛伴胀满，连及两胁，兼见嗳气、吞酸者，证属肝气犯胃，宜加按揉肝俞、胆俞、期门、阳陵泉穴。

2）上腹部隐痛，泛吐清水，喜暖恶凉，按之痛缓，神疲乏力者，证属脾胃虚寒，宜加按揉章门、内关、大肠俞。

3）胃痛急性发作者，宜先在其背部阿是穴及脾俞、胃俞处，用较重的按揉法与点法连续刺激 2～5 分钟左右，待疼痛明显缓解后，再行其他治疗。

5. 疗程：每日 1 次，15 次为 1 疗程。各疗程之间间隔 5～7 天。

慢 性 胃 炎

慢性胃炎是以胃粘膜非特异性炎症为主要病理变化的慢性胃病。其临床特点是长期反复发作的上腹疼痛或胀闷感。本病属中医"胃痛"、"痞症"等范畴。

【临床表现】

本病发展缓慢，常反复发作。浅表性胃炎多表现为饭后上腹部感觉不适，有饱闷及压迫感，嗳气后自觉舒服，有时还有恶心、呕吐及一时性胃痛；萎缩性胃炎则主要表现为食欲不振，饭后饱

tis is mainly manifested by poor appetite, fullness and distention after meal, dull pain in upper abdomen and the general symptoms of weakness such as anemia, emaciation, tiredness, and diarrhea; hypertrophic gastritis has pantothenate symptoms. Gastroscopy is helpful to confirming the diagnosis.

TREATMENT

This disease needs a long course of treatment with a massage therapy. It should be distinguished from gastritic cancer, gastritic ulcer and duodenal ulcer. In the course of treatment, the patient should avoid taking gastric mucosa-stimulating medicines, cultivate a good habit of diet and a good way of life, and avoid eating excess-cold and pungent food.

1. Manipulation: Pushing with one-finger meditation, rubbing, pressing kneading, obliquely-pulling, etc.

2. Location of Points: Zhongwan (Ren 12), Qihai (Ren 6), Neiguan (P 6), Pishu (UB 20), Weishu (UB 21), Ganshu (UB 18), Zusanli (St 36), etc.

3. Operation

1) The patient is in supine position with upper limbs naturally put at two sides of the body respectively and the hip and knee slightly flexed. The doctor rubs with palm the upper abdomen (a little bit to the left) clockwise for 300—500 times. Talc powder may be used as a medium and the manipulation should be light, soft and continuous.

2) The posture is the same as the mentioned above. The doctor pushes with one finger from Zhongwan (Ren 12) upwards to Shangwan (Ren 13). The pushing should be slow and last for 3—5 minutes.

3) With the middle finger, the doctor vibrates Zhongwan (Ren 12) for 3—5 minutes.

4) The doctor press-kneads Qihai (Ren 6) with the thumb or the middle finger for 2—3 minutes.

5) The patient is in supine position, with lower limbs stretched straight, relaxes the whole body and the doctor press-kneads

胀，上腹部钝痛以及贫血、消瘦、疲倦和腹泻等全身虚弱症状，肥厚性胃炎，有泛酸症状。胃镜检查能帮助确诊。

【治疗】

推拿治疗本病，疗程较长。本病应注意与胃癌、胃十二指肠溃疡等病相鉴别。治疗期间，患者应避免服用对胃粘膜有刺激的药物，养成良好的饮食及生活习惯，避免食用过热、过冷及辛辣之品。

1．手法：一指禅推、摩、按、揉、斜扳等。

2．取穴：中脘、气海、内关、脾俞、胃俞、肝俞、足三里等。

3．操作

1）患者仰卧，两上肢自然放于体侧，微屈髋膝，以掌摩法在上腹部稍偏左，顺时针摩动300～500次，可用滑石粉为介质，手法宜轻柔不滞。

2）体位姿势同上，以一指推法自中脘穴向上脘穴推动，推动时移动宜缓慢，推3～5分钟。

3）以中指振法振中脘穴3～5分钟。

4）以拇指或中指按揉气海穴2～3分钟。

5）患者仰卧位，两下肢伸直，全身放松，以拇指按揉足三里

Zusanli (St 36) with the thumb for 3—5 minutes.

6) The patient is in prone position, the waist and back revealed and coated with Chinese holly leaf. The doctor, standing to his right, scrubs the lateral parts of the spine and waist with right palm or minor thenar eminance focusing on Pishu (UB 20) and Weishu (UB 21), till the heat produced penetrates the abdomen and then with empty palm lightly pats the lower chest and upper waist for 5—10 minutes.

7) The operator stands behind the sitting patient, grasps Jianjing (GB 21) with two hands, press-kneads Shousanli (LI 10), Neiguan (P 6) and Hegu (LI 4) of the upper limbs in an orderly way, 30—50 times for each point; then foulages and shakes upper limbs; finally foulage-rubs costal regions from above to below for 3—5 times.

4. Modification of Manipulation according to Different Syndromes

1) In the case of a dull pain in gastric cavity, joy for hot and pressing, anorexia, gastric distension and fullness after meal, sallow complexion and weakness, which is called dificiency of qi of the spleen and stomach, also press-knead Pishu (UB 20), Weishu (UB 21), Zhangmen (Liv 13) and Neiguan (P 6).

2) In the case of distending pain, fullness and discomfort in the stomach especially after meals, wandering pain radiating to hypochondria and aggravated by emotional upset, frequent eructation, relieved when there is wind from bowels, acid regurgitation and vomitus, which is called stagnation of qi of liver and stomach, also press-knead Qimen (Liv 14), Ganshu (UB 18), Yanglingquan (GB 34) and Taichong (Liv 3).

3) In the case of burning pain in the gastric cavity which occurs now and then, exacerbation in the afternoon or in hunger, remission on food-entry, dry mouth with bitter taste, vexation and irritability, and poor appetite, which is called stomach-heat and *yin*-difficiency, also press-knead Yanglingquan (GB 34), Neiguan (P 6) Weishu (UB 21) in addition.

穴3～5分钟。

6）患者俯卧位，暴露腰背部，医者站于患者右侧，在腰背部涂以冬青膏，以右手掌或小鱼际擦腰背脊柱两侧，重点在脾俞、胃俞部，以热渗透至腹部为宜。再以空掌轻轻拍击下胸、上腰部5～10下。

7）患者坐位，医者站其身后，用双手拿肩井，并依次按揉两上肢手三里、内关、合谷穴，每穴30～50次，搓抖上肢，最后搓摩胁肋，自上而下3～5遍。

4. 随证加减

1）胃脘部隐隐作痛，喜热喜按，纳呆，饭后胃部胀满，面黄乏力，证属脾胃气虚，宜加按揉脾俞、胃俞、章门、内关等穴。

2）胃脘胀痛，饱闷不适，食后尤甚，痛无定处，攻撑连胁，遇情志不遂则重，嗳气频作，得矢气则舒，或吞酸、呕恶，证属肝胃气滞，宜加按揉期门、肝俞、阳陵泉、太冲等穴。

3）胃脘呈烧灼样疼痛，痛不定时，下午或空腹较重，得食稍缓，口干苦，心烦易怒，纳食量少，证属胃热阴虚，宜加按揉阴陵泉、内关、胃俞等穴。

5. Course of Treatment: Once a day, 15 times as one course; with an interval of 5—7 days between two courses.

Gastroptosis

Gastroptosis means that the stomach position is abnormal because of a ptosis. The degree of ptosis varies and gastroptosis is sometimes accompanied by ptoses of other internal organs, mostly seen in leptosomatic and asthemic types. TCM calls this disease *"zhongqi xiaxian"* (sinking of qi of middle-jiao).

CLINICAL MANIFESTATIONS

This disease is mainly manifested as emaciation, listlessness, poor appetite, tasteless eating, distension and discomfort in gastric cavity especially after food-entry in left abdomen, tenesmic sensation, intestinal gurgling sound, splashing sounds in the stomach, joy for holding-up and pressing of lower abdomen, or frequent vomitus and eructation, and remission in supine position. An x-ray barium meal examination of gastrointestinal tract is helpful to confirming the diagnosis.

TREATMENT

Massage therapy has a curative effect on gastroptosis, especially mild gastroptosis; support of stomach should be added in the treatment of a serious gastroptosis.

1. Manipulation: Pushing with one-finger meditation, rubbing, holding-up, grasping, and pressing-kneading.

2. Location of Points: Qihai (Ren 6), Guanyuan (Ren 4), Pishu (UB 20), Weishu (UB 21), Zusanli (St 36) and Jianjing (GB 21).

3. Operation

1) The patient is in supine position, with upper limbs naturally put on two sides of the body respectively and lower limbs stretched straight. The doctor pushes with one-finger meditation from Guanyuan (Ren 4) to xiphoid process for 3 to 5 minutes. The movement shonld be slow.

5．疗程：每日1次，15次为1疗程。各疗程之间间隔5～7天。

胃 下 垂

胃下垂是指胃的位置异常，发生下垂。下垂的程度差别较大，且往往合并有其他内脏下垂，多见于瘦长无力型者。本症属中医"中气下陷"范畴。

【临床表现】

患者多表现为消瘦，乏力，胃纳减少，食而无味，胃脘胀闷不舒，食后更甚，尤以左小腹为甚，似有物下坠，肠鸣作响，胃内有振水音，下腹部喜托按，常有呕吐、嗳气，但平卧后减轻。X线胃肠钡餐检查可帮助确诊。

【治疗】

推拿治疗胃下垂，对下垂较轻者疗效较好。下垂严重者治疗时宜加用胃托。

1．手法：一指禅推、摩、托、拿、按揉等。

2．取穴：气海、关元、脾俞、胃俞、足三里、肩井等。

3．操作

1）患者仰卧，上肢自然放于体侧，下肢伸直，医者以一指禅推法，自关元穴向剑突穴推动，移动应缓慢，推3～5分钟。

2) The positioning is the same as mentioned above. The doctor holds up and rubs clockwise with the manipulation of palm-rubbing from lower waist to upper abdomen for 300—500 times; then with palm lateral lightly strikes the straight muscles of the abdominal region, with such a force that there is a reaction of abdominal muscular contraction. The frequency of hitting which lasts 2—3 minutes should be slow, 20—30 times per minute.

3) The doctor press-kneads Zusanli (St 36) with the thumb for 3 to 5 minutes.

4) With one hand holding the patient's ankle, the doctor holds up the knee with another hand and makes the patient have unilateral genuflexion and hip-flexion; expiration for genuflexion and inspiration for hip-flexion; 20—30 times each side.

5) The patient, in a sitting position, puts the bent left arm and elbow on the lumbosacral portion. The doctor, with four right fingers combined and the palm upward, enters fingertips into the Geguan (UB 46) and Yixi (UB 45) on the inferior border inside the scapula, and from the oblique-above part enters the gap between scapula and chest wall about 2—3 cun deep; meanwhile, the left hand, proping the shoulder front, pushes and kneads backwards with force, the two hands exerting forces in opposite directions and in a closing-approaching way. In 1 or 2 minutes this way, the patient will have a sensation of stomach-lifting, then slowly the doctor withdraws his right hand. The operation should be repeated 3 to 5 times.

6) The patient, sitting on a chair, faces and holdes the chair back and discloses the waist and back region. The doctor coats the two laterals of the spine with Chinese holly leaf ointment, and scrubs from the minor thenar eminence till there is penetrating heat.

7) The doctor lifts and grasps Jianjing (GB 21) with two hands for 3—5 times; then press-kneads Shousanli (LI 10), Neiguan (P 6) and Hegu (LI 4); finally foulage-rubs

2）体位姿势同上，医者以掌摩法自下腹部向上腹部逆时针托摩 300～500 次。然后以侧掌轻轻捶击两侧腹直肌，用力以引起腹部肌肉收缩反应为度。频率宜缓慢，20～30 次/分，捶 2～3 分钟。

3）医者以拇指按揉足三里穴 3～5 分钟。

4）医者一手握住踝部，一手托住膝部做单侧屈膝屈髋活动，屈髋时呼气，伸髋时吸气。一侧做 20～30 次。

5）患者取坐势，将左臂和肘弯曲放于腰骶部。医者以右手四指并拢，掌心向上，指尖由肩胛骨内下缘之膈关、谚谚穴处插入，向斜上方直入肩胛——胸壁间隙约 2～3 寸左右；同时左手抵在其肩前方用力向后方推按，两手相对用力呈合拢之势，这样 1～2 分钟后，患者即有胃上提之感，随之慢慢将右手退出，如此反复 3～5 次。

6）患者坐位，前扶椅背，暴露腰背皮肤，在脊柱两侧涂以冬青膏，以小鱼际行擦法，以热深透为度。

7）医者先以两手提拿肩井穴 3～5 下，然后按揉手三里、内

costal regions from above to below for 2 or 3 times.

4. Course of Treatment: Once a day, 15 times as one course; at an interval of 3—5 days between two courses.

In addition to massage therapy of this disease, a cooperation with the therapeutic exercise will be more effective. Steps are the following:

1) Genuflexion and buttocks raising: Take a supine position, with genuflexion, and the foot bottom treading the bed, and do buttocks raising. Just now only let the two shoulders and foot bottoms touch the bed. When the buttocks are raised, contracts the anus tightly for about 1 minute. Relax the contracted anus back to normal state and redo it after a short rest. This should be repeated for 4—9 times.

2) Sitting-up: Lie on the back, stretch lower limbs straight and keep them close to each other, with two hands grasping each other on occiput, heave by abdominal muscles and raise the body upwards slowly into sitting position, then lie down slowly returning to original position. This should be repeated 6—8 times.

3) Standing upside down on the shoulder and back: Lie on the back, raise the feet high next to the wall, with buttocks next to the wall as much as possible, hold up Yaoyan(Extra) with two hands, and assume the posture of standing upside down on the shoulder and back. At this moment, only the shoulder touches the bed and the foot bottoms touch the wall. Having finished this, make abdominal respiration for one minute. Redo it after a rest of lying-down. Repeat the above continuously for 4 or 5 times.

4) Adducting abdominal muscles and raising two legs: Lie on the back, stretch lower limbs straight and keep them close to each other, raise the lower limbs slowly at the same time by abdominal muscles, and keep the raising for a period of time. Slowly put them down to original position. Redo it after a short break. Repeat the above continuously for

关、合谷，最后搓摩胁肋，由上而下 2～3 次结束。

4．疗程：每日1次，15次为1疗程。各疗程之间间隔3～5天。

本病除推拿治疗外，适当配合医疗体操，收效更佳。步骤如下：

1）屈膝抬臀　仰卧、屈膝，足底踏着床面，做臀部抬起的动作。此时仅两肩及两足底着床。臀部抬起后，将肛门缩紧，并持续1分钟左右。放下还原，休息片刻再做。连续做4～9次。

2）仰卧起坐　仰卧，两下肢伸直靠紧，两手在枕部相握，以腹肌用劲，慢慢把身体上部抬起成坐位，然后再缓缓躺下还原。连续做6～8次。

3）肩背倒立　仰卧，两足贴墙高高翘起，臀部尽量靠近墙边，两手紧托腰眼，做肩背倒立姿势。此时，仅肩部着床，足底踏在墙上。倒立后，做腹式呼吸，持续1分钟左右。躺下休息片刻再做。连续做4～5次。

4）收腹双抬腿　仰卧，两下肢伸直靠紧。以腹肌用劲，慢慢把两下肢同时抬起，并尽可能地维持一段时间。慢慢放下还

4 to 6 times.

5) Rubbing–kneading–upholding abdomen with two palms: Lie on the back, with two palms overlapped and put tightly onto the lower abdomen; rub–knead the whole abdomen, by way of right lower abdomen, upwards, across upper abdomen and turn to the left. No force is needed in downward operating; upwards, hold up the abdomen while rubbing–kneading. A constant rubbing–kneading–upholding of 30—50 times is needed.

Gastrointestinal Neurosis

Gastrointestinal neurosis is a series of disturbances of gastrointestinal function caused by dysfunction of vegetative nervous system because of the disturbance of higher nervous activity. This disease is mainly manifested in adolescence and adulthood, in more females than males. It falls into the categories of *"ou tu"* (vomitus), *"bian mi"* (constipation) and *"xie xie"* (diarrhea) in TCM.

CLINICAL MANIFESTATIONS

1. Gastric Neurosis: Mainly marked by discomfort or distension and pain in upper abdomen, vomiting after meal, sour regurgitation, eructation and poor appetite. TCM divides it into two types:

1) Deficiency of the Spleen-*yang* and Stomach-*yang*: Fullness in gastric cavity, retching, frequent eructation, or vomiting with poor digestion, cool limbs, light–coloured urine, pale tongue with whitish and smooth coating, deep and slow pulse.

2) Dificiency of the Liver-*yin* and Stomach-*yin*: Vexation and retching, gastric discomfort with acid regurgitation, aversion to dryness and sweet odour, dry mouth and much thirst but drinking little, poor appetite, oppilation, deep-red tongue with little or uncoated coating, wiry, thready, rapid and feeble pulse.

2. Intestinal Neurosis: Mainly marked by abdominal distension and pain, diarrhea, constipation, etc. TCM divides

原。稍休息再做，连续做 4～6 次。

5）双掌摩、揉托腹部　仰卧，双掌重叠紧贴下腹部，循顺时针方向摩揉全腹，自下腹起，经右下腹向上，横过上腹部，转向左侧，向下时不用力，向上时边摩揉边上托，连续摩揉上托30～50次。

胃肠神经官能症

胃肠神经官能症是一种因高级神经活动障碍所致的植物神经系统功能失常，从而引起一系列胃、肠道功能紊乱症状。本病多见于青壮年，女多于男。属中医"呕吐"、"便秘"、"泄泻"等范畴。

【临床表现】

1．胃神经官能症：主要表现为上腹部不适感或胀痛，饭后呕吐，反酸，嗳气，食欲不振等。中医辨证可分为以下两型：

1）脾胃阳虚型：胸脘痞满，干呕，嗳气频作，或呕吐不消化食物，四肢发凉，小便清长。舌质淡，苔白滑，脉沉迟。

2）肝胃阴虚型：虚烦干呕，胃脘嘈杂，恶闻香燥，口干欲饮，但饮水不多，食欲不振，便秘。舌质红绛，苔少或无苔，脉弦细数无力。

2．肠神经官能症：主要表现为腹胀、腹痛、腹泻及便秘等。

it into two types:

1) Stagnation of *Qi*: Abdominal distension and wandering pain, sometimes diarrhea or constipation, mucous stool, no remission after diarrhea, reddish tongue with thin and whitish or smooth coating, wiry and uneven pulse.

2) Insufficiency of *Qi* and Body Fluid: Thinness and weakness, listlessness, dizziness and dry throat, short breath and sweating, low voice, oppilation or weakness after defecation, reddish tongue with denudation of central coating, thready, uneven or feeble pulse.

TREATMENT

Massage therapy has a fast and curative effect on gastrointestinal neurosis. But before treatment, tumours and gastrointesinal organic pathological change should be negated. In the course of treatment, a rationally-adjusted diet is needed. Avoid eating pungent, raw, cold and hard-to-digest food, have ease of mind, and coordinate with corresponding physical exercises to build up health.

1. Manipulation: Rubbing, pushing with one-finger meditation, scrubbing, pressing, kneading, obliquely-pulling or rotating.

2. Location of Points: Huatuojiaji (Extra), Weishu (UB 21), Pishu (UB 20), Dachangshu (UB 25), Zhongwan (Ren 12), Liangmen (St 21), Tianshu (St 25), Guanyuan (Ren 4) and Zusanli (St 36).

3. Operation

1) The patient is in a supine position, with the upper limbs naturally put on the two sides of the body respectively, and the lower limbs slightly flexing the knee and hip. The doctor, sitting to the right of the patient, rubs the abdomen with palm-rubbing manipulation clockwise and counterclockwise for 200—300 times respectively; focusing on upper abdomen in the case of gastric neurosis; focusing on lower abdomen in the case of intestinal neurosis.

2) The patient is in the same position as mentioned above.

中医辨证可分为以下两型：

1）气滞型：腹部胀痛，痛无定处，时有腹泻或便秘，大便带粘液，泻后痛不减。舌质淡红，苔薄白或滑，脉弦涩。

2）气津亏虚型：形瘦无力，精神萎靡，头晕咽干，气短汗出，声音低微，大便秘结或便后乏力。舌质淡红，苔多中间剥脱，脉细涩或虚软无力。

【治疗】

推拿治疗胃肠神经官能症，见效快，疗效好。但治疗前应排除肿瘤及胃肠器质性病变。治疗期间应合理调节饮食，避免食用辛辣、生冷及难消化食物，保持心情舒畅，并配合适当的体育锻炼，以增强体质。

1．手法：摩、一指禅推、擦、按、揉、斜扳或旋转等。

2．取穴：夹脊、胃俞、脾俞、大肠俞、中脘、梁门、天枢、关元、足三里等。

3．操作

1）患者仰卧，两上肢自然放于体侧，两下肢微屈膝髋。医者坐于患者右侧，以掌摩法摩腹部。胃神经官能症患者以摩上腹部为主，肠神经官能症患者以摩小腹部为主。顺、逆时针各摩200～300次。

2）体位姿势同上，以一指禅推法，推中脘、梁门、上脘、天

With the manipulation of one-finger pushing meditation, the doctor pushes Zhongwan (Ren 12), Liangmen (St 21), Shangwan (Ren 13), Tianshu (St 25), Qihai (Ren 6) and Guanyuan (Ren 4); the first two points for gastric neurosis, the last two for intestinal neurosis; 2 or 3 minutes for each point.

3) The patient is in a supine position and stretches the lower limbs, to have Zusanli (St 36) press-kneaded by the thumb for 2 or 3 minutes.

4) In a prone position, the patient discloses his waist and back, coats the two laterals of the spine with Chinese holly leaf ointment and rubs with minor thenar eminance and from the lower chest to sacrum till the heat becomes penetrating. The rubbing focuses on the part between the lower chest and waist in the case of gastric neurosis; waist and sacrum in the case of intestinal neurosis.

4. Modification of Manipulation according to Different Sydromes

1) Dificiency of the Spleen-*yang* and Stomach-*yang*: Separately push Tanzhong (Ren 17) and two costal arches for 30—50 times as well. Horizontally scrub the upper abdomen till there occurs penetrating hot.

2) Dificiency of the Liver-*yin* and Stomach-*yin*: Also press-knead Ganshu (UB 18), Pishu (UB 20), Weishu (UB 21), Neiguan (P 6) and Sanyinjiao (SP 6).

3) Stagnation of *Qi*: Additionally press-knead Yanglingquan (GB 34) and Taichong (Liv 3). Separately push Zhongwan (Ren 12).

4) Insufficiency of *Qi* and the Body Fluid: Also pinch the spine, knead and rub the region around the umbilicus, lightly lift and grasp abdominal muscles.

5. Course of Treatment: Once every two days, 3—5 times as one course.

Oppilation

Oppilation refers to constipation, prolongation of the

枢、气海、关元穴。胃神经官能症患者推前两穴，肠神经官能症患者推后两穴，每穴推 2～3 分钟。

3）患者仰卧，下肢伸开，以拇指按揉足三里穴 2～3 分钟。

4）患者俯卧，暴露腰背部，在脊柱两侧涂以冬青膏，以小鱼际部自下胸段至腰骶部擦，以热深透为度。胃神经官能症以擦下胸段下腰段为主，肠神经官能症以擦腰骶部为主。

4．随证加减

1）脾胃阳虚者，宜加分推膻中及两肋弓部 30～50 次。横擦上腹部以透热为度。

2）肝胃阴虚者，宜加按揉肝俞、脾俞、胃俞、内关、三阴交等穴。

3）气滞者，宜加按揉阳陵泉、太冲，分推中脘等。

4）气津亏虚者，宜加捏脊、揉摩脐周，轻轻提拿腹肌等。

5．疗程：隔日 1 次，3～5 次为 1 疗程。

便　　秘

便秘是指大便秘结不通，排便时间延长，或虽有便意，而排

period of defecation, or the fact one has the desire to defecate, but it is hard to defecate. Oppilation can be found in various diseases. It is mainly caused by the abnormal conduction of large instetine, and too long the retention period of feces within the instetine, and too much moisture absorbed that results in desiccative and solid feces.

CLINICAL MANIFESTATIONS

1) Type of Gastroinstetinal Tract Dryness–heat: Feces are dry and hard to defecate. Scybala can be touched in the abdomen. It is accompanied with foul smell in the mouth, dark urine, restlessness, dizziness, dryness of the throat, reddened tongue with yellow fur and forceful slippery pulse.

2) Type of Stagnation of *Qi*: Constipation, the desire to confecate but with difficulty, thus leading to general discomfort, hypochondriac pain or fullness of the abdomen, frequent eructation, thin and white fur, taut and uneven pulse.

3) Type of Deficiency of both *Qi* and Blood: Constipation, dizziness, dryness of the throat, palpitation, shortness of breath, listlessness, emaciation and pale lips, hypodynamia with sweating after defecation, denudation of central tongue fur, thready and uneven or feeble pulse,

4) Type of Concretion of Severe Pathogenic Cold: Astrigent and difficult defecation, light–coloured urine, warmless extremities, slight pain in the abdomen but comfort in pressing, white and moist fur, deep and slow pulse.

TREATMENT

Massage therapy has a peculiar effectiveness on constipation. Meanwhile, the patient should eat more vegetables with much fiber, avoid eating pungent and stimulating food, cultivate the habit of regular defecation.

1. Manipulation: Pushing with one–finger meditation, rubbing, pressing–kneading, pushing, scrubbing, etc.

2. Location of Points: Zhongwan (Ren 12), Tianshu (St 25), Guanyuan (Ren 4), Zusanli (St 36), Chengshan (UB 57)

便困难而言。本症可见于多种病证中。主要是由于大肠传导功能失常，粪便在肠内停留时间过久，水分被过多吸收，而致粪质干燥、坚硬所致。

【临床表现】

1．胃肠燥热型　大便干结，小腹部可触及燥屎硬块，口臭尿赤，心烦头昏，咽干。舌质红，苔黄，脉滑实。

2．气机郁滞型　大便秘结，欲便不能，周身不舒，胸胁或腹中胀满，嗳气频作。舌苔薄白，脉弦涩。

3．气血亏虚型　大便秘结，头晕咽干，心悸气短，精神萎靡，形瘦唇白，便后乏力汗出。舌苔中间剥脱，脉细涩或虚软无力。

4．阴寒凝结型　大便艰涩难出，小便清长，四肢不温，腹部微痛，按之则舒。舌苔白滑，脉沉迟。

【治疗】

推拿对便秘有独特疗效。同时，患者宜多食纤维多的青菜，忌食辛辣刺激食品，并养成定时排便习惯。

1．手法：一指禅推、摩、按揉、推、擦等。

2．取穴：中脘、天枢、关元、足三里、承山、大肠俞、八

Dachangshu (UB 25), and Baliao (UB 31—34).

3. Operation

1) The patient who is in prone position naturally puts his two lower limbs on the two sides of his body respectively, with the two lower limbs slightly flexing the knee and hip. The doctor, sitting to the right of the patient, pushes left downwards from Zhongwan (Ren 12) to Tianshu (St 25) with light and soft one–finger–pushing manipulation for 3—5 minutes, focusing on the two points. Then, with palm–rubbing, the operator rubs for 200—300 times from the left upper abdomen to the left lower abdomen.

2) The patient is in a prone position with the two lower limbs stretched. The doctor presses and kneads with the thumb for 2 or 3 minutes from Zusanli (St 36) to Shangjuxu (St 37).

3) The patient, in prone position, is coated with talcum powder on the gastrocnemius muscles. The Chengshan (UB 57) point is pushed for 150-200 times by the palmar sides of the two thumbs from above to below.

4) The patient is still in a prone position. The doctor presses and kneads Dachangshu (UB 25) with his two thumb tips for 1—2 minutes.

4. Modification of Manipulation according to Different Syndromes

1) Type of Gastroinstetinal Tract Dryness–heat: The doctor also uplift–grasps Tianshu (St 25) with the thumb, the fore finger and the middle finger 3 to 5 times, scrubs horizontally Baliao (UB 31—34) till they become penetratedly hot; uplift–grasps the two Jianjing (GB 21) 3—5 times.

2) Type of Stagnation of Qi: The doctor pushes in addition Tanzhong (Ren 17), press–kneads Ganshu (UB 18), Danshu (UB 19), Qimen (Liv 14), Yanglingquan (GB 34) and Taichong (Liv 3), scrubs–obliquely two hypochodriac regions till they become slightly warm.

3) Type of Deficiency of both Qi and Blood: The doctor

髎等。

3．操作

1) 患者仰卧，两上肢自然放于体侧，两下肢微屈膝髋。医者坐于患者右侧，以轻柔的一指禅推法，自中脘穴向左下推动至天枢穴，重点推中脘与天枢穴，推3～5分钟。然后以掌摩法自左上腹摩向左下腹部，摩200～300次。

2) 患者仰卧，两下肢伸开，医者以拇指端自足三里穴按揉至上巨虚穴2～3分钟。

3) 患者俯卧，在两小腿腓肠肌处敷以滑石粉，以两拇指腹自上而下推承山穴150～200次。

4) 患者仍俯卧，医者以两拇指端按揉两大肠俞1～2分钟。

4．随证加减

1) 胃肠燥热型宜加拇、食、中三指提拿天枢穴3～5次，以小鱼际横擦八髎穴以透热为度，提拿两肩井穴3～5次。

2) 气机郁滞型宜加分推膻中，按揉肝俞、胆俞、期门、阳陵泉、太冲等穴，斜擦两胁肋部，以感微热为度。

3) 气血亏虚型宜加平推脊柱两侧，捏脊，按揉气海、脾俞、

also flat –pushes the two sides of the spine, pinches the spine, presses and kneads Qihai (Ren 6), Pishu (UB 20) and Weishu (UB 21) till they become aching and distending.

4) Type of Concretion of Severe Pathogenic Cold: The doctor also flat–pushes the scapula horizontally, scrubs horizontally Baliao (UB 31—34), rubs obliquely the lower abdomen till they become penetratedly hot, and presses and kneads Shenshu (UB 23) and Mingmen (Du 4).

Asthma

Asthma is manifested as rapid breathing, wheezing with noises, and even mouth–opening, shoulders–lifting and difficulty in prone positioning. Bronchial wheezing is a rooted chronic disease, which is a syndrome with constant attacks; the syndrome characterized by dyspnea is often accompanied with various kinds of acute and chronic diseases. Bronchial wheezing is always accompanied by dyspnea, thus it is called "*xiao chuan*" in TCM.

CLINICAL MANIFESTATIONS

1. Excess Syndromes:

1) Attack of Wind–cold on the Lung: Marked by rapid breathing and stuffiness in the chest, accompanied with cough, thin and whitish sputum and no thirst; at the beginning it is usually accompanied with chills, headache, pantalgia, no sweating, etc. It is also marked by thin and whitish fur of the tongue, floating and tense pulse.

2) Attack of Wind–heat on the Lung: Marked by short breath, wheezing, nares flaring, cough, yellowish, sticky and thick sputum, thirst, preference for cold drink, tightness of the chest, restlessness, sweating, fever and flushed face in severe cases, reddened tongue with yellow fur, rapid and floating pulse.

3) Stagnation of Phlegm in the Lung: Marked by shortness of breath, cough, copious, thicky and greasy sputum, uncomfortable expectoration, even laryngeal rales, feeling of

胃俞，以酸胀为度。

4）阴寒凝结型宜加横向平推肩胛部，横擦八髎穴，斜擦下腹部，均以热深透为度，按揉肾俞、命门穴。

哮　　喘

哮喘以呼吸急促，喘鸣有声，甚至张口抬肩，难以平卧为特征。哮有宿根，为一种经常发作性的病证；喘则多并发于各种急慢性疾病中。哮必兼喘，故一般多哮喘并称。

【临床表现】

1. 实证

1）风寒袭肺：喘急胸闷，伴有咳嗽，痰稀薄，色白，口不渴，初起多兼恶寒、头痛、身痛、无汗等表症。舌苔薄白，脉浮紧。

2）风热犯肺：喘促气粗，甚则鼻翼扇动，咳嗽痰黄而粘稠，口渴喜冷饮，胸闷烦躁，汗出，甚则发热面红。舌质红，苔黄，脉浮数。

3）痰浊阻肺：气喘咳嗽，痰多粘腻，咯出不爽，甚则喉中

stuffiness and tightness in the chest, nausea, anorexia, tastelessness in the mouth, white and greasy tongue fur and slippery pulse.

4) Impairment of the Lung Caused by Stagnation of Qi: Caused by stagnation of qi due to constant worrying and mental stimulus, manifested as sudden rapid breath, discomfort in the throat, even pain in the chest, probably accompanied with insomnia, palpitation, etc; it is also marked by thin and whitish fur and taut pulse.

2. Deficiency Syndromes

1) Deficiency of the Lung: It is marked by rapid breathing, shortness of breath, weak voice, feeble cough, spontaneous sweating, aversion to wind or unsmooth throat, dry mouth, flushed face, reddened tongue and feeble pulse.

2) Deficiency of the Kidney: It is marked by constant rapid breathing, long puffing and short drawing, stronger gasp on slight exertion, thin body, lassitude, difficulty in maintaining breathing, sweating, cold limbs, blue face, even dropsy, unsmooth urine, palpitation, mental restlessness, pale tongue, deep and thready pulse.

TREATMENT

Massage therapy has good curative effect on asthma to remit its symptom. The treatment before the attack will be helpful to its prevention.

1. Manipulation: Flat–pushing, pressing, kneading, lifting–up and grasping.

2. Location of Points: Tanzhong (Ren 17), Tiantu (Ren 22), Jianjing (GB 21), Feishu (UB 13), Geshu (UB 17) and Shenshu (UB 23).

3. Operation

1) The patient is in a prone position, naturally stretching his limbs. The doctor, sitting to the right of the patient, slowly pushes with one finger from Tiantu (Ren 22) to Tanzhong (Ren 17) for 2 or 3 minutes, then pushes with two fingers

痰鸣，胸中满闷，恶心纳呆，口淡无味。舌苔白腻，脉滑。

4）气郁伤肺：平素忧思气结，复因精神刺激，突然呼吸短促，咽中不适，甚则胸痛，可伴有失眠、心悸等症。舌苔薄白，脉弦。

2．虚证

1）肺虚：喘急气短，言语无力，咳声低弱，自汗恶风，或咽喉不利，口干面红。舌质偏红，脉软弱。

2）肾虚：喘促日久，呼长吸短，动则喘息更甚，形瘦神疲，气息难续，汗出肢冷面青，甚则肢体浮肿，小便不利，心悸不安。舌质淡，脉沉细。

【治疗】

推拿治疗哮喘，对缓解症状有较好疗效。若能在发作前治疗，对防止发作有一定效果。

1．手法：平推、按、揉、提拿等。

2．取穴：膻中、天突、肩井、肺俞、膈俞、肾俞等。

3．操作

1）患者仰卧，四肢自然伸开，医者坐于患者右侧，以一指推法从天突穴缓慢推向膻中穴，往返推动2～3分钟，再以两拇

from Tanzhong to its two sides for 200—300 times.

2) The patient is in a sitting position. The doctor lifts and grasps the patient's cervical part with the thumb and the fingers for 1 or 2 minutes, then flat-pushes the chest and back, obliquely pushes the two costal regions till the heat produced becomes penetrating.

3) The doctor presses and kneads Feishu (UB 13) and Geshu (UB 17) with the tips of the thumbs and the middle finger till they become aching and swelling.

4) The doctor lift-grasps Jianjing (GB 21) on the two shoulders for 3—5 minutes.

5) The doctor first flat-pushes the upper arm and the forearm and then lift-grasps them and Hegu (LI 4).

6) The doctor restores the patient's fingers, foulages and shakes the upper limbs.

7) The shoulders are rotated forwards and backwards for 3 circles respectively.

4. Modification of Manipulation according to Different Syndromes

1) Attack of Wind-cold on the Lung: Also grasping Fengchi (GB 20) and straightly-scrubbing both sides of the spine.

2) Attack of Wind-heat on the Lung: pressing-kneading Fengmen (UB 12), grasping Fengchi (GB 20), straightly-rubbing the neck of urinary bladder on the back as well.

3) Stagnation of Phlegm in the Lung: In addition, pressing-kneading Fenglong (St 40) and Zusanli (St 36).

4) Impairment of the Lung Caused by Stagnation of Qi: Also pressing-kneading Qimen (Liv 14), Ganshu (UB 18), Yanglingquan (GB 34) and Taichong (Liv 3).

5) Deficiency of the Lung: Additionally, focusing on horizontally pushing the upper part of the front chest and the back, digital pressing and kneading Feishu (UB 13) and Geshu (UB 17), Pressing and kneading Taiyuan (Lu 9) and Taixi (K 3).

6) Deficiency of the Kidney: Focusing on flatpushing the

指从膻中穴向两旁分推200～300次。

2）患者坐位，医者以拇指及其他四指提拿颈 项 部 1 ～ 2 分钟，然后平推胸背，斜推两胁，均以透热为度。

3）以拇指或中指端按揉肺俞、膈俞，以酸胀为度。

4）提拿两侧肩井穴 3 ～ 5 次。

5）平推然后提拿上臂、前臂，提拿合谷穴。

6）理手指，搓抖上肢。

7）摇膀子前后各 3 周。

4．随证加减

1）风寒袭肺型，宜加拿风池，直擦脊柱两侧。

2）风热犯肺型，宜加按风门，拿风池，直擦背部膀胱经。

3）痰浊阻肺型，宜加按揉丰隆、足三里等穴。

4）气郁伤肺型，宜加按揉期门、肝俞、阳陵泉、太冲穴。

5）肺虚型，宜重点横推前胸上部及背部，点按揉肺俞、膈俞穴，加按揉太渊、太溪两穴。

6）肾虚型，宜重点平推腰骶部，按揉肾俞、命门、太溪穴。

sacral portion, pressing–kneading Shengshu (UB 23), Mingmen (Du 4) and Taixi (K 3).

5. Course of Treatment: Once a day; for excess syndromes, 6 times as one course; for the deficiency type, 12 times. The interval between two courses is from 5 to 7 days.

Headache

Headache is a kind of clinically common subjective symptom. It can be accompanied by various kinds of acute and chronic diseases. This section will mainly discuss some symptoms characterised mainly by headache.

CLINICAL MANIFESTATIONS

1. Headache due to Exopathy

1) Headache due to Pathogenic Wind-cold Pathogen: frequent headache, pain extending to the nape and back, aversion to cold and wind, joy for head-binding, no thirst, thin and whitish tongue fur, floating and tense pulse.

2) Headache due to Pathogenic Wind-heat: distension and pain in the head, fever, aversion to wind, thirst with desire to drink, dark urine, reddened tongue with thin and yellow fur, floating and rapid pulse.

3) Headache due to Pathogenic Summer-heat and Dampness: strong binding pain in the head, lassitude of limbs, poor appetite, fullness in the epigastric region, fever, sweating, dysphoria, thirst, greasy fur and slippery pulse.

2. Headache due to Internal Injury

1) The Liver-*yang* Headache: Headache with intermittent dizziness, dysphoria, irritability, insomnia, bitter taste, reddened tongue with thin and yellowish fur, taut and forceful pulse.

2) Headache due to Stagnation of Phlegm: Headache with dizziness, fullness in the epigastric region, vomiting, abundant expectoration, whitish and greasy fur, slippery or taut and slippery pulse.

3) Headache due to Deficiency of Blood: Headache and

5. 疗程：每日 1 次。实证 6 次为 1 疗程，虚证12次为 1 疗程。各疗程之间间隔 5～7 天。

头　痛

头痛是一种临床常见的自觉症状，可出现在多种急、慢性疾病中。本篇仅讨论以头痛为主要症状的一些证侯。

【临床表现】

1. 外感头痛

1）风寒头痛　头痛时作，痛连项背，恶风寒，常喜裹头，口不渴。舌苔薄白，脉浮紧。

2）风热头痛　头胀痛，发热恶风，口渴欲饮，小便黄。舌质黄，苔薄黄，脉浮数。

3）暑湿头痛　头痛如裹，肢体倦怠，脘闷纳呆，身热汗出，心烦口渴。舌苔腻，脉滑。

2. 内伤头痛

1）肝阳头痛　头痛而眩，心烦易怒，睡眠不宁，口苦。舌质红，苔薄黄，脉弦有力。

2）痰浊头痛　头痛昏蒙，胸脘满闷，呕恶痰涎。舌苔白腻，脉滑或弦滑。

3）血虚头痛　头痛头晕，遇劳加剧，神疲乏力，心悸气短，

dizziness which become intense with slight labour, weakness, dysphoria, palpitation, shortness of breath, pale complexion, pale tongue with thin and whitish fur, thready and feeble pulse.

4) Headache due to Deficiency of the Kidney: Headache with a sensation of emptiness inside the head, dizziness, weakness and lassitude in loins and legs, emission, leukorrhagia, tinnitus, insomnia, reddened tongue with little fur, thready and feeble pulse.

TREATMENT

Massage has a great remitting effect on headache, especially on headache due to cold, migraine and muscular contraction headache.

1. Manipulation: Pushing with one-finger meditation, lifting-grasping, wiping, flat-pushing, pressing-kneading, etc.

2. Location of Points: Yintang (Extra 1), Jingming (UB 1), Taiyang (Extra 2), Fengchi (GB 20), Feishu (UB 13), Ganshu (UB 18) and Shenshu (UB 23).

3. Operation

1) The patient is in a sitting position. The doctor, sitting behind the patient, lift-grasps the cervical point with the thumb and the four fingers from below to above for 30 ~ 50 times.

2) Wipe the forehead and superciliary arch in two directions, digital pressing Jingming (UB 2), wipe Yingxiang (LI 20), Renzhong (DU 26) and Chengjiang (Ren 24) in two directions for 3 ~ 5 times respectively. This should be repeated 3 times.

3) Sweep the temple for 30 to 50 times.

4) Grasping with the five fingers along the five channels of Du, Taiyang and Shaoyin from front to back. This should be repeated for 3—5 times.

5) Flat-push the chest and back till they become penetratedly hot; grasp Jianjing (GB 21), the upper arms, forearms; foulage-shake the upper limbs; rotate the shoulders forwards

面色㿠白。舌质淡，苔薄白，脉细弱无力。

4）肾亏头痛　头痛且空，每兼眩晕，腰膝酸软，神疲乏力，遗精带下，耳鸣失眠。舌红少苔，脉细无力。

【治疗】

推拿对缓解头痛有较好的疗效，尤其对感冒、偏头痛、肌收缩性头痛，疗效尤佳。

1．手法：一指禅推、提拿、抹、平推、按揉等。

2．取穴：印堂、睛明、太阳、风池、肺俞、肝俞、肾俞等。

3．操作

1）患者坐位，医者站其身后，以拇指和其他四指自下而上提拿颈项部30～50次。

2）分抹前额、眉弓，点睛明，分抹迎香、人中、承浆，各3～5次，反复3遍。

3）扫散两颞部30～50次。

4）以五指自前向后沿督脉、太阳、少阴五条经线拿，反复3～5遍。

5）平推胸背，以热透为度；拿肩井、上臂、前臂；搓抖上

and backwards for 3 circles respectively.

4. Modification of Manipulation according to Different Syndromes

1) Headache due to Wind-cold Pathogen: Also press and knead Feishu (UB 13) and Dazhu (UB 11); straightly scrub the channel of the bladder at the two sides of the spine till they become penetratedly hot and slightly sweating. Press and knead Quchi (LI 11) and Hegu (LI 4) till they become aching and distending.

2) Headache due to Wind-heat Pathogen; Additionally, push Dazhui (Du 14) with one-finger meditation for 3~5 minutes; pat and hit the Bladder Channels at the two sides of the spine till the skin becomes reddish.

3) Headache due to Pathogenic Summer-heat: Also pat and hit the Bladder Channels at the two sides till the skin becomes reddish, and pinch Yintang (Extra 1) and nuchal region till there appears slight blood stasis in the skin.

4) The Liver-*yang* Headache: In addition, push Qiaogong, sweep the temple, obliquely-push two costal regions, press-knead Ganshu (UB 18), Yanglingquan (GB 34) and Taichong (Liv 3).

5) Headache due to Stagnation of Phlegm: Also press-knead Pishu (UB 20), Weishu (UB 21), Zusanli (St 36) and Fenglong (St 40), rub the abdomen, push Zhongwan (Ren 12) and Qihai (Ren 6) with one-finger meditation.

6) Headache due to Deficiency of Blood: Additionally pinch the spine for 3 to 5 times, press-knead Xinshu (UB 15), Geshu (UB 17) and Zusanli (St 36), rub the abdomen, push Zhongwan (Ren 12) and Qihai (Ren 6) with one-finger meditation.

7) Headache due to the Kidney Deficiency: Also flat-push the lumbosacral portion, press-knead Shenshu (UB 23) and Mingmen (Du 4); rub the abdomen, push Qihai (Ren 6) and Guanyuan (Ren 4) with one-finger meditation.

5. Course of Treatment: Once a day, 3 times as one course

股；摇膀子前后各3周。

4. 随证加减

1）风寒头痛，加按揉肺俞、大杼穴，直擦脊柱两侧膀胱经线，以热透微汗为度。按揉曲池、合谷穴，以酸胀为度。

2）风热头痛，加一指禅推大椎穴3～5分钟，拍击脊柱两侧膀胱经，以皮肤微红为度。

3）暑湿头痛，加拍击两侧膀胱经，以皮肤微红为度。并用捏法将印堂及项部皮肤捏至皮肤轻度瘀血。

4）肝阳头痛，宜加推桥弓，扫散颞部，斜推两胁，按揉肝俞、阳陵泉、太冲穴。

5）痰浊头痛，宜加按揉脾俞、胃俞、足三里、丰隆，摩腹，一指禅推中脘、天枢等穴。

6）血虚头痛，宜加捏脊3～5遍，按揉心俞、膈俞、足三里穴，摩腹，一指禅推中脘、气海等穴。

7）肾亏头痛，宜加平推腰骶部，按揉肾俞、命门，摩腹，一指禅推气海、关元穴。

5. 疗程：每日1次。外感头痛3次为1疗程，内伤头痛10

for headache due to exopathy and 10 times as one course for the headache due to internal injury.

Common Cold

Common cold, caused by expathogen, is a disease seen in four seasons, especially in winter and spring. Clinically it is manifested as symptoms of headache, sore-throat, nasal obstruction, running nose, aversion to wind and fever.

CLINICAL MANIFESTATIONS

1. Wind-cold Type: aversion to cold and fever, anhidrosis, aching in four limbs, nasal obstruction, running watery discharge, itching of the throat, cough, watery and thin sputum, thin and whitish fur, floating or floating and tense pulse.

2. Wind-heat Type: fever, slight aversion to wind, inhibited sweating, distension and pain in the head, cough, thick and yellowish sputum, sore-throat, dry mouth, thin and yellow fur, floating and rapid pulse.

TREATMENT

1. Manipulation: Pushing with one-finger meditation, pressing, kneading, wiping, grasping, etc.

2. Location of Points: Fengchi (GB 20), Fengfu (Du 16), Tianzhu (UB 10), Fengmen (UB 12), Feishu (UB 13), Yintang (Extra 1), Taiyang (Extra 2), Touwei (St 8), Baihui (Du 20) and Hegu (LI 4).

3. Operation

1) The doctor stands posterior-lateral to the sitting patient, with one hand proping the forehead of the patient. The other hand repeatedly operates one-finger meditation pushing or pressing-kneading along the line from Fengchi (GB 20) directly downwards to Dazhui (Du 14) for 3~5 times; then from Fengchi (GB 20) downwards, along the line connecting Tianzhu (UB 10), Dazhu (UB 11) and Fengmen (UB 12) for 3~ 5 times. The operating time should be longer at each point.

2) The doctor, standing anterior-lateral to the patient,

次为 1 疗程。

感　冒

感冒是四季常见的外感疾病，尤以冬、春两季为多见。临床症状以头痛、咽痛、鼻塞、流涕、恶风、发热等为特征。

【临床表现】

1．风寒型　恶寒发热，无汗，头痛，四肢酸痛，鼻塞，流清涕，喉痒，咳嗽，吐痰清稀。舌苔薄白，脉浮或浮紧。

2．风热型　身热，微恶风，汗出不畅，头胀痛，咳嗽，咯痰稠黄，咽痛，口干。舌苔薄黄，脉浮数。

【治疗】

1．手法：一指禅推法、按、揉、抹、拿等。

2．取穴：风池、风府、天柱、风门、肺俞、印堂、太阳、头维、百会、合谷等。

3．操作

1）患者取坐位，医者站在其后外侧，一手扶持其前额，另一手以一指禅推法或按揉法，沿风府直下至大椎一线，反复操作3～5遍；再沿风池向下，经天柱、大杼、风门一线，反复操作3～5遍，凡经穴位处操作时间略长。

2）医者位于其前外侧，一手扶持其枕后部；另一手用一指

with one hand props his occipitoposterior portion and with the other hand repeatedly operates one-finger meditation pushing or pressing-kneading along the line from Yintang (Extra 1), Shenting (Du 24), Touwei (St 8) to Taiyang (Extra 2) and the line from Yintang (Extra 1), Yangbai (BG 14) to Taiyang (Extra 2) for 3~5 times.

3) The doctor, standing right in front of the patient, operates wiping with the fingerprint regions of the two thumbs for 3~5 times repeatedly, from Yintang (Estra 1), by way of supercil'ary arch, to superciliary end; from midfront, by way of Yangbai (GB 14), to Taiyang (Extra 2); from Shenting (Du 24), by way of Touwei (St 8) and Jiaosun (SJ 20) and along the the two temples, to Fengchi (GB 20).

4) The doctor, standing posterior-lateral and posterior to the patient, grasps Fengchi (GV 20) and the major tendons of the neck first, then Jianjing (GB 21).

5) The doctor repeatedly operates one-finger meditation pushing or pressing-kneading in an orderly way in Fengmen (UB 12), Jianjing (GB 21) and Fishu (UB 13) for one minute each, finally ends the operation with grasping Jianjing (GB 21) and Hegu (LI 4).

4. Modification of Manipulation according to Different Syndromes

1) Wind-cold Type: Also push the interscapular region with the manipulation of palm-pushing till it becomes hot.

2) Wind-heat Type: Push with one-finger meditation or press-knead Dazhui (Du 14) nip-knead Hegu (LI 14) as well.

3) Nasal Obstruction: In addition, knead and press Yingxiang (LI 20)

4) Sore and Swelling Throat: Also nip Shaoshang (Lu 11) and Shangyang (LI 1), finger-knead submaxillary Ashi point.

5) Inhibited Sputum: Additionally knead Tiantu (Ren 22) and Tanzhong (Ren 17).

5. Course of Treatment: Once a day, 3 times as one course;

禅推法或按揉法，沿印堂、神庭、头维、太阳一线与印堂、阳白至太阳一线，各反复操作 3～5 遍。

3）医者站在患者正前方，用双手拇指罗纹面，从印堂沿眉弓至眉外梢；从额中经阳白至太阳，从神庭，经头维、角孙沿两颞至风池，用抹法分别操作 3～5 遍。

4）医者位于患者后外侧及后方，拿风池及项后大筋，再拿肩井。

5）用一指禅推法或按揉法，依次在风门、肩井、肺俞穴上各操作1分钟，最后以拿肩井、合谷结束治疗。

4. 随证加减

1）风寒型，加用掌推法推肩胛间区，以热为度。

2）风热型，加一指禅推或按揉大椎穴，掐揉合谷。

3）鼻塞不通，加揉、按迎香。

4）咽喉肿痛，加揉少商、商阳，指揉颌下阿是穴。

5）咳嗽不爽，加揉天突、膻中。

5. 疗程：每日1次，3次为1疗程。各疗程之间间隔1天。

with an interval of one day between two courses.

Essential Hypertension

Essential hypertension is a common clinical syndrome mainly characterized by the increase of arterial pressure of the systemic circulation. It is generally believed to be a hyhertension for people below 40 years old if the systolic pressure is over 18.7 kPa (140 mm Hg) and the diastolic pressure is over 12 kPa (90 mm Hg); for people of 40~59 years old, over 20/12 kPa (150/90 mmHg); for people over 60 years old, over 21.3/12 kPa(160/90 mm Hg). Clinically, hypertension is mainly manifested by headache, dizziness, fullness of head, etc. In TCM it falls into categories of *"tou tong"* (headache), *"xuan yun"* (dizziness), *"jing ji"* (palpitation due to fright) and *"shi mian"* (insomnia).

CLINICAL MANIFESTATIONS

Based on the development of the disease and the degree of seriousness, we can divide hypertension into two types: benigh hypertension and accelarated hypertension. In the primary stage of benigh hypertension, there are symptoms of headache, dizziness, insomnia, hypomnesis, palpitation and tinnitus, but mostly no organic changes of blood vessels and the heart, brain, kidney, etc. In the middle stage, the above-mentioned symptoms become more serious and there may appear temporary aphasia, hemiparalysis, polyuria, red blood cells and cast in urine. On the electrocardiogram left ventricular hypertrophy and strain can be seen. In the later stage, in addition to the ever increasing of blood pressure, benigh hypertension is marked by symptoms and physical signs of dysfunction of the heart, brain and kidney. Accelarated hypertension is mainly manifested as fast development of the disease, a constant diastolic pressure over 17.3 kPa, and physical signs of fundus bleeding, oozing and papilledema.

TREATMENT

Massage therapy is mainly curative for benigh hypertension

高 血 压 病

高血压病是一种常见的，以体循环动脉血压增高为主的临床症候群。一般认为,40岁以下收缩压超过 18.7 kPa（140 毫米汞柱）、舒张压超过 12 kPa（90 毫米汞柱），40～59 岁的人超过 20/12kPa（150/90 毫米汞柱），60 岁以上的人超过 21.3/12 kPa（160/90毫米汞柱），则认为患高血压。临床主要表现为头痛、头晕、头胀等,属中医"头痛"、"眩晕"、"惊悸"、"失眠"等范畴。

【临床表现】

根据本病的病程进展快慢及病势的轻重程度，可分为缓进型与急进型两类。缓进型高血压早期可见头痛、头晕、失眠、记忆力减退、心悸、耳鸣等症状，多无血管和心、脑、肾等器官的器质性改变。中期可见上述症状加重，甚则出现一时性失语、偏瘫、多尿、尿中出现红细胞、管型等，心电图可见左室肥大与劳损。后期除血压持续升高外，表现为心、脑、肾功能不全症状及体征。急进型高血压主要表现为病情进展迅速，舒张压常持续在 17.3 kPa 以上，并有眼底出血、渗出和视神经乳头水肿等体征。

【治疗】

推拿主要适宜于治疗缓进型高血压，对缓解各种症状有明显

to reimt the various symptoms, especially for primary hypertension if there is a constant therapy, in such case, by function of nerve reflex and humoral regulation, the inhibited activites of cerebral cortex can be increased to regulate the function of vasomotor center, bringing about hypotension and blood pressure decreasing of small arteries. Subsequently the symptoms may remit or disappear.

1. Manipulation: Pushing with one-finger meditation, lifting-grasping, pressing-kneading, arching-pushing with elbow and rubbing.

2. Location of Points: Fengchi (GB 20), Dazhui (Du 14), Huantiao (GB 30), Baihui (Du 20) and Qiaogong.

3. Operation

1) Standing behind the patient, the doctor lift-grasps the cervical portion for 30~50 times.

2) With the mainipulation of thumb-straight-pushing, the doctor pushes the left and right Qiaogong from above to below for 30~50 times each side.

3) With the manipulation of one-finger pushing, the doctor repeatedly and alternatively pushes from Yintang (Extra 1), by way of superciliary arch, to Taiyang (Extra 2), then to Touwei (St 8), Shuaigu (GB 8), Fubai (GB 10) and Naokong (GB 19), for 3~5 minutes.

4) With the thumb and the four fingers, the doctor grasps from the front of the head, along the channels of Du, Shaoyang and Taiyang, to the back of the head for 3~5 times.

5) With the manipulation of one-finger pushing, the doctor pushes Dazhui (Du 14) for 3~5 minutes.

6) The doctor sits to the right of the patient who is in a supine position, and rubs the abdomen clockwise for 5 ~7 minutes.

7) The patient in lateral-lying posision, the doctor elbow-motions Huantiao (GB 30) for 5~7 minutes.

8) The patient is in a prone position, with the waist and

效果，尤其对早期高血压病，若能坚持治疗，可通过神经反射及体液调节等作用，增加大脑皮质的抑制过程，达到调节血管运动中枢的机能，使小动脉的张力降低和血压下降，从而使症状减轻或消失。

1. 手法：一指禅推、提拿、按揉、肘运、摩等。

2. 取穴：风池、大椎、环跳、百会、桥弓等。

3. 操作

1）患者坐位，医者站其身后，提拿颈项部30～50次。

2）以拇指直推法，推左、右桥弓穴，自上而下每侧30～50次。

3）以一指推法自印堂沿眉弓推至太阳，再推至头维、率谷、浮白、脑空，两侧交替，反复推3～5分钟。

4）以五指自前头部沿督脉、少阳、太阳经线拿至后头部3～5次。

5）以一指推法推大椎穴3～5分钟。

6）患者仰卧，医者坐其右侧，顺时针摩腹5～7分钟。

7）患者侧卧，医者以肘部肘运环跳穴5～7分钟。

8）患者俯卧，在腰骶部涂以冬青膏，以小鱼际横擦腰骶部，

sacrum coated with Chinese holly leaf ointment. With minor thenar eminance the doctor horizontally-scrubs the waist and sacrum till they become penetratedly hot.

9) With the thumb, the doctor pushes Yongquan (K 1) for 3∼5 minutes.

4. Course of Treatment: Once a day, 10 times as one course; with an interval of 2 or 3 days between two courses.

Mastitis

Mastitis, which is called "*ru yong*" (acute mastitis) in TCM, is mostly seen in breast feeding women, especially primiparae. At the beginning, the redness, heat and swelling in breasts are accompanied with general symptoms of fever, aversion to cold and headache. A long-standing case may have suppuration and ulceration. The acute mastitis in pregnancy is called "*neichui ruyong*" (acute mastitis during pregnancy); "*waichui ruyong*" (postpartum manstitis) in breast feeding period in TCM.

CLINICAL MANIFESTATIONS

Local Symptoms: Tumefection and pain in breasts, slight pressure pain or mass in the affected part, reddish surface with slight heat, and there will be suppuration in a short time.

General Symptoms: Lymphadenectasis of axillary fossa of the affected side, fever, aversion to cold, headache, red tongue with thin and yellow fur, slippery and rapid pulse. In blood routine examination, the total number of WBC can be seen increased and classified neutrophlic granulocyte a bit more.

TREATMENT

Massage therapy has a better curative effect on primary mastitis. The sooner the treatment, the better the effectiveness. In the case of suppuration or diabrosis, there should be operative incision and drainage.

1. Manipulation: Rubbing, kneading, pressing and grasping.
2. Location of Points: Ruzhong (St 17), Rugen (St 18), Tianchi (P. 1), Tianxi (Sp 18), Shidou (Sp 17), Fengchi

以透热为度。

9）以拇指推涌泉穴 3～5 分钟。

4．疗程：每日 1 次，10 次为 1 疗程。各疗程之间间隔 2～3 天。

乳 腺 炎

乳腺炎，中医称之为"乳痈"。多见于哺乳期的妇女，尤以初产妇最为多见。初起乳部嫩红肿痛，同时伴有发热、恶寒、头痛等全身症状，日久化脓溃烂。乳痈发于妊娠期称为"内吹乳痈"，发于哺乳期的称为"外吹乳痈"。

【临床表现】

局部表现：乳房肿胀、疼痛，患部轻度压痛或有肿块，表面微热或微红，短期内可成脓。

全身症状：常有同侧腋窝淋巴结肿大，发热，恶寒，头身痛，舌质红，苔薄黄，脉滑数。血常规可见白细胞总数增多，分类嗜中性粒细胞偏高。

【治疗】

推拿治疗本病，以早期为佳。治疗越早，疗效越好。若已成脓或溃破，宜手术切开引流排脓。

1．手法：摩、揉、按、拿等。

2．取穴：乳中、乳根、天池、天溪、食窦、风池、肩井、合

(BG 20), Jianjing (GB 21), Hegu (LI 4), Ganshu (UB 18), Feishu (UB 13), Weishu (UB 21), etc.

3. Operation

1) The patient is in a sitting or supine position, with the affected breast coated with a little liquid paraffin or vaseline. The doctor, with his four fingers combined, pushes light from around the breast to the nipple; he mustn't press with force or rotating-press, but operates with positive pressure to push out the stagnating milk. While pressing and rubbing, the nipple may be picked slightly by hand for several times to expand the lactiferons duct of the nipple.

2) The doctor, sitting to the right of the patient who is in a supine position, rubs the abdomen clockwise with palm for 3~5 minutes, then repeatedly pushes with thumb from Zhongwan (Ren 12) to Tianshu (S5 25) for 2 or 3 minutes.

3) The doctor, standing behind the sitting patient, grasps Fengchi (GN 20) with the thumb and four fingers for 5~10 times, then slightly lift-grasps Jianjing (GB 12) for 3~5 times.

4) The patient in a sitting position, the doctor press-kneads Ganshu (UB 18), Pishu (UB 20) and Weishu (UB 21) with the thumb till there's an aching and distension sensation.

The manipulation throughout the operation should be soft and slow. Roughness is forbidden.

4. Course of Treatment: One or two times a day till the recovery of the disease.

Dysmenorrhea

Before or after menstruation or in the menstrual period, some women have pain in the lower abdomen, waist and sacrum, which is even unbearable, accompanied with symptoms of pale face, dripping cold sweat in the head and face, cold clammy extremities, nausea and vomiting. The troubles that go with menstrual cycles are called dysmenorrhea.

谷、肝俞、肺俞、胃俞等。

3．操作

1）患者坐位或仰卧，先在患侧乳房涂上少许液状石蜡或凡士林，医者以四指并拢由乳房四周轻轻向乳头方向推动，不要用力按压或旋转按压，而是沿着乳腺管的方向，施以正压，把瘀滞的乳汁逐步推出。在按摩的同时可以用手轻轻揪乳头数次，以扩张乳头部的输乳管。

2）患者仰卧，医者坐于其右侧，以手掌顺时针方向摩腹3～5分钟。然后以拇指自中脘穴推至天枢穴反复2～3分钟。

3）患者正坐，医者站其身后，以拇指和其他四指拿风池穴5～10次，然后轻轻提拿肩井穴3～5次。

4）患者正坐，以拇指按揉肝俞、脾俞、胃俞，以酸胀为度。

全过程手法宜轻柔和缓，切忌粗暴。

4．疗程：每日1次或2次，病愈为止。

痛　经

妇女在行经前后，或正值行经期间，小腹及腰骶部疼痛，甚至剧痛难忍，并伴有面色苍白、头面冷汗淋漓、手足厥冷、泛恶呕吐等症状，随月经周期而发作者，称为"痛经"，亦称"经行腹痛"。

CLINICAL MANIFESTATIONS

1. Stagnancy of *Qi* and Blood Stasis: Distending pain in the lower abdomen before or during menstruation, dripping and oligomenorrhea, dark menses, blood with clots, relief of pain with the discharge of clots, distension in sternocostal part and breasts, purplish and dim tongue with ecchymosis on tne border, deep and taut pulse.

2. Menorrhalgia due to Cold-dampness: Lower abdominal pain before or during menstruation which may cause pain in waist and spine which can be relieved by heat, scanty menstruation, dark menses with clots, aversion to cold and loose stools, white and greasy tongue, deep and tight pulse.

3. Dysmenorrhea due to Deficiency of *Qi* and Blood: Lingering pain in the lower abdomen during and after menstruation, remission of the pain on pressing, pale, thin and watery menorrhea, pale complexion, lassitude, pale tongue with thin and whitish fur, and feeble thready pulse.

4. Dysmenorrhea due to Deficiency of the Liver and Kidney: Dull pain in the lower abdomen after menstruation, pale oligomenorrhea, aching of the waist, paravertebral musculature of the back, dizziness and tinnitus, reddish tongue, deep and thready pulse.

TREATMENT

Massage therapy has a curative effect on dysmenorrhea, which may be before, during or after the menstruation. During menstruation, manipulation should be light and soft to avoid such abnormality as abundant menses.

1. Manipulation: Pushing with one-finger meditation, rubbing, pressing-kneading, scrubbing, etc.

2. Location of Points: Qihai (Ren 6), Guanyuan (Ren 4), Baliao (UB 31—34), Shenshu (UB 23), Zhangmen (Liv 13), Qimen (Liv 14), Zusanli (St 36), Sanyinjiao (Sp 6), Yanglingquan (GB 34), etc.

3. Operation

1) The patient is in a supine position, with the upper

【临床表现】

1. 气滞血瘀型　经前或经期小腹胀痛，行经量少，淋漓不畅，血色紫黯有血块，块下则疼痛减轻，胸胁乳房作胀。舌质紫黯，舌边或有瘀点，脉沉弦。

2. 寒湿凝滞型　经前或经行小腹冷痛，甚则牵连腰脊疼痛，得热则舒，经行量少，色黯有瘀块，畏寒便溏。苔白腻，脉沉紧。

3. 气血虚弱型　经期或经净后，小腹绵绵作痛，按之痛减，经色淡，质清稀，面色苍白，精神倦怠。舌质淡，苔薄白，脉虚细。

4. 肝肾亏损型　经后小腹隐痛，经来色淡量少，腰脊酸楚，头晕耳鸣。舌质淡红，脉沉细。

【治疗】

推拿治疗痛经，疗效较好。治疗可在经前，亦可在经期或经后。在经期治疗，手法宜轻柔，以防引起月经过多等不良情况。

1. 手法：一指禅推、摩、按揉、擦等。

2 取穴：气海、关元、八髎、肾俞、章门、期门、足三里、三阴交、阳陵泉等。

3. 操作

1) 患者仰卧，两上肢自然放于体侧，下肢微屈膝、髋，医者

limbs naturally put on two sides of the body respectively and lower limbs slightly flexing the knee and hip. The doctor, sitting to his right, first rubs the abdomen clockwise and counterclockwise for 5—10 minutes; then with one-finger meditation pushing slowly pushes Qihai (Ren 6) and Guanyuan (Ren 4) to and fro for 3—4 minutes.

2) The patient is still in a supine position with his two lower limbs stretched. The doctor presses and kneads Xuehai (Sp 10), Sanyinjiao (Sp 6) for 1 or 2 minutes at each point till there's an aching and distending sensation.

3) With the waist and sacrum coated with Chinese holly leaf ointment and the patient is in prone position, the doctor scrubs waist and sacrum with palm minor thenar eminance till they become penetratedly hot.

4. Modification of Manipulation according to Different Syndromes

1) Stagnancy of *Qi* and Blood Stasis: Also obliquely push costal regions and press-knead Zhangmen (Liv 13), Qimen (Liv 14), Ganshu (UB 13), Yanglingquan (GB 34) and Taichong (Liv 3).

2) Menorrhalgia due to Cold and Dampness: In addition obliquely–scrub the lower abdomen and press-knead Sanyinjiao (Sp 6), Taichong,(Liv 3) and the Baliao (UB 31—34) till there is an aching and distending sensation.

3) Dysmenorrhea due to Deficiency of *Qi* and Blood: Pinch the spine, push Zhongwan (Ren 12) with one-finger meditation and intervally-press knead Pishu (UB 20) Weishu (UB 21) and Zusanli (St 36) as well.

4) Dysmenorrha due to Deficiency of the Liver and Kidney: Additionally palm-vibrate the lower abdomen for 5—10 minutes and pressknead Ganshu (UB 18), Shenshu (UB 23) and Mingmen (Dn 4) till there is aching and distending sensation.

5. Course of Treatment: Once a day or every two days, 3 times as one course; with an interval of 3—5 days between two

坐其右侧，先顺、逆时针摩腹各 5～10 分钟。继以一指禅推法推气海、关元穴往返缓慢移动，推 3～5 分钟。

2）患者仍仰卧，两下肢伸开，以拇指按揉血海、三阴交，每穴 1～2 分钟，以酸胀为度。

3）患者俯卧，在腰骶部涂以冬青膏，以手掌小鱼际直擦腰骶部，以热深透为度。

4. 随证加减

1）气滞血瘀型 宜加斜推两胁，按揉章门、期门、肝俞、阳陵泉、太冲穴。

2）寒湿凝滞型 宜加斜擦少腹、按揉三阴交、太冲、八髎穴，以酸胀为度。

3）气血虚弱型 宜加捏脊，一指禅推中脘穴，按揉脾俞、胃俞、足三里穴。

4）肝肾亏虚型 宜加掌振小腹部 5～10 分钟，按揉肝俞、肾俞、命门，以酸胀为度。

5. 疗程：每日或隔日 1 次，3 次为 1 疗程。各疗程之间间

courses.

Myopia

After parallel rays are deflected by the eyeball dioptric system (which includes cornea, aqueous humor, lens and vitreous body), the aggregated focus is before retina, thus causing a normal close vision but vague distant vision. This is called myopia, "*neng jin que yuan zheng*" (myopia) in TCM.

CLINICAL MANIFESTATIONS

A slight myopia (less than 3 diopters), though with a vague distant vision, sees things in a shorter distance clearly. A moderate myope (3 to 6 diopters), with an increased vagueness of distant vision, often squints. When a serious myope (more than 6 diopters), with an increased vagueness of near vision, writes or works in case of short distance, the distance between eyeballs and objects becomes shorter and shorter; and after a long-time working, there'll appear near vision-decreasing and some vision tiredness symptoms such as eye distension and headache.

TREATMENT

Massage therapy has a curative effect on juvenile slight myopia, esp. on pseudomyopia. Myopes with more than 2 diopters should wear glasses, and massage therapy may go along with eye exercises.

1. Manipulation: Pushing with one-finger meditation, pressing-kneading and grasping.

2. Location of Points: Jingming (UB 1), Zanzhu (UB 2), Sizhukong (SJ 23), Sibai (St 2), Fengchi (GB 20), Dazhui (Du 14), Yifeng (one *cun* behind Yifeng point), Ganshu (UB 18) and Guangming (GB 37).

3. Operation

1) Standing behind the sitting patient, the doctor liftgrasps the cervical part for 30—50 times with his thumb and the other fingers; then press-kneads Yiming (Extra) for about

隔3～5天。

近 视 眼

平行光线经过眼球屈光系统(包括角膜、房水、晶状体和玻璃体)屈折后，集合焦点在视网膜之前，致使视近物正常，视远物模糊不清者，则称为近视眼。中医称之为"能近怯远症"。

【临床表现】

轻度近视眼(3个屈光度以下)，虽然看远处的物体模糊不清，但看近处的物体却毫无影响。中度近视眼(3～6个屈光度)，看远物模糊的程度加重，患者常喜眯眼视物。高度近视者（6个屈光度以上），远视力更加模糊，书写或做其他近距离工作时，眼球与目标的距离越来越短，工作久后将会出现近视力减退及眼胀、头痛等视力疲劳症状。

【治疗】

推拿治疗青少年轻度近视效果良好，尤其对假性近视，疗效更佳。2个屈光度以上的近视患者，应该配戴眼镜。在推拿治疗的过程中，可配合做眼保健操。

1. 手法：一指禅推、按揉、拿等。

2. 取穴：睛明、攒竹、丝竹空、四白、风池、大椎、翳明、(翳风穴后1寸)、肝俞、光明等。

3. 操作

1）患者坐位，医者站其身后，以拇指及其他四指提拿颈项部30～50次，然后以拇指按揉翳明穴约1分钟以酸胀为度。再以拇

one minute with his thumb till there's an aching and distending sensation; then pushes Dazhui (Du 14) for 2 or 3 minutes with the manipulation of thumb-pushing; finally press-kneads Ganshu (UB 18) till there's a sensation of aching and distension.

2) Flatly push the neck and back till they become penetratedly hot.

3) The doctor, standing in front of the patient, pushes with the manipulation of one-finger pushing, around the orbit in a "∞" way for 3—5 minutes; then digital presses Jingming (UB 1), Shangming (point intersuperciliary point, below upper orbit) and Sibai (St 2) till there's a sensation of aching and distension.

4) Lift-grasp Jianjing (GB 21) and Hegu (LI 4).

5) The patient, in a supine position, press-kneads Shangming point for 1 or 2 minutes with the thumb till it becomes aching and distending.

4. Modification of Manipulation according to Different Syndromes

1) In the case of dizziness, nausea and vomiting, also wipe the forehead in two directions and press-knead Neiguan (P 6) and Waiguan (SJ 5).

2) In the case of aching, distending and dry eyes, press-knead Baihui (Du 20) and push Qiaogong point on the two laterals as well.

5. Course of Treatment: Once a day, 6 times as one course; with an interval of 3—5 days between two courses.

Dysraphism of Glottis

Dysraphism of glottis means that the glottal gap is over 1 mm wide. It is also called "phonasthenia" or "myasthenia", in TCM it is called "*shiyin*" (myasthenia), mostly seen in singers, actors and professional voiceusers.

一指推法推大椎穴2～3分钟。按揉肝俞，以酸胀为度。

2）平推颈背部，以热深透为度。

3）医者站于患者前面，以一指推法沿眼眶四周呈"∞"推动，推3～5分钟，然后以拇指端点按睛明、上明（眉弓中点、眶上缘下）、四白，以酸胀为度。

4）提拿肩井、合谷穴。

5）患者仰卧，以拇指按揉上明穴1～2分钟，以酸胀为度。

4．随证加减

1）伴有头晕、恶心、呕吐者，宜加分抹前额，按揉内、外关。

2）兼有两眼酸胀干涩者，宜加按揉百会，推两侧桥弓。

5．疗程：每日1次，6次为1疗程。各疗程之间间隔3～5天。

声门闭合不全

声门裂隙超过1毫米，称为声门闭合不全，又称"发声无力症"、"喉肌无力症"等。中医称之为"失音"。多见于声乐和戏剧演员以及职业用嗓者。

CLINICAL MANIFESTATION

In the case of a slight dysraphism, high vocalization is difficult, vocalization is short and mute, accompanied with dry throat and foreign body sensation. In case of a serious dysraphism, there's unfluent vocalization, crackling and hoarseness, accompanied with pharyngeal pain and sensation of sticky sputum. In indirect laryngoscopy, dysraphism of glottis varies in degrees and froms.

TREATMENT

Massage therapy has a reliable effect on this disease. In the course of treatment, forbid high vocalization and long-time talking ,eating pungent and stimulating food. If necessary, a temporary vocalization-forbiddence is needed.

1. Manipulation: Pushing with one-finger meditation, grasping, kneading, etc.

2. Location of Points: Lianquan (Ren 23), Renying (St 9), Shuitu (S5 10), Fengchi (GB 20), Fengfu (Du 16) and Yamen (Du 15).

3. Operation

1) The doctor, standing anterior-lateral to the sitting patient, pushes with the manipulation of one-finger meditation pushing from Lianquan (Ren 23) to Renying (St 9) and Shuitu (St 10) for 10 minutes, focusing on laryngeal protuberance. The manipulation should be light, soft and slow. Roughness is forbidden.

2) The doctor stands behind the patient, with the thumb and the four fingers, grasps the cervical part, focusing on Fengchi (GB 20); then pushes repeatedly with the thumb from Fengfu (Du 16) to Yamen (Du 15) for 2—3 minutes; finally press-kneads sternocleidonastoid muscles on the two laterals for 3—5 minutes with the first, middle and ring fingers.

4. Course of Treatment: Once a day, 5 times as one course.

【临床表现】

轻度闭合不全患者，发高音费力，发声不持久，声音变喑，同时伴有咽喉部干燥及异物感。重度闭合不全患者，发音不扬，出现破音，甚至声音嘶哑，伴有喉痛、痰粘感。间接喉镜检查，可见声门不同程度及不同形态的闭合不全。

【治疗】

推拿治疗本病，疗效可靠。治疗期间应避免高音、持久的讲话，必要时应短期禁发声，避免食用辛辣、刺激之品。

1. 手法：一指禅推、拿、揉等。

2. 取穴：廉泉、人迎、水突、风池、风府、哑门等。

3. 操作

1）患者坐位，医者站其侧前方，以一指禅推法，自廉泉推向人迎、水突穴，重点在喉结周围推之，约推10分钟。手法宜轻揉和缓，切忌粗暴。

2）医者站于患者身后，以拇指和其他四指提拿颈项部，重点拿风池穴，然后以拇指从风府推至哑门反复2～3分钟。最后以两手食、中、无名三指轻轻按揉两侧胸锁乳突肌3～5分钟。

4. 疗程：每日1次，5次为1疗程。

Chapter Three

Child Massage

Section 1

Common Manipulations

Child massage consists of a series of convenient and effective manipulations for treating children's diseases which took shape gradually in the course of long medical practice in accordance with the characteristics of children's physique, physiology, pathology and the forms and positions of the specific points. Children have inferior adaptability to outside irritations and poor ability to resist the attack of disease due to incomplete function of the *zang-fu* organs andtenderness of muscles and skin. Therefore, child massage puts more emphasis on softness, smoothness, steadiness, correctness and painlessness compared with the requirements of the manipulations for adults. Clinically, apart from the manipulations with strong stimulation needed for the treatment of infantile convulsion and syncope, all the other manipulations for children in general cases must be soft, slow, and moderate in strength, natural in changing of movement, appropriate in the extent of mobilizing the function of the manipulations and exclusive of excessive exertion of force. The treatment should not go beyond the desirable state that the affected children feel no pain and discomfort. Otherwise, their crying and struggling caused thereof will render the treatment unable to proceed. So, a doctor with rich experience often completes his manipulations while teasing and joking with the infantile patients. What is more, some medium such as talcum

第 三 章

小 儿 推 拿

第一节　常用手法

小儿推拿手法是根据小儿的形体、生理、病理以及特定穴位的形态和位置等特点，经过长期的医疗实践逐步形成的一套便于操作并且能有效地治疗小儿疾病的推拿手法。由于小儿脏腑机能尚未完善且肌肤娇嫩，所以接受外界刺激的能力较低，抵抗疾病的能力较差，故小儿推拿手法与成人推拿手法的要求相比，更强调轻柔、平稳、着实、正确与无痛。临床上，除治疗惊风、昏厥等症时需要用强力的刺痛性手法外，在通常情况下，其手法用力应轻柔缓和，用力大小要适度、深透，动作变化要自然流畅，手法作用要适达病所，不可竭力攻伐。在治疗过程中，以不使患儿感到疼痛不适为度，否则，会引起患儿哭闹、挣扎而使治疗无法进行。故经验丰富的医生，常在与患儿的逗笑、嬉戏中完成手法操作。

powder, ginger juice, the mixture of Chinese onion and ginger juice, peppermint water and egg white must be used in the course of massage so as to make the operation easier, the skin smoother and the treatment more effective.

In addition to the traditionally-called "the eight manipulations for children", namely, pressing, palm-rubbing, nipping, motioning, kneading, pushing, foulaging and rotating, there are still some other commonly used manipulations: grasping, piching, sqeezing, pounding, etc. Among all these manipulations, pressing, palm-rubbing, kneading, rocking and grasping are done basically the same way as those for adults. The only difference lies in that the intensity, frequency, direction and extent of the manipulations must be adjusted according to the characteristics of children. Although some of the manipulations bear the same names as those of the manipulations for adults, taking pushing for example, it is operated in entirely different ways. And some of the manipulations, taking motioning for example, only fit infants, not adults. As for the manipulations used for both children and adults, please refer to the related part in Section 1 of Chapter II in this book. Introduced here are only some other manipulations commonly used for children.

1. Straight-Pushing Manipulation

This manipulation means that the doctor pushes the point straightly with the radial or fingerprint surface of his thumb, or the flat of the index and middle fingers (Fig. 3—1).

ESSENTIALS OF MANIPULATION

The finger cushion used must be close to the skin of the point, operating from the beginning of the linear point to the end or from one point to another. The movement must be done straightly without obliquity. The strength used must be steady. You can't operate heavily only on the middle way while operate slightly at the beginning and the end. The operation can be a bit heavier but not too heavy. Otherwise, it will be diffi-

另外，许多小儿推拿的手法在操作时要使用介质，如滑石粉、姜汁、薄荷水、葱姜汁、鸡蛋清等，以方便操作，滑润皮肤，并增强疗效。

小儿推拿手法，除传统推拿学所称"小儿推拿八法"即按、摩、掐、运、揉、推、搓、摇八种手法外，常用的还有拿、捏、挤、捣等手法。其中，按、摩、揉、搓、摇、拿六法的术式与成人推拿手法基本相同，只是在具体应用时，其手法的强度、频率、方向以及动作的幅度要根据小儿的特点做适当的调整。有的手法如推法虽然在名称上和成人手法一样，但具体操作方法却完全不同。有些手法，如运法只用于小儿，而不用于成人。与成人推拿相同的手法术式，请参阅本书第二章第一节的有关内容。这里仅将其他几种小儿推拿常用手法介绍如下。

1. 直推法

以拇指桡侧面或罗纹面，或用食中二指指面，在穴位上做直线推动，称为"直推法"（图3-1）。

【动作要领】

操作时，着力指面要与穴位皮肤贴紧，从线状穴位的起点至终点，或从一个穴点向另一个穴点施术。推移的轨迹一定要沿直线进行，不得斜曲，同时，用力要着实。自起点至终点，用力的强度要均匀，不可只在中间用力，而在两端轻轻带过。用力可稍重，但又不要压得太重，因如果压得太重，会使动作滞涩，甚至

cult to operate smoothly, and the skin may be damaged. In addition, pushing method must be done with medium, 200-300 times in one minute.

CLINICAL APPLICATION

This manipulation is the most common one for children. It is suitable for all the linear points in the body and the case which requires the doctor to push from one point to another. Clinically, the doctor may use one hand to push along or against the course of the channel in one direction. It has the function of treating asthenia and reducing sthenia. Pushing along the point back and forth has the function of regulating *yin* and *yang*, improving the function of *zang*-organs and *fu*-organs. The doctor may push straightly in one direction along one line such as Kai Tianmen alternatively using two thumbs. Straight-pushing is considered the most commonly used manipulation for children in clinical practice.

2. Parting-pushing, Meeting-pushing

Pushing from the point to both its lateral sides using the radial or fingerprint surface of the two thumbs or the cushions of index and middle fingers is called "parting-pushing"; (Fig. 3–2) otherwise, pushing from two sides to meet at the center of the point is called "meeting-pushing" (Fig. 3–3).

ESSENTIALS OF MANIPULATION

The strength produced by the two hands must be even. No matter whether you push transversely or obliquetly, your hand movement must be straight. In some special cases such as separating *yin-yang*, you must do it with one hand slightly and the other hand heavily. In a word, the manipulation with the two hands must be coordinate.

CLINICAL APPLICATION

Parting-pushing is suitable for operating on the head, face, chest, abdomen, and back. Meeting-pushing is mainly suitable for *yin-yang* points on the hands, rarely used on other

擦破皮肤。此外，用推法时要使用介质，其频率每分钟 200～300次。

【临床应用】

本法是小儿推拿最常用的手法，适用全身所有线状穴位以及需要从一个穴点推向另一个穴点的情况。临床应用时，可以单手做顺经或逆经的单方向用力直推，有补虚泻实的治疗作用；也可沿直线在穴位上用力来回直推，有调和阴阳、脏腑功能的作用。另外，也可用双手拇指在一条路线上向同一方向交替直推，如开天门。可以说，直推法是小儿推拿临床使用频度最高的一种手法。

2. 分推法、合推法

用两手拇指桡侧或罗纹面，或用食、中指二指面，自穴位向两侧分推的操作方法称"分推法"（图3-2）。反之，如从穴位两端向中间推动，则称为"合推法"（图3-3）。

【动作要领】

操作时，双手用力要均匀一致，推动的方向无论是横向的或作"八"形的斜向分推，移动的轨迹都要保持直行。在某些特殊情况下，如在分阴阳时，有时双手用力要根据需要一轻一重。总之，双手动作要配合协调。

分推法主要适用于头面部、胸腹部与背部；合推法主要用于

parts.

3. Pinching

The manipulation which is done by using the cushions of the thumb, index and middle fingers (or the thumb and radial side of the middle part of arcuated index fingers) together to lift up the skin of the massaged region and move forwards while twisting the skin with two hands alternatively, is called pinching (Fig. 3–4).

ESSENTIALS OF MANIPULATION

During operation the skin on the child's back must be fully exposed and a right amount of talcum powder should be used in order to protect the skin. The strength for lifting must be moderate, and the pinching should not be so tight as to cause pain. The twirling must be in a straight way, and twisting or curving must be avoided.

CLINICAL APPLICATION

Clinically, the manipulation used for children on his spinal point is called "the spine pinching therapy". Please see the detailed introduction in Section 2 of this chapter "the Spine Pinching Method"

4. Arc-pushing

The manipulation which is done by the radial or fingerprint surface of the thumb or the cushion of the index or middle finger, and which reguires the doctor to push lightly in an arching or circling way around a point, is called arc-pushing (Fig. 3–5).

ESSENTIALS OF MANIPULATION

The strength used must be light and the speed of pushing must be slow. The rubbing should be soft and gentle and move along the operating line on the surface of the skin in a circling way. The strength used is much lighter than that for palm-rubbing. The frequency is 80–100 times in one minute.

CLINICAL APPLICATION

This manipulation which is light and slow is suitable for

推手阴阳穴，其他部位很少应用。

3．捏法

用拇指指面与食、中二指指面或用拇指指面与屈曲成弓状的食指中节桡侧面同时用力，将施术部位的皮肤挟持拿紧后向上提起，并双手交替捻动向前移动的手法，称为"捏法"（图3-4）。

【动作要领】

操作时，患儿背部的皮肤要充分暴露，并涂以适量的滑石粉，以保护皮肤。提拿的力量要适度，不可挟持得太紧，以免引起疼痛。捻动时要沿直线前进，不可拧转或歪斜。

【临床应用】

本法在小儿推拿临床应用中，主要用于在背穴上操作，称"捏脊疗法"。具体应用方法，详见本章第二节脊穴之后介绍的"捏脊法"。

4．运法

用拇指指面或桡侧面，也可用食指或中指指面，在一定穴位上作弧形或环形的轻轻推摩，称为"运法"（图3-5）。

【动作要领】

本法在操作时，用力宜轻，推运的速度要稍慢，不能太快。只是在体表沿着操作路线做轻柔缓和的摩擦旋绕，其用力较摩法为轻。操作频率为每分钟80～100次。

【临床应用】

本法轻柔缓和，多用于在手掌的特定穴位操作，如运八卦等。

the special points on the palm, such as arc-pushing Bagua. It performs the functions of dredging the muscles, tendons and channels and promoting blood circulation. It is often used to treat wind-heat cold, alternate attacks of chills and fever, dyspepsia, abdominal distention, borborygmus, etc.

5. Nipping

The manipulation which is done by the finger nails to irritate the point forcefully is called nipping (Fig. 3-6).

ESSENTIALS OF MANIPULATION

The manipulating point is the finger nail of the thumb. The essentials of the manipulation are just the same as the pressing manipulation. As the old saying goes "pressing by fingernail is nipping". The strength must be increased gradually. Attention must be paid to avoiding skin damage. Nipping-forcefully 3-5 times is necessary for each treatment.

CLINICAL APPLICATION

This is one of the manipulations with strong stimulation. It plays the roles of causing resuscitation and restoring consciousness, relieving convulsion, reducing fever, removing restlessness, and arresting spasm and pain. It is often used as the first aid manipulation to treat fainting spell. It proves effective in treating fainting spell, infantile convulsion, tic of limbs and high fever. The manipulation is often used along with kneading after nipping forcefully in order to relieve local pain and discomfort.

6. Squeezing

This manipulation is done by gripping the skin round the point with thumbs and index fingers together to lift the skin and then squeeze-press the point in opposite position in order to make the local part round the point become ecchymosis (Fig 3-7).

它具有宣通筋络、调和血脉的功能，常用于治疗风热感冒、寒热往来、食积不化、腹胀肠鸣等病证。

5. 掐法

用指甲重刺激穴位的方法称为"掐法"（图3-6）。

【动作要领】

掐法的着力点为拇指的指甲，其动作要领与按法同，故古人有"爪按为掐"的说法。操作时要逐渐用力，注意不要掐破皮肤，每次治疗重掐3～5次即可。

【临床应用】

本法为强刺激手法之一，具有开窍醒神、镇惊止掐、退热除烦、解痉止痛之功效。它常用作昏厥的急救手法，对昏厥、惊风、四肢抽搐、高热等症有良效。应用本法时，常在重掐局部后再用揉法，以缓解局部疼痛、不适之感。

6. 挤法

用两手拇、食指同时将穴位周围的皮肤挟持并轻轻提起，再相对用力挤压穴位，以使穴点处局部产生瘀斑的手法，称为"挤法"（图3-7）。

ESSENTIALS OF MANIPULATION

When operating, the gripping strength of the two hands on the skin round the point must not be too great, but it is necessary to squeeze and press the skin round the point in the direction towards the center, 4–5 times each treatment until ecchymosis appears.

CLINICAL APPLICATION

Squeezing-pressing can be done on the points to get spotted ecchymosis, it can also be done along the channel with the ecchymosis arranged in lines. This manipulation is often used on the points of Taiyang (Extra 2), Yintang (Extra 1) on the head, and the neck, chest, abdomen and back. It plays the roles of dispersing and relieving superficial syndrome, inducing menstruation to relieve mental depression, and dispelling localized nodule of soft tissues. It is mainly used to treat summer-heat, wind-cold due to exogenous evils, headache, nausea vomiting, seasickness, carsickness, etc.

7. Pounding

This manipulation is operated by the tip of the middle finger or the joint of the index and middle fingers, pounding at the certain points or parts regularly (Fig. 3–8).

ESSENTIALS OF MANIPULATION

The doctor uses his wrist joint as the center of the movement, pounding the point with elastic coordinate strength given by the wrist joint just like a dragonfly skimming the surface of the water. The doctor must move his hand away soon after pounding the point with moderate strength. Pound 10–15 times for each treatment. The essentials of the manipulation of the wrist joint can be seen in the part of striking-pounding manipulation" in Section 1 of Chapter Two.

CLINICAL APPLICATION

Though the strength given is less than the strength introduced in "striking-pounding manipulation" for adults, it is

【动作要领】

操作时，双手挟持穴位周围皮肤的力量不要太重，而主要是用力向中间挤压穴位处的皮肤。每次治疗重复挤压 4～5 次，以局部出现皮下出血的瘀斑为度。

【临床应用】

操作时，可按穴点做点状挤压，也可在身上循经络连续挤压出多个瘀斑瘀点、并使之排列成行。本法多用于头部的太阳、印堂等穴，以及颈项、胸腹及背部。有发散解表、通经疏郁、消散筋结之功效，主要用于治疗暑热、外感风寒、头痛、恶心呕吐、晕船晕车等病证。

7．捣法

用中指指端或用食指、中指屈曲后的近侧指间关节突起部为着力点，在一定的穴位或部位上做有节律地点击，称为"捣法"（图3-8）。

【动作要领】

操作时，要以腕关节为活动中心，用腕关节发出的富有弹性的协调力量来点击穴位，犹如蜻蜓点水，点击后旋即抬起术手，不要用力太重。每次治疗捣击 10～15 次即可。有关腕关节的动作要领，可参阅本书第二章第一节"击点法"中部分内容。

【临床应用】

本法用力虽较成人推拿手法中介绍的"击点法"为轻，但实为

one of the strong irritating manipulation of child massage. It has the functions of dredging the obstruction, expelling pathogenic cold, relieving pain and tranquilizing the mind. It is often used to treat infantile convulsion, fever, restlessness with fear, tic of limbs, etc.

Section 2

Commonly-used Points

Apart from the acupuncture points on the fourteen regular channels and *qixue* (extra-ordinary poir ts) introduced in Section 4 of Chapter One, there are some special points used for children. The characteristics of the points are: firstly, most points are not on the line of the fourteen regular channels; secondly, most of the points are distributed under elbow joints and knee joints of the limbs, especially on the palm and dorsum of the hand. As an old saying goes: "All the channels and collaterals of children converge in the hands." Because of the active *yang* at the extremities, they are sensitive to the stimuli from outside and liable to accept and transmit the stimuli to *zang*-organs and *fu*-organs in the body, and can produce curative effect. Additionally, the points used for children are divided into point form, linear form and reginal form, which are specially used for child massage, but rarely used for adults. These points are called special points in massage for children (Fig. 3–9, 3–10).

The effective points used in massotherapy for children have been found and named gradually since the Ming Dynasty. Up to now there are about 160 special points which can be looked up in books. There may be as many as 200 points including those in the operated parts for duplicate manipulations. Generally, the points used commonly in clinical practice, are

小儿推拿中一种具有较强刺激作用的手法。具有开导闭塞、祛寒止痛、镇惊安神的功能，常用于治疗惊风、发热、惊惕不安、四肢抽搐等病证。

第二节　常用穴位

小儿推拿临床用穴除了本书第一章第四节所介绍的十四经穴与奇穴外，尚有一些小儿推拿专用的特定穴位。这些穴位具有以下特点：一是多数穴位的位置不在十四经经络线上，二是多数分布在四肢的肘膝关节以下，尤多位于手掌与手背。古人谓"小儿百脉汇于两掌"，其四肢末梢的阳气比较活跃，因而对于手法等外界刺激的感觉亦较敏感，且易于接受并传递这些刺激至体内有关脏腑，从而发挥治疗作用。另外，小儿推拿特定穴的形态有点状、线状与面状之分。这些穴位在成人推拿中基本不被采用，只为小儿推拿所专用，故称为小儿推拿特定穴位（图3-9.3-10）。

自明代以来，小儿推拿的有效治疗穴点不断被发现并逐渐被定名。至今，有文献可查的特定穴已有 160 个左右，如果再加上复式手法的操作部位，则可达 200 个之多。但一般在临床上常用的穴位有 50～60 个左右，现将最常用的 54 个小儿推拿特定穴位

only about 50–60. Here are introduced 54 special points commonly used in massage for children.

1. Points on the Head and Face

Tianmen

Location: the part above the line between the eyebrows up to the anterior hair line.

Manipulation: Pushing straightly with radial surface or face of thumbs alternatively from below to above is called "opening Tianmen", also known as "pushing Zanzhu" (Fig. 3–11).

Frequency: 30–50 times.

Function: dispelling wind, relieving exterior syndrome, causing resuscitation and restoring consciousness, tranquilizing and allaying excitement.

Indication: fever, headache, cold without sweating or with obstructed sweating, listlessness, vigilance and restlessness.

Kangong

Location: along the eyebrow from the beginning to the end.

Manipulation: Parting-pushing from the beginning to the end of the eyebrow with the thumbs is called "pushing Kangong" (Fig. 3–12).

Frequency: 30–50 times.

Function: promoting diaphoresis, expelling superficial evils, restoring consciousness, improving vision, relieving headache.

Indication: fever due to exogenous evils, headache, dizziness, conjunctival congestion with pain, infantile convulsion.

Taiyang (Extra 2)

Location: in the depression about 1.0 cun posterior to the midpoint between the lateral ends of the eyebrows and the outer canthus

Manipulation: Pushing straightly backward with the radial surface of the two thumbs is called "pushing Taiyang". Knead-

介绍如下：

1. 头面部穴位

天门

位置：两眉中间直上，至前发际成一条直线。

操作：用两拇指桡侧面或两拇指指面自下而上交替直推，称为"开天门"，亦称"推攒竹"（图3-11）。

次数：30～50次。

作用：疏风解表，开窍醒神，镇静安神。

主治：发热，头痛，感冒无汗，或汗出不畅，精神萎靡，惊惕不安等。

坎宫

位置：自眉头起沿眉弓向眉梢成一横线。

操作：用两拇指自眉头向眉梢作分推，称为"推坎宫"（图3—12）。

次数：30～50次。

作用：发汗解表，醒脑明目，止头痛。

主治：外感发热，头痛，头晕，目赤痛，惊风。

太阳

位置：在眉梢与目外眦连线中点，向后约一寸凹陷中。

操作：用两拇指桡侧自前向后直推，称为"推太阳"；用中指

ing with the middle finger is called "kneading Taiyang" (Fig. 3–13). Kneading in the direction of the eye means reinforcing, in the direction of the ear means reducing.

Frequency: 30–50 times.

Function: dispersing wind, relieving exterior syndrome, clearing away pathogenic heat, improving the vision, relieving headache.

Indication: cold, fever, headache, infantile convulsion, conjunctival congestion with pain.

Erhougaogu

Location: in the depression inferior to postauditory process and superior to retroauricular hairline.

Manipulation: Kneading Erhougaogu with thumbs or tips of middle fingers is called "kneading Erhougaogu" (Fig 3–14).

Frequency: 30–50 times.

Function: relieving exterior syndrome by means of diaphoresis, tranquilizing convulsion and restlessness.

Indication: cold due to pathogenic wind, headache, infantile convulsion, restlessness. Pushing Zanzhu, Kangong, kneading Taiyang and Erhougaogu are called "the four major manipulations", used coordinatively to treat cold, headache, dizziness, redness, swelling and pain of the eye.

Renzhong (Du 26)

Location: at the junction of the superior 1/3 and middle 2/3 of the philtrum.

Manipulation: Nipping Renzhong (Du 26) with the nail of the thumb is called "nipping Renzhong" (Fig. 3–15).

Frequency: 5 times or stop immediately after the patient comes to himself.

Function: restoring consciousness, causing resuscitation.

Indication: infantile convulsion, syncope, tic.

Yingxiang (LI 20)

Location: 0.5 *cun* lateral to the midpoint of the lateral

端揉，称为"揉太阳"（图3-13）。向眼方向揉为补，向耳方向揉为泻。

次数：30～50次。

作用：疏风解表，清热明目，止头痛。

主治：感冒，发热，头痛，惊风，目赤痛。

耳后高骨

位置：耳后入发际高骨下凹陷中。

操作：用两拇指或中指端揉，称为"揉耳后骨"（图3-14）。

次数：30～50次。

作用：发汗解表，镇惊除烦。

主治：伤风感冒，头痛，惊风抽搐，烦躁不安。

以上推攒竹、推坎宫、揉太阳、揉耳后高骨四法合称为"四大手法"，可协同治疗感冒，头痛，头晕，目赤肿痛病证等。

人中

位置：在人中沟的上1/3与下2/3的交界处。

操作：用拇指甲掐之，称为"掐人中"（图3-15）。

次数：掐5次，或醒后即止。

作用：醒神开窍。

主治：惊风，昏厥，抽搐。

迎香

位置：鼻翼外缘中点旁开0.5寸，鼻唇沟中。

border of ala nasi, in the nasolabial groove.

Manipulation: Pushing-kneading up and down along the edge of the upper nasal bone at both sides of the nose with separated index and middle fingers is called "kneading Yingxiang", also known as "Huangfeng Rudong (wasp entering its comb)". Kneading-slightly into the child's nostrils with the index and middle fingers is also called "wasp entering its comb" (Fig. 3–16). The effect is just as the same as the former.

Frequency: 20–30 times.

Function: relieving superficial syndrome by means of diaphoresis, clearing the nasal passage, promoting the dispersing function of the lung.

Indication: cold due to pathogenic wind, stuffed running nose, chronic rhinitis.

Tianzhugu

Location: The straight line from the middle of the hairline to Dazhui (Du 14).

Manipulation: Pushing Tianzhugu with the thumb or the index and middle fingers straightly downward is called "pushing Tianzhugu" (Fig. 3–17), or scraping with a spoon dipped with some water.

Frequency: scraping 100–500 times or till lihgt ecchymoma appears.

Function: lowering the adverse flow of qi, stopping vomiting, expelling wind and clearing away coid.

Indication: vomiting, nausea, stiffness of the neck, fever, sore throat, infantile convulsion.

2. Points on the Chest and Abdomen

Tiantu (Ren 22)

Location: at the center of the suprasternal fossa.

Manipulation: Pressing or kneading Tiantu with the index or the tip of the middle finger is called "pressing or kneading Tiantu"

操作：以食、中两指分开，在鼻翼两侧鼻骨边缘处，上下推揉之，称为"揉迎香"，又称"黄蜂入洞"。若以食、中二指轻入患儿两鼻孔揉之，亦称黄蜂入洞(图3-16)。功效与前者相同。

次数：20～30次。

作用：发汗解表，通鼻窍，宣通肺气。

主治：伤风感冒，鼻塞流涕，慢性鼻炎等。

天柱骨

位置：项后发际正中至大椎穴成一直线。

操作：用拇指或食、中二指自上而下直推，称为"推天柱骨"(图3-19)；或用汤匙边蘸水自上而下刮。

次数：推100～500次，或刮至皮下轻度瘀血为度。

作用：降逆止呕，祛风散寒。

主治：呕吐，恶心，项强，发热，咽痛，惊风等。

2．胸腹部穴位

天突

位置：胸骨上窝正中。

操作：用食指或中指端按或揉，称为"按天突"或"揉天突"(图

(Fig. 3–18). Pinching-squeezing the point with the thumb and the index finger is called "pinching-squeezing Tiantu".

Frequency: press and knead 10–15 times each. Pinch and squeeze till stasis of blood with red-purple colour appears.

Function: regulating the flow of qi, resolving phlegm lowering the adverse flow of qi, relieving asthma, stopping vomiting.

Indication: stuffiness in the chest, cough with dyspnea, accumulation of phlegm with rapid breathing, nausea, vomiting, sore throat.

Tanzhong (Ren 17)

Location: On the anterior midline at the level with the fourth intercostal space, midpoint between the two nipples.

Manipulation: Kneading with the tip of the middle finger is called "kneading Tanzhong" (Fig. 3–19). Pushing-side-wise with the two hands from the point to the left and right nipples is called "parting-pushing Tanzhong" (Fig 3–20). Pushing down from the castal incisures of the sternum to xiphoid process with the index and middle fingers is called "pushing Tanzhong".

Frequency: pushing or kneading 100–200 times.

Function: soothing the chest, regulating the flow of qi, relieving cough and reducing sputum.

Indication: stuffiness in the chest, rale, cough, dyspnea, vomiting, nausea, hiccup, etc.

Rugen (St 18)

Location: 0.2 *cun* below the breast.

Manipulation: kneading with the tip of the index or middle finger is called "kneading Rugen" (Fig. 3–21).

Frequency: 100–200 times.

Function: soothing the liver, regulating the circulation of qi, resolving sputum and relieving cough.

Indication: stuffiness in the chest, chest pain, cough, dyspnea,

3—18）。用两手拇，食指捏挤天突穴，称"捏挤天突"。

次数：按、揉均为 10～15 次；捏挤至皮下淤血呈红紫 色 为度。

作用：理气化痰，降逆平喘，止呕。

主治：胸闷，咳喘，痰壅气急，恶心，呕吐，咽痛等。

膻中

位置：前正中线，平第四肋间隙处，相当于两乳之间连线的中点。

操作：以中指端揉称为"揉膻中"（图3-19）；以两拇指自穴中向两旁分推至乳头名"分推膻中"（图3-20）；用食、中二指自胸骨切迹向下推至剑突名"推膻中"。

次数：推或揉均为 100～200 次。

作用：宽胸理气，止咳化痰。

主治：胸闷，痰鸣，咳嗽，气喘，恶心，呕吐，呃逆等。

乳根

位置：乳下 2 分。

操作：以食指或中指端揉之，称为"揉乳根"（图3-21）。

次数： 100～200 次。

作用：舒肝理气，化痰止咳。

主治：胸闷，胸痛，咳嗽，气喘。

Rupang

Location: 0.2 *cun* lateral to the breast.

Manipulation: Kneading Rupang with the index or middle finger is called "kneading Rupang". Clinically, it is often used in the combination with Rugen. The doctor uses his index and middle fingers at the same time (Fig. 3-21).

Frequency: 100-200 times.

Function: soothing the chest oppression, regulating the flow of *qi*, relieving cough and reducing sputum.

Indication: stuffiness in the chest, cough, rale, vomiting.

Xielei (Hypochondrium)

Location: from the two hypochondria under the armpits to Tianshu (St. 25).

Manipulation: Ask the sick child to raise his hands or put the hands on the shoulder. The doctor uses both of his palms to do foulaging-rubbing manipulation from the hypochondria under the armpits to Tianshu. It is called "foulaging-rubbing Xielei", also known as "foulaging-rubbing while touching strings" (Fig. 3-22).

Frequency: 100-300 times.

Function: keeping the adverse *qi* downwards, reducing sputum, relieving stuffiness in the chest and mass in the abdomen.

Indication: stuffiness in the chest, hypochondriac pain, abdominal distention, phlegm-dyspnea, rapid breathing, infantile malnutrition, hepatosplenomegaly.

Fu (Abdomen)

Location: On the abdomen.

Manipulation: Parting-pushing obliquely down with the face of the thumbs or ribbed surface of the index, middle, ring and little fingers simultaneously from Zhongwan (Ren 12) (midpoint between the xiphoid process and navel) point to both sides is called "parting-pushing Fu yin-yang" (Fig. 3-24). Rubbing the abdomen with the palm or the four fingers is called "rubbing the abdomen" (Fig. 3-23). Palm-rubbing

乳旁

位置：乳外旁开 2 分。

操作：以食指或中指端揉，称为"揉乳旁"。临床多乳根、乳旁配合应用，以食、中二指同时操作(图3-21)。

次数：100～200次。

作用：宽胸理气，止咳化痰。

主治：胸闷，咳嗽，痰鸣，呕吐。

胁肋

位置：从腋下两胁至天枢处。

操作：令患儿两手抬起，或放于肩上，医者以两手掌从患儿两胁腋下搓摩至天枢处，称为"搓摩胁肋"，又称"按弦走搓摩"(图3-22)。

次数：100～300次。

作用：顺气，化痰，除胸闷，开积聚。

主治：胸闷，胁痛，腹胀，痰喘气急，疳积，肝脾肿大等。

腹

位置：腹部。

操作：用两手拇指面或食、中、无名和小指指腹，同时自中脘穴(剑突与肚脐连线的中点)斜下向两旁分推，称为"分推腹阴阳"(图3-24)；用掌或两指摩腹部，称为"摩腹"(图3-23)。逆时

adversely means reinforcing, otherwise, means reducing.

Frequency: parting-pushing abdominal *Yin-Yang* 100–200 times, palm-rubbing *Fu* for 5 minutes.

Function: regulating *qi*, promoting digestion, lowering the adverse flow of *qi*, relieving vomiting, strengthening the spleen and stomach.

Indication: abdominal pain, abdominal distention, indigestion, nausea, vomiting, food retention in stomach, and anorexia. The effect of parting-pushing *Fu Yin-Yang* is good at regulating the stomach and *qi*, lowering the adverse flow of *qi*, and relieving vomiting. So it is often used to treat abdominal distention, nausea and vomiting. Palm-rubbing the abdomen is good at strengthening the spleen and promoting digestion. So it is often used to treat indigestion, anorexia, etc. In addition, palm-rubbing abdomen with reducing manipulation can be used to treat constipation.

Umbilicus (Shenque Ren 8)

Location: in the center of the umbilicus.

Manipulation: Kneading it with the tip of the middle finger or the root of the palm is called "kneading the umbilicus" (Fig. 3–25). Rubbing it with the palm or the index, middle, ring and little fingers is called "rubbing the umbilicus" (Fig. 3–26). Kneading-rubbing it counterclockwise means reinforcing, otherwise means reducing. But if you do it half clockwise and half counterclockwise, it means uniform reinforcing-reducing manipulation. Kneading-shaking it with the thumb and the index, middle fingers by holding the umbilicus is also called "kneading the umbilicus". Pinching-squeezing the region around the umbilicus with the thumb and index finger till light stasis of blood appears is called "pinching-squeezing the umbilicus".

Frequency: kneading 100–300 times, rubbing 5 minutes.

Function: warming *yang*, dispelling cold, replenishing and restoring *qi* and blood, strengthening the spleen and stomach, relieving dyspepsia.

针方向摩为补，顺时针方向摩为泻。

次数：分推腹阴阳 100～200 次；摩腹 5 分钟。

作用：理气消食，降逆止呕，健脾和胃。

主治：腹痛，腹胀，消化不良，恶心，呕吐，积滞，厌食等。

分推腹阴阳善于和胃理气，降逆止呕，多用于治疗腹胀、恶心、呕吐；摩腹偏于健脾消食，多用于消化不良、积滞、厌食等。此外，摩腹用泻法还可用于治疗便秘。

脐（神阙）

位置：即肚脐中。

操作：用中指端或掌根揉之，称为"揉脐"（图3-25）；用手掌或食、中、无名，小指摩，称"摩脐"；逆时针方向揉摩为补，顺时针方向揉摩为泻（图3-26），顺时针和逆时针各半为平补平泻；用拇指和食、中二指抓住肚脐抖揉，亦称"揉脐"；以拇食指捏挤脐四周，至轻度瘀血为止，称为"捏挤肚脐"。

次数：揉 100～300 次；摩 5 分钟。

作用：温阳散寒，补益气血，健脾和胃，消食导滞。

Indication: abdominal distention, abdominal pain, dyspepsia, constipation, borborygmus, vomiting and diarrhea.

Dantian (Elixir Field)

Location: on the lower abdomen, between 2 and 3 *cun* under the umbilicus.

Manipulation: Kneading, rubbing it with the ribbed surface of thumb or middle finger or palm area of index, middle, ring and little fingers is called "kneading-Dantian" or "rubbing Dantian" (Fig. 3–27). Kneading and rubbing it counterclockwise means reinforcing, otherwise means reducing. Parting-pushing down from the umbilicus with the face of the thumb or the center of the palm is called "pushing Dantian". Pressing it with the face of the thumb or the middle finger or the palm which pressed lightly and slowly during respiration while moving with the movement of the abdomen during inspiration, is called "pressing Dantian".

Frequency: 100–300 times.

Function: reinforcing the kidney, strengthening the body resistance, warming *yang*, dispelling cold, separating the useful from the waste.

Indication: pain in the lower abdomen, diarrhea, enuresis, prolapse of rectum, hernia, uroschesis, scanty dark urine, weakness.

Dujiao

Location: lateral to the umbilicus, on the strong tendons of both sides of the abdomen (In other words, it is 2 *cun* below and 2 *cun* lateral to the umbilicus).

Manipulation: Grasping the abdominal tendons on both sides with the thumb, index and middle fingers of the two hands at the same time in depth is called "grasping Dujiao" (Fig. 3–28). Pressing it with the middle finger is called "pressing Dujiao".

Frequency: 3–5 times.

Function: relieving abdominal pain, dispelling abdominal distention, strengthening the spleen and stomach, regulating the

主治：腹胀，腹痛，食积，便秘，肠鸣，呕吐，腹泻。

丹田

位置：小腹部（脐下 2 寸与 3 寸之间）。

操作：用拇指或中指指腹或用食、中、无名和小指四指指面揉、摩，称为"揉丹田"或"摩丹田"（图3-27）。逆时针方向揉、摩为补，顺时针方向揉、摩为泻；用拇指面或掌心自脐向下直推，称为"推丹田"；用拇指指腹或中指指腹或手掌按丹田部，呼气时轻压慢按，吸气时略随腹壁而起，称"按丹田"。

次数：100～300 次。

作用：培肾固本，温阳散寒，泌别清浊。

主治：小腹痛，腹泻，遗尿，脱肛，疝气，尿潴留，小便短赤，体虚。

肚角

位置：脐旁，腹部两侧大筋（另一种说法是在脐下 2 寸 旁 开 2 寸）。

操作：用双手拇、食、中三指同时向深处拿双侧肚筋，称为"拿肚角"（图3-28）；用中指端按，称为"按肚角"。

次数：3～5 次。

作用：止腹痛，消腹胀，健脾和胃，理气消滞。

flow of qi, promoting digestion.

Indication: abdominal pain, diarrhea, abdominal distention, dysentry, constipation.

Pressing-intervally or pressing-digging Dujiao are the main manipulation to relieve abdominal pain. It can also be used to treat abdominal pain caused by any other reasons, especially good at treating abdominal pain caused by cold and indigestion.

3. Points on the Lumbodorsal Area

Jianjing (GB 21)

Location: midway between Dazhui (DU 14) and the acromion.

Manipulation: Lifting-grasping the scapulo-tendon symmetrically with the thumb and index, middle fingers heavily is called "grasping Jianjing"(Fig. 3–29). Pressing on the point with middle finger is called "pressing Jianjing". Nipping-pressing the patient's Jianjing with middle finger of left hand while grasping the patient's index and ring fingers, which are forced to be straight and swaying with thumb, index and middle fingers of right hand is called "general ending manipulation".

Frequency: pressing or grasping 5 times each.

Function: removing obstruction in qi and blood circulation, relieving superficial syndrome by means of diaphoresis.

Indication: cold, infantile convulsion, raising disorder of the upper limbs. This can also be used as ending manipulation.

Dazhui (Du 14)

Location: Below the spinous process of the 7th cervical vertebra.

Manipulation: Kneading it with the thumb or middle finger is called "kneading Dazhui" (Fig. 3–30); pinching the skin with the thumb and index fingers, or holding the skin with the middle part of the bent index and middle fingers along with the movement of holding and going off is called "lifting-pinching

主治：腹痛，腹泻，腹胀，痢疾，便秘。

按、拿肚角是止腹痛的要法，对各种原因引起的腹痛均可应用，特别是对寒痛、伤食痛效果尤佳。

3. 腰背部穴位

肩井

位置：在大椎穴与肩峰连线之中点。

操作：用拇指与食、中二指对称用力提拿肩筋，称为"拿肩井"（图3-29）；用中指端按其穴，称为"按肩井"；以左手中指掐按患儿肩井，右手拇、食、中三指拿患儿食指和无名指，使其伸直摆动，称为"总收法"。

次数：按、拿均为 5 次。

作用：宣通气血，发汗解表。

主治：感冒，惊厥，上肢抬举不利。本法可作为结束手法。

大椎

位置：第七颈椎棘突下。

操作：用拇指或中指端揉，称为"揉大椎"（图3-30）；用拇、食指指端捏住皮肤或以屈曲的食、中指中节夹住皮肤，用力作一拉

Dazhui", which is also known as "pulling Dazhui"; pinching the skin with the thumbs and index fingers, and squeezing in opposite direction is called "pinching-squeezing Dazhui."

Frequency: kneading 20–30 times, lifting-pinching and squeezing-pinching till stasis of blood appears.

Function: clearing away pathogenic heat and relieving exterior syndrome.

Indication: cold, fever, stiffness of neck, cough. Lifting-pinching manipulation is effective for whooping cough.

Feishu (UB 13)

Location: 1.5 *cun* lateral to the lower border of the spinous process of the 3rd thoracic vertebra.

Manipulation: Kneading it with the tips of the thumbs orindex and middle fingers is called "kneading Feishu" (UB 13) (Fig 3–31). Pushing from the inner border of the scapula in the direction from above to below with radial surface or faces of thumbs is called "pushing Feishu" or "parting-pushing scapula" (Fig. 3–32).

Frequency: kneading 50–100 times, pushing 100–300 times.

Function: clearing away pathogenic heat, promoting the dispersing function of the lung, soothing chest oppression, regulating the flow of *qi*, restoring *qi* and relieving cough.

Indication: cough, asthma, rale, stuffiness and pain in the chest, fever.

Ji (Spine)

Location: the straight line between Dazhui (Du 14) and Changqiang (Du 1).

Manipulation: Pushing straightly it with faces of index and middle fingers from above to below is called "pushing the spine" (Fig. 3–33). Pinching it from below to above is called "pinching spine" (Fig. 3–34)

Frequency: pushing 100–300 times, pinching 3–5 times.

Function: pushing the spine plays the roles of clearing away

一放动作，称为"提捏大椎"，亦称"扯大椎"；用两手拇、食指捏起皮肤相对用力挤，称为"挤捏大椎"。

次数：揉 20～30 次；提捏，挤捏至皮下瘀血为度。

作用：清热解表。

主治：感冒，发热，项强，咳嗽。其中，提捏法对百日咳有一定疗效。

肺俞

位置：第三胸椎棘突下，旁开 1.5 寸处。

操作：用两拇指或食、中两指端揉，称为"揉肺俞"（图3-31）；用两手拇指桡侧或拇指面分别自肩胛骨内缘从上而下推动，称为"推肺俞"或"分推肩胛骨"（图3-32）。

次数：揉 50～100 次；推 100～300 次。

作用：清热宣肺，宽胸理气，补虚止咳。

主治：咳嗽，哮喘，痰鸣，胸闷、胸痛，发热等。

脊

位置：大椎至长强成一条直线。

操作：用食、中二指指面自上而下直推，称为"推脊"（图3-33）；用捏法自下而上，称为"捏脊"（图3-34）。

次数：推脊 100～300次；捏脊 3～5 遍。

作用：推脊能清热泻火、通便。捏脊能调阴阳、补气血、和

pathogenic heat, purging pathogenic fire and relaxing the bowels. Pinching spine plays the roles of regulating *yin* and *yang*, invigorating *qi* and blood, regulating the *zang*-organs and *fu*-organs, clearing and activating the channels and collaterals, reinforcing the primordial *qi*, promoting appetite, and improving health.

Indication: Pushing the spine can be used to treat cold, fever, constipation, vomiting and acute infantile convulsion. Pinching the spine can be used to treat infantile malnutrition, diarrhea, abdominal pain, chronic infantile convulsion, infantile anorexia, muscular emaciation, etc.

Annex: Pinching Spine Manipulation

Manipulation

① Put some medium on the child's back, massage lightly along the middle of spine from above to below for 3 times, to the make muscle relax and, *qi* and blood blow freely.

② Lift-grasp the skin heavily with the palmar face of the thumb which is held out against the skin, index and middle fingers, and twist forword with two hands alternatively; or bend the index finger, and apply its radial surface against the skin part. Lift-grasp the skin heavily with it and the thumb and twist forward, with the two hands moving alternatively, from the end of coccyx to Dazhui point.

③ While pinching for the second or third time, lift up the skin heavily with the thumbs, index and middle fingers or with the thumb, index finger after 2—3 movements of pinching. Sometimes you can hear the sound "*Ka*". Some corresponding *Shu* points on the back can be lifted according to the cases.

④ At last, press, knead Shenshu (UB 23) (1.5 *cun* lateral to the lower border of the spinous process of the 2nd lumbar vertebra) several times to end the treatment.

Clinical Application

The manipulation used singly is called "pinching spine

脏腑、通经络、培元气、促进饮食、增强体质。

主治：推脊善治感冒、发热、便秘、呕吐、急惊风等。捏脊可用于治疗疳积、腹泻、腹痛、慢惊风、小儿厌食症、肌肉消瘦等。

附：捏脊法

操作：①先在患儿背部涂些介质，由上而下沿脊柱正中轻轻按摩三遍，使肌肉松弛，气血流畅。

②用拇指指面顶住皮肤，食、中指前按，三指同时用力提拿皮肤，双手交替捻动向前；或食指屈曲，用食指中节桡侧顶住皮肤，拇指向前按，两指同时用力提拿皮肤，双手交替捻动向前，一从尾骨端直到大椎穴为止。

③捏第二或第三遍时，每捏2～3下即以双手拇、食、中三指或拇、食二指用力将皮肤向上提一次，有时可听到"咔"的响声，可根据具体的病情，重提几处相应的背部俞穴。

④最后用两拇指按揉肾俞穴（第二腰椎棘突下，旁开1.5寸，左右各一）数次，结束治疗。

临床应用：本法单用称为"捏脊疗法"，因对积滞有较好的治

therapy". It is also called "pinching therapy for indigestion" because it is effective for treating digestive disorders and malnutrition of children. The manipulation can also be used to treat infantile anorexia, infantile malnutrition and diarrhea, with good effect. It is also suitable for children's health care, and for insomnia, enterogastric disorder and irregular menstruation in adults. If the manipulation is used together with pinching-kneading or pushing Sihengwen, it will be more effective in treatment of infantile malnutrition.

Qijiegu

Location: the line from the fourth lumbar vertebra to caudal vertebra.

Manipulation: ① push-up Qijiegu: push straightly from coccyx up to the fourth lumbar vertebra with the radial surface of thumb or ribbed surface of index and middle fingers (Fig. 3—35).

② push-down Qijiegu: Push from the fourth lumbar vertebra to the end of coccyx with the radial surface of the thumb or the faces of index and middle fingers (Fig. 3–35).

Frequency: 100—300 times.

Function: Pushing-up Qijiegu plays the roles of warming *yang* and relieving diarrhea; pushing-down Qijiegu plays the role of expelling pathogenic heat to loosen the bowels.

Indication: Pushing-up Qijiegu can be used to treat diarrhea of asthenia-cold type, persistent dysentry, enuresis, and prolapse of rectum. Pushing-down Qijiegu can be used to treat constipation due to heat in the bowel, dysentry, and abdominal distention.

Guiwei

Location: at the end of caudal vertebra.

Manipulation: Kneading it with tip of thumb or middle finger is called "kneading Guiwei" (Fig. 3—36).

Frequency: 100—300 times.

Function: relieving diarrhea and relaxing the bowels.

疗作用，故又称"捏积疗法"。本法对小儿厌食症、疳积、泄泻等症均有很好的治疗效果，并可用于小儿保健，以及成人失眠、肠胃病、月经不调等证。若本法与掐、揉或推四横纹合用，对治疗疳积、腹泻等证效果更佳。

七节骨

位置：从第四腰椎至尾椎骨端成一直线。

操作：①推上七节骨：用拇指桡侧面或食、中二指指腹，自尾骨端直上，向第四腰椎直推（图3-35）。

②推下七节骨：用拇指桡侧面或食、中二指指腹自第四腰椎推至尾骨端（图3-35）。

次数：100～300次。

作用：推上七节骨能温阳止泻，推下七节骨可泻热通便。

主治：推上七节骨用于治疗虚寒性腹泻、久痢、遗尿、脱肛；推下七节骨则用于治疗肠热便秘、痢疾、腹胀。

龟尾

位置：尾椎骨端。

操作：用拇指指端或中指端揉，称为"揉龟尾"（图3-36）。

次数：100～300次。

作用：止泻，通便。

Indication: diarrhea, dysentry, constipation, prolapse of rectum, enuresis.

4. Points on the Upper Limds

Pijing

Location: on the red-white border of the radial surface of the thumbs, the straight line from the finger tip to the end.

Manipulation: Pushing from the tip of the thumb to the root with the child's thumb bent slightly is called "reinforcing Pijing" (Fig. 3—37), while pushing from the root to the tip of the thumb which keeps straight is called "clearing Pijing". Pushing back and forth plays the role of uniform reinforcing-reducing. It is called "clearing-reinforcing Pijing". Reinforcing, clearing and clearing-reinforcing Pijing are all called "pushing Pijing".

Frequency: 100—500 times.

Function: Reinforcing Pijing plays the roles of strengthening the spleen and stomach, invigorating qi and enriching the blood. Clearing Pijing plays the roles of clearing away damp-heat, resolving phelgm and relieving vomiting. Clearing-reinforcing Pijing plays the role of eliminating indigested food.

Indication: Reinforcing Pijing is mainly used to treat debility, anorexia, emaciation of muscle, lassitude and indigestion. Clearing Pijing is mainly used to treat jaundice, dampness-phlegm syndrome, hematochezia, nausea, vomiting, diarrhea, dysentry, constipation, etc. Clearing-reinforcing Pijing can be used to treat fullness in the stomach, acid regurgitation, anorexia, diarrhea, vomiting, etc. Reinforcing Pijing is often used for children with weak spleen and stomach. Clearing manipulation can be used for strong children.

Ganjing

Location: at the end part of the index finger of the palm area.

Manipulation: Pushing from the fingerprint at the end

主治：腹泻，痢疾，便秘，脱肛，遗尿。

4．上肢部穴位

脾经

位置：在拇指桡侧赤白肉际，自指尖至指根成一条直线。

操作：使患儿微屈拇指，自指尖推向指根为补，称为"补脾经"（图3—37）；使患儿拇指伸直，自指根推向指尖为 清，称 为"清脾经"；来回推为平补平泻，名"清补脾经"。补脾经、清脾经和清补脾经统称为"推脾经"。

次数：100～500次。

作用：补脾经能健脾胃、补气血；清脾经善清湿热、化痰涎、止呕吐；清补脾经则能消食滞。

主治：补脾经主治体质虚弱、食欲不振、肌肉消瘦、精神萎靡、消化不良等症；清脾经善治黄疸、湿痰、便血、恶心、呕吐、腹泻、痢疾、便秘等症；清补脾经可用于治疗饮食停滞引起的胃脘痞满、吞酸恶食、腹泻、呕吐等症。

小儿脾胃较弱，脾经多用补；体壮邪实者，方可用清。

肝经

位置：在食指掌面末节。

操作：用推法自食指掌面末节指纹起向指尖推为清，名"清

part of the index finger on the palm surface to finger tip is called "clearing Ganjing" (Fig. 3—38). It is also known as "calming the liver". Pushing from the end part plays a role of reinforcing, called "reinforcing Ganjing". Clearing Ganjing and reinforcing Ganjing are called "pushing Ganjing".

Frequency: 100—500 times.

Function: Clearing Ganjing plays the roles of calming the liver and removing fire from the liver, relieving depression, removing restlessness, and relieving convulsion and spasm. Reinforcing Ganjing plays the roles of nourishing *yin*, calming the liver, regulating *qi*, and enriching the blood.

Indication: infantile convulsion, conjunctival congestion, restlessness, dysphoria with feverish sensation in chest, palms and soles, bitter taste, dry throat, dizziness, headache, tinnitus, etc. The Liver Channel should be heat-cleared other than reinforced. If the liver is weak and needs reinfo rcing, reducing must be given after reinforcing or by reinforcing Shenjing instead, called "nourishing the kidney and liver".

Xinjing

Location: at the end part of the middle finger on palm surface.

Manipulation: Pushing from the transverse crease near the fingerprint of the middle finger to finger tip is called "clearing Xinjing" (Fig. 3—39), while pushing in the opposite direction called "reinforcing Xinjing". Clearing Xinjing, reinforcing Xinjing are called "pushing Xinjing."

Frequency: 100—500 times.

Function: Clearing Xinjing plays the roles of clearing away heat and purging pathogenic fire in the heart; reinforcing Xinjing plays the roles of enriching the heart-blood and nourishing the heart to calm the mind.

Indication: Clearing Xinjing can be used to treat pyrexia with delirium, dysphoria with feverish sensation in the chest, palms and soles, oral ulceration, difficulty and dark urine, and

肝经"(图3—38)，亦称为"平肝"；反之为补，名"补肝经"。清肝经、补肝经统称为"推肝经"。

次数：100～500次。

作用：清肝经能平肝泻火，解郁除烦，息风镇惊；补肝经可养阴镇肝，和气生血。

主治：惊风，目赤，烦躁不安，五心烦热，口苦咽干,头晕,头痛，耳鸣等。

肝经宜清不宜补。若肝虚确需补时则应补后加清，或以补肾经代之，称为"滋肾养肝法"。

心经

位置：在手中指掌面末节。

操作：用推法自中指掌面末节指纹起推向指尖为清，称为"清心经"(图3—39)；反之为补，名"补心经"。清心经、补心经统称为"推心经"。

次数：100～500次。

作用：清心经能清热泻心火；补心经能补益心血，养心安神。

主治：清心经可用于治疗高热神昏，五心烦热，口舌生疮，

frightening with restlessness; reinforcing Xinjing can be used to treat deficiency of heart blood, sweating, listlessness, restlessness, and sleeping with eyes open. Xinjing should be cleared rather than reinforced. If reinforcing manipulation is used, clearing must be added or reinforcing Pijing can be used instead.

Feijing

Location: at palm surface of the end of the ring finger.

Manipulation: Pushing from the transverse crease near the fingerprint of the ring finger to its tip is called "clearing Feijing" (Fig. 3—40); pushing in the opposite direction is called "reinforcing Feijing". Clearing Feijing and reinforcing Feijing are called "pushing Feijing".

Frequency: 100—500 times.

Function: Clearing Feijing plays the roles of promoting the dispersing function of the lung, clearing away pathogenic heat, dispelling wind, relieving exterior syndrome, relieving cough and reducing sputum. Reinforcing Feijing plays the roles of replenishing and restoring the lung-qi.

Indication: Clearing Feijing can be used to treat cold, fever, cough, dyspnea, rale, stuffiness in the chest, etc. Reinforcing Feijing can be used to treat cough due to insufficiency of the lung-qi, shortness of breath, pale face, spontaneous perspiration, chillness and prolapse of rectum.

Shenjing

Location: from the tip of little finger to the root of palm, on the palm aspect of the little finger, slightly towards ulna.

Manipulation: Pushing from the palm root to the tip of the little finger is called "reinforcing Shenjing" (Fig. 3—41); pushing in an opposite direction is called "clearing Shenjing". Clearing and reinforcing shenjing are called "pushing Shenjing".

Frequency: 100—500 times.

Function: Reinforcing Shenjing plays the roles of tonifying the kidney, and strengthening the brain, muscles and bones; clearing Shenjing, clearing away heat and diu-

小便赤涩、惊惕不安等症；补心经则用于治疗心血不足、汗出无神、心烦不安、睡卧露睛等。

心经宜清不宜补。需用补法时，可补后加清，或以补脾经代之。

肺经

位置：在手无名指掌面末节。

操作：用推法，自无名指掌面末节指纹起推至指尖为清，称为"清肺经"（图3—40）；反之为补，名"补肺经"。清肺经、补肺经统称为"推肺经"。

次数：100～500次。

作用：清肺经能宣肺清热，疏风解表，止咳化痰；补肺经能补益肺气。

主治：清肺经可用于治疗感冒、发热、咳嗽、气喘、痰鸣、胸闷等症；补肺经则用于治疗肺气虚损之咳嗽、气短、面白、自汗、畏寒以及脱肛等症。

肾经

位置：在小指掌面稍偏尺侧，自小指尖直至掌根。

操作：用推法，自掌根推至小指尖为补，名"补肾经"（图3—41）；反之为清，称为"清肾经"。补肾经和清肾经统称为"推肾经"。

次数：100～500次。

作用：补肾经能补肾益脑，强健筋骨；清肾经则能清热利

resis.

Indication: Reinforcing Shenjing can be used to treat congenital defect, weakness due to chronic disease, chronic diarrhea due to kidney deficiency, polyuria, enuresis, sweating due to debility, dyspnea, etc. Clearing Shenjing can be used to treat heat in the urinary bladder, dark urine, etc. Shenjing is often reinforced and when it needs to be heat-cleared, clearing Xiaochang is often used instead.

Dachang

Location: the edge of the radial surface of the index finger, or the straight line from the tip of the finger to the part which is between the thumb and the index finger.

Manipulation: Pushing straightly from the tip of the finger to the end with radial surface of the thumb of the right hand is called "reinforcing Dachang", also known as "pushing-laterally Dachang" (Fig. 3—42). Pushing in the opposite direction is called "reducing Dachang". Pushing-to-and-fro is called "clearing Dachang." Reinforcing, reducing and clearing Dachang are called "pushing Dachang".

Frequency: 100—500 times.

Function: Reinforcing Dachang plays the roles of astringing intestine and relieving diarrhea by warming the middle-*jiao*. Clearing the large intestine plays the roles of clearing the intestine, clearing away damp-heat, and relieving intestinal stasis. Clearing Dachang plays the roles of clearing away liver-fire and gallbladder-fire, and relaxing the bowel.

Indication: Reinforcing Dachang can be used to treat diarrhea of asthenia-cold type, and prolapse of rectum. Clearing Dachang can be used to treat fever, abdominal pain, dysentry, indigestion and diarrhea due to dampheat. Reducing Dachang can be used to treat bitter taste and dry throat, constipation, pain in the chest and hyppochondrium, and red and swollen anus. The manipulation is rarely used clinically at present. Clearing Ganjing is often used for the

尿。

主治：补肾经可用于治疗先天不足，久病体虚、肾虚久泻、多尿、遗尿、虚汗、喘息等症；清肾经则用于治疗膀胱蕴热、小便赤涩等症。

肾经多用补法，需用清法时多以清小肠代之。

大肠

位置：在食指桡侧缘，指尖至虎口成一直线。

操作：医者用右手拇指桡侧面，自指尖直推至指根为补，称为"补大肠"，亦称"侧推大肠"(图3—42)；反之为泻，名"泻大肠"；来回推为清，名"清大肠"；补大肠、泻大肠、清大肠，统称为"推大肠"。

次数：100～500次。

作用：补大肠能涩肠固脱，温中止泻；清大肠则善于清肠腑，除湿热，导积滞；泻大肠则能泻肝胆之火，通便。

主治：补大肠可用于治疗虚寒性腹泻，脱肛等；清大肠则治疗湿热、食积滞留肠道所致的身热，腹痛，痢下赤白，湿热泄泻等；泻大肠可用于口苦咽干，大便秘结，胸胁疼痛，肛门红肿。

patient with liver-fire and gallbladder-fire.

Xiaochang

Location: on the ulnar edge of the little finger, the straight way from the tip of little finger to the end.

Manipulation: Pushing from the tip of the finger to the end is called "reinforcing Xiaochang" (Fig. 3—43). Otherwise, it is called "clearing Xiaochang". Reinforcing and clearing Xiaochang are called "pushing Xiaochang".

Frequency: 100—500 times.

Function: Reinforcing Xiaochang plays the roles of nourishing *yin* and treating asthenia. Clearing Xiaochang plays the roles of clearing away pathogenic heat and inducing diuresis, and separating the useful from the waste.

Indication: Clearing Xiaochang is often used to treat scanty dark urine, anuresis, and watery diarrhea. Reinforcing Xiaochang is used to treat hectic fever in the afternoon, polyuria, and enuresis.

Shending

Location: on the tip of the little finger.

Manipulation: Pressing and kneading with tips of the thumb, index or middle finger is called "kneading Shending" (Fig. 3—44).

Frequency: 100—500 times.

Function: astringing primordial *qi*, consolidating superficial resistance to stop perspiration.

Indication: spontaneous perspiration, night sweat, infantile metopism, etc.

Sihengwen

Location: on the cross-striation area of the first finger joint of the index, middle, ring, and little fingers on the palm.

Manipulation: Nipping with the nail of the thumb in proper order followed by kneading is called "nipping-kneading Sihengwen" (Fig. 3—45). Pushing from the cross-striation area of the index finger to the cross-striation area of the little

目前，此法临床较少应用，肝胆火旺者多用清肝经。

小肠

位置：小指尺侧边缘，自指尖到指根成一直线。

操作：从指尖直推向指根为补，称为"补小肠"（图3—43）；反之则为清，称为"清小肠"。补小肠和清小肠统称为"推小肠"。

次数：100～500次。

作用：补小肠能滋阴补虚；清小肠则能清热利尿，泌别清浊。

主治：清小肠多用于治疗小便短赤不利、尿闭、水泻等症；补小肠则用于治疗午后潮热、多尿、遗尿等症。

肾顶

位置：小指顶端。

操作：以拇指、食指或中指端按揉之，称为"揉肾顶"（图3—44）。

次数：100～500次。

作用：收敛元气，固表止汗。

主治：自汗、盗汗，解颅等症。

四横纹

位置：掌面食、中、无名、小指第一指间关节横纹处。

操作：用拇指甲依次掐之，继以揉之，称为"掐揉四横纹"

finger with the four fingers side by side is called "pushing the Sihengwen."

Frequency: nipping-kneading 5 times for each, pushing 100—300 times.

Function: Nipping-kneading Sihengwen plays the roles of reducing fever, relieving restlessness, removing blood stasis, and dispersing accumulation of pathogen. Pushing Sihengwen plays the roles of regulating *qi* and blood, and relieving flatulence and fullness.

Indication: infantile malnutrition, abdominal distention and pain, derangement of *qi* and blood, indigestion, infantile convulsion, dyspnea, and cracked lips. Additionally, in coordination with pinching the spine and inserting Sihengwen with a filiform needle or three-edged needle can produce a good result in treating infantile malnutrition.

Xiaohengwen

Location: at the cross-striation area of metacarpophalangeal articulation of the index, middle, ring and little fingers on the palm aspect.

Manipulation: Nipping with the nail of the thumb in proper order followed be kneading is called "nipping-kneading Xiaohengwen" (Fig. 3—45). Pushing Xiaohengwen back and forth from the index to the little finger with the radial surface of the thumb is called "pushing Xiaohengwen".

Frequency: nipping-kneading 5 times for each, pushing 100—300 times.

Function: reducing fever, relieving distention, removing blood stasis, and dispersing accumulation of pathogen.

Indication: cracked lips, aphthae, fever, restlessness, abdominal flatulence.

Zhang xiaohengwen

Location: at the edge of ulnar palm print, the end of the little finger on the palm aspect.

Manipulation: pressing-kneading with the tip of the

（图3—45）；四指并拢，从食指横纹处推向小指横纹处，称为"推四横纹"。

次数：掐揉各5次，推100～300次。

作用：掐揉四横纹能退热除烦，消瘀散结。推四横纹则能调中行气，和气血，消胀满。

主治：疳积、腹胀腹痛、气血不和、消化不良、惊风、气喘、唇裂。

此外，用毫针或三棱针点刺本穴，并配合捏脊治疗疳积效果甚佳。

小横纹

位置：掌面食、中、无名、小指掌指关节横纹处。

操作：以拇指甲依次掐之，继而揉之，称为"掐揉小横纹"（图3—45）；以拇指桡侧从食指到小指在小横纹上往返推之，称为"推小横纹"。

次数：掐揉各5次，推100～300次。

作用：退热，消胀，消瘀散结。

主治：唇裂、口疮、发热、烦躁、腹胀等。

掌小横纹

位置：掌面小指根下，尺侧掌纹头。

操作：用中指或拇指端按揉，称为"揉掌小横纹"（图3—46）。

middle finger or thumb is called "kneading Xiaohengwen of palm" (Fig. 3—46).

Frequency: 100—500 times.

Function: clearing away pathogenic heat, dispersing accumulation of pathogen, soothing the chest oppression, promoting the dispersing function of the lung, resolving sputum and relieving cough.

Indication: dyspnea and cough due to heat and phlegm, aphthae, slobbering, pneumonia, whooping cough.

Weijing

Location: on the red-white border of the radial surface of the major thenar eminence.

Manipulation: Pushing from the root of the palm to the end of the thumb with the thumb or the index and middle fingers is called "clearing Weijing" (Fig. 3—47).

Frequency: 100—500 times.

Function: clearing damp-heat in the spleen and stomach, promoting digestion, lowering the adverse flow of qi, relieving vomiting.

Indication: nausea, vomiting, hiccup, eructation, excessive thirst and desire for food, hematemesis and nosebleeding, etc.

Banmen

Location: on the flat area of the major thenar eminence of palm.

Manipulation: Kneading on flat area at the central point of the major thenar eminence with thumb or index finger is called "kneading Banmen" or "arc-pushing Banmen" (Fig. 3—48). Pushing from the end of the thumb to the cross striation of wrist with the radial surface of the thumb is called "pushing from Banmen to the cross striation" (Fig. 3—49). Otherwise, it is called "pushing from the cross striation to Banmen" (Fig. 3—50).

Frequency: 100—500 times.

Function: Kneading Banmen plays the roles of strength-

次数：100～500 次。

作用：清热散结，宽胸宣肺，化痰止咳。

主治：痰热喘咳、口舌生疮、流涎、肺炎、百日咳等症。

胃经

位置：大鱼际桡侧赤白肉际。

操作：用拇指或食、中指自掌根推向拇指根，称为"清胃经"（图3—47）。

次数：100～500 次。

作用：清脾胃湿热、消食积、降逆止呕。

主治：恶心、呕吐、呃逆、嗳气、烦渴善饥、吐血、衄血等症。

板门

位置：手掌大鱼际之平面。

操作：用拇指或食指在大鱼际平面的中点上揉之，称为"揉板门"或"运板门"（图3—48）；用拇指桡侧自拇指根推向腕横纹，称为"板门推向横纹"（图3—49）；反之，称为"横纹推向板门"（图3—50）。

次数：100～500 次。

ening the spleen and regulating the stomach, relieving dyspepsia, and putting *qi* in motion. Pushing from Banmen to the cross striation plays the role of relieving diarrhea. Pushing from the cross striation to Banmen plays the role of relieving vomiting.

Indication: dyspepsia, abdominal flatulence, anorexia, vomiting, diarrhea, dyspnea, eructation, etc.

Neilaogong (P8)

Location: in the center of the palm at the midpoint between the bent middle and ring finger.

Manipulation: Kneading with the tip of the index or middle finger is called "kneading Neilaogong" (Fig. 3—51). Pinching, arc-pushing from the root of the little finger through Xiaohengwen of palm, Xiaotianxin to Neilaogong is called "arc-pushing Neilaogong" also known as "fishing for the moon in the water" (Fig. 3—52).

Frequency: 100—300 times by kneading and motioning.

Function: Kneading Neilaogong plays the roles of clearing away sthenic heat in the Heart Channel and relieving restlessness. Motioning Neilaogong plays the role of clearing away asthenic heat in the Heart and Kidney Channel.

Indication: Fever, excessive thirst, aphthae, erosion of gum, asthenia-type restlessness with heat in the interior.

Neibagua

Location: On plam surface. Taking the center of the palm as the center of a circle and 2/3 from the center of the circle to the cross striation of the middle finger as the radius, draw a circle. The circle is Bagua point.

Manipulation: Arc-pushing clockwise is called "Arc-pushing Neibagua" or "Arc-pushing Bagua". The manipulation should be gentle at the root of the middle finger (Fig. 3—53).

Frequency: 100—300 times.

Function: soothing chest oppression, regulating the flow of *qi* and eliminating phlegm, removing food retention and promoting digestion.

作用：揉板门能健脾和胃、消食化滞、运达上下之气；板门推向横纹能止泻；横纹推向板门可止呕。

主治：食积、腹胀、食欲不振、呕吐、腹泻、气喘、嗳气等症。

内劳宫

位置：掌心中，屈指时中指、无名指之间中点。

操作：用食指或中指端揉，称为"揉内劳宫"（图3—51）；自小指根掐运起，经掌小横纹，小天心至内劳宫，名"运内劳宫"，亦称"水底捞明月"（图3—52）。

次数：揉、运均为100～300次。

作用：揉内劳宫能清心经实热而除烦；运内劳宫则能清心肾经虚热。

主治：发热、烦渴、口疮、齿龈糜烂、虚烦内热等症。

内八卦

位置：在手掌面，以掌心为圆心，从圆心至中指根横纹约2/3处为半径，画一圆圈，此圆即为八卦穴。

操作：用运法，顺时针方向运，称为"运内八卦"或"运八卦"，在运至中指根位置时轻轻而过（图3—53）。

次数：100～500次。

作用：宽胸利膈，理气化痰，行滞消食。

Indication: cough with phlegm-dyspnea, stuffiness in the chest with anorexia, abdominal distention, vomiting, diarrhea, loss of appetite.

Xiaotianxin

Location: in the depression of the intersection point of major thenar eminence and minor thenar eminence at the root of palm.

Manipulation: Kneading with the tip of the middle finger is called "kneading Xiaotianxin" (Fig. 3—54). Nipping with the nail of the thumb followed by kneading with it is called "nipping-kneading Xiaotianxin". Striking with the tip of the middle finger or the flexed finger joint is called pounding Xiaotianxin".

Frequency: Kneading 100—500 times, nipping 5—10 times; pounding 20—50 times.

Function: Kneading Xiaotianxin plays the roles of clearing away pathogenic heat, relieving convulsion, reducing diuresis and improving vision. Nipping-kneading and pounding Xiaotianxin play the roles of relieving convulsion and tranquilizing the mind.

Indication: Kneading Xiaotianxin can be used to treat conjunctival congestion with pain, aphthae, convulsion with restlessness, scanty dark urine, scleroderma neonatorum, jaundice, enuresis, edema, sore furunde, and measles with incomplete eruption. Nipping-kneading and pounding Xiaotianxin are suitable for convulsion, night cry, restlessness, strabismus, somnambulism, etc.

Nipping and pounding to the left can be used for the patient with right-strabismus, and vice versa. The massagist can nip and strike downward for the patient with superduction. Otherwise, upward.

Zongjin

Location: On the middle of the cross striation, at the palm surface of the wrist.

Manipulation: Kneading with the thumb or middle finger is

主治：咳嗽痰喘，胸闷纳呆，腹胀，呕吐泄泻，食欲不振。

小天心

位置：在掌根，大小鱼际交接之中点凹陷中。

操作：用中指端揉，称为"揉小天心"（图3—54）；用拇指甲掐，继而揉之，称为"掐揉小天心"；以中指尖或屈曲的指间关节捣，称为"捣小天心"。

次数：揉100～500次。掐5～10次；捣20～50次。

作用：揉小天心可清热、镇惊、利尿、明目；掐揉小天心能镇惊安神；捣小天心有镇惊安神之功。

主治：揉小天心可用于治疗目赤肿痛、口舌生疮、惊惕不安、小便短赤、新生儿硬皮症、黄疸、遗尿、水肿、疮疖、疹出不透等证。掐揉、捣小天心适用于惊风抽搐、夜啼、惊惕不安、斜视、夜游症等证。

用于治疗斜视时，右斜视者，向左掐、捣；左斜视者，则向右掐、捣，用于惊风目翻，目上翻者，向下掐、捣；目下翻者，则向上掐、捣。

总筋

位置：在手腕掌侧横纹中点。

操作：以拇指或中指揉之，称为"揉总筋"（图3—55）；用拇

called "kneading Zongjin" (Fig 3—55). Nipping with the nail of the thumb is called "nipping Zongjin". Grasping with the thumb on the point and the index finger on the back of the wrist, with the other hand holding the patient's four fingers and shaking them is called "grasping Zongjin".

Frequency: Kneading 100—300 times, grasping 3—5 times.

Function: clearing away pathogenic heat in the heart channel, removing obstruction and relieving spasm, and activating *qi* in the body.

Indication: infantile convulsion, spasm, night cry, aphthae, hectic fever, toothache, and borborygmus with vomiting and diarrhea.

Dahengwen (Yinchi, Yangchi)

Location: at the cross striation of the wrist, on the palmar aspect. Yangchi is near the thumb, Yinchi is near the little finger.

Manipulation: Pushing-separately from Zongjin to both sides with the two thumbs is called "parting-pushing Dahengwen", also known as "separating Yinchi-Yangchi" (Fig. 3—56). Pushing-jointly from Yinchi and Yangchi to Zongjin is called "meeting-pushing Yinchi-Yangchi."

Frequency: 30—50 times.

Function: balancing *yin* and *yang*, regulating *qi* and blood, promoting digestion, eliminating phlegm and removing obstruction.

Indication: alternating episodes of chills and fever, diarrhea, vomiting, dysentery, abdominal distention, indigestion, persistent fever, restlessness, infantile convulsion, spasm, and abundant expectoration.

When the manipulation of "separating Yinchi-Yangchi" is done, the doctor must do it heavily on Yinchi point for the patient with sthenic-heat syndrome, while for the patient with asthenia-cold syndrome, heavily on Yangchi

指甲掐之，称为"掐总筋"；以拇指按穴位上，以食指按手腕背部对合拿之，另一手握其四指摇动，称为"拿总筋"。

次数：揉100～300次；拿3～5次。

作用：清心经热，散结止痉，通调周身气机。

主治：惊风、抽掣、夜啼、口舌生疮、潮热、牙痛、肠鸣吐泻等症。

大横纹（阴池、阳池）

位置：仰掌，手腕掌侧横纹。近拇指端为阳池，近小指端为阴池。

操作：用两手拇指自掌后横纹中（总筋）向两旁分推，称为"分推大横纹"，又称"分阴阳"（图3—56）；自两旁（阴池、阳池）向总筋合推，称为"合推阴阳"。

次数：30～50次。

作用：平衡阴阳，调和气血，消食积，化痰散结。

主治：寒热往来，腹泻，呕吐，痢疾，腹胀，食积，身热不退，烦躁不安，惊风，抽搐，痰涎壅盛。

分阴阳，操作时实热证阴池宜重分，虚寒证则阳池宜重分。

point.

Shixuan (Extra 30)

Location: on the tips of the ten fingers, about 0.1 *cun* distal to the nails.

Manipulation: Nipping the ten points in turn with the nail of the thumb is called "nipping Shixuan" (Fig. 3—57).

Frequency: 5 times for each point or stop immediately after the patient comes to.

Function: clearing away pathogenic heat, restoring consciousness and inducing resuscitation.

Indication: acute fever with convulsion, spasm, heat syndromes of the heart, restlessness and trance.

Ershanmen

Location: in the depression on both sides of the caput of the third ossa metacarpi on the dorsum of the hand.

Manipulation: Nipping with the nail of the thumb is called "nipping Ershanmen". "Kneading with the corner of the thumb or with the index and middle fingers is called "kneading Ershanmen" (Fig. 3—58).

Frequency: nipping 5 times, kneading 100—500 times.

Function: relieving superficial syndrome by means of diaphoresis, reducing fever, relieving asthma.

Indication: convulsion, fever with anhidrosis, cold, phlegm-dyspnea, difficult respiration, acute convulsion, facial hemiparalysis.

Erma

Location: in the depression of the metacarpophalangeal articulationes of the ring and little finger on the dorsum of the hand.

Manipulation: Kneading with the thumb or the middle finger is called "kneading Erma". Nipping with the nail of the thumb is called "nipping Erma" (Fig. 3—59).

Frequency: nipping 3—5 times, kneading 100—500 times.

十宣

位置：在手十指的尖端，距指甲约0.1寸。

操作：以拇指甲依次掐之，称为"掐十宣"(图3—57)。

次数：各掐5次或醒后即止。

作用：清热，醒神，开窍。

主治：急热惊风，抽搐，心热，烦躁不安，精神恍惚。

二扇门

位置：在手背三掌骨头两侧凹陷处。

操作：用拇指甲掐，称为"掐二扇门"；用拇指偏峰或食、中二指揉，称为"揉二扇门"(图3—58)。

次数：掐5次；揉100～500次。

作用：发汗透表，退热平喘。

主治：惊风抽搐，身热无汗，伤风感冒，痰喘气粗，呼吸不畅，急惊风，口眼歪斜。

二马

位置：手背无名指及小指掌指关节后陷中。

操作：用拇指或中指揉之，称为"揉二马"；用拇指甲掐，称为"掐二马"(图3—59)。

次数：掐3～5次；揉100～500次。

Function: nourishing *yin*, reinforcing the kidney, promoting the circulation of *qi* and removing the obstruction, and inducing diuresis for treating stranguria.

Indication: fever of deficiency type and cough with dyspnea, scanty dark urine and dribbling urination, abdominal pain, weakness, stranguria, prolapse of rectum, enuresis, indigestion, toothache, teethgrinding while sleeping, dyspnea.

Wailaogong

Location: On the dorsum of hand, opposite to Neilaogong.

Manipulation: Kneading with the index or the middle finger is called "kneading Wailaogong" (Fig. 3—60). Kneading after nipping with the nail of thumb is called "nipping-kneading Wailaogong".

Frequency: Nipping 5 times, kneading 100—500 times.

Function: warming *yang*, expelling cold, invigorating the vital function to treat hypofunction of the spleen with sinking symptoms, relieving superficial syndrome by means of diaphoresis.

Indication: common cold of wind-cold type, abdominal pain, abdominal distention, borborygmus, diarrhea, dysentery, prolapse of rectum, enuresis, cough, dyspnea, hernia, etc.

Yiwofeng

Location: in the depression in the middle of the transverse crease of the wrist on the dorsum of hand.

Manipulation: Kneading with the tip of the thumb or the middle finger is called "kneading Yiwofeng" (Fig. 3—61). Kneading after nipping with the nail of the thumb is called "nipping-kneading Yiwofeng."

Frequency: nipping 3—5 times, kneading 100—300 times.

Function: dispersing pathogenic wind-cold, promoting *qi* of exterior and interior, warming the spleen and stomach to promote the flow of *qi*, relieving pain due to arthralgia-syndrome, and relieving rigidity of the joints.

Indication: invasion by wind, cold, abdominal pain, borborygmus, arthralgia and acute and chronic convulsion.

作用：滋阴补肾，顺气散结，利水通淋。

主治：虚热喘咳，小便短赤淋沥，腹痛，体虚，淋证，脱肛，遗尿，消化不良，牙痛，睡时磨牙，喘促。

外劳宫

位置：在手背面，与内劳宫相对。

操作：用食指或中指揉，称为"揉外劳宫"（图3—60）；用拇指甲掐，继而揉之，称为"掐揉外劳宫"。

次数：掐5次；揉100～500次。

作用：温阳散寒，升阳举陷，发汗解表。

主治：风寒感冒、腹痛、腹胀，肠鸣、腹泻、痢疾、脱肛、遗尿、咳嗽、气喘、疝气等病证。

一窝风

位置：在手背腕横纹正中凹陷中。

操作：用拇指或中指端揉之，称为"揉一窝风"（图3—61）；用拇指甲掐，继而揉之，称为"掐揉一窝风"。

次数：掐3～5次；揉100～300次。

作用：发散风寒，宣通表里，温中行气，止痹痛，利关节。

主治：伤风，感冒，腹痛，肠鸣；关节痹痛，急慢惊风。

Boyangchi

Location: 3 *cun* posterior to Yiwofeng, between the ulna and radius on the dorsal aspect of the forearm.

Manipulation: Kneading after nipping with the nail of the thumb is called "nipping-kneading Boyangchi" (Fig. 3—62).

Frequency: nipping 3—5 times, kneading 100—300 times.

Function: relieving headache, relaxing the bowels and inducing urination.

Indication: cold, headache, constipation, dark urine.

Sanguan

Location: the straight way from the transverse crease of the wrist to the transverse crease of the elbow, on the radial aspect of the forearm.

Manipulation: Pushing from the transverse crease of the wrist to elbow with the radial surface of the thumb or the faces of the index and middle fingers is called "pushing Sanguan" (Fig. 3—63). Pushing from the radial surface of the thumb to the elbow, with the child's thumb bent, is called "pushing Sanguan heavily".

Frequency: 100—500 times.

Function: warming *yang*, dispelling cold, invigorating *qi* and promoting blood circulation, aud relieving superficial syndrome by means of diaphoresis.

Indication: all kinds of cold of insufficiency type such as deficiency of both *qi* and blood, weakness after illness, insufficiency of *yang* and cold extremities, myasthenia of limbs, as well as abdominal pain, diarrhea, mascular eruption and miliaria alba, measle with incomplete appearance of rash es, infantile acroparalysis, etc.

Liufu

Location: at the ulnar part of the forearm, the straight way from the transverse crease of the elbow to the wrist.

Manipulation: Pushing from the transverse crease of the elbow to the wrist with the faces of the thumb or index and middle fingers is called "reducing Liufu" or "pushing Liufu" (Fig 3–64).

膊阳池

位置：在手背一窝风之后 3 寸处，前臂背侧，尺、桡骨之间。

操作：用拇指甲掐，继而揉之，称为"掐揉膊阳池"（图3—62）。

次数：掐 3 ～ 5 次；揉 100～300 次。

作用：止头痛，通大便，利小便。

主治：感冒，头痛，便秘，尿赤。

三关

位置：在前臂桡侧，腕横纹至肘横纹成一条直线。

操作：用拇指桡侧面或食中二指指面自腕横纹推向肘 横 纹，称为"推三关"（图3—63）；屈患儿拇指，自拇指桡侧端推向肘，称为"大推三关"。

次数：100～500 次。

作用：温阳散寒，益气活血，发汗解表。

主治：一切虚寒症，如气血虚弱、病后体虚、阳虚肢冷、四肢无力，以及虚寒性腹痛、腹泻、斑疹白痦、疹出不透、小儿肢体瘫痪。

六腑

位置：前臂尺侧，自肘横纹至腕横纹成一条直线。

操作：用拇指面或食、中二指指面自肘横纹推向腕横纹，称为"退六腑"或"推六腑"（图3—64）。

Frequency: 100-500 times.

Function: Clearing away pathogenic heat, cooling blood, detoxicating.

Indication: all kinds of sthenic-heat syndrome such as high fever, restlessness, thirst and desire for cold water, infantile convulsion, thrush, swollen and rigid tongue, double tongue, sore throat, mumps, pyogenic infections and dysentery of heat type.

Tianheshui

Location: the straight way from the transverse crease of wrist to the elbow, in the middle of medial aspect of the forearm.

Manipulation: ① Pushing from the [transverse crease of wrist to the elbow with the faces of the index and middle fingers is called "clearing Tianheshui" (Fig. 3-65).

② Pushing from Neilaogong point to the transverse crease of the elbow with the faces of the index and middle fingers is called "pushing Tianheshui heavily".

③ Arc-pushing Neilaogong, then grasp the child's clenched four fingers with the left hand. Striking the points one by one from Neiguan (P 6), Jianshi (P 5) along Tianhe upward to Hongchi with the tips of index and middle fingers is called "crossing Tianhe while beating the horse" (Fig. 3-66).

④ Pour some cold water on the area of the large transverse crease, then push slowly to Hongchi with the faces of the index and middle fingers, pat with the four fingers of the two hands, giving a puff on Tianhe point. The manipulation is called "leading water to the Tianhe".

Frequency: 100-300 times for each mentioned above.

Function: clearing away pathogenic heat and relieving exterior syndrome, removing fire from the heart, relieving restlessness, moistening the lung and resolving phlegm.

Indication: all kinds of heat syndrome such as fever due to exogenous pathogenic factors, internal-heat syndrome, hectic fever, restlessness, thirst, swollen and rigid tongue, double tongue infantile convulsion, phlegm-dyspnea, cough, etc.

次数：100～500次。

作用：清热，凉血，解毒。

主治：一切实热证，如高热、烦躁、口渴饮冷、惊风、鹅口疮、木舌、重舌、咽痛、腮腺炎、肿毒、热痢等症。

天河水

位置：在前臂内侧正中，自腕横纹至肘横纹成一直线。

操作：①用食、中二指指面自腕横纹推至肘横纹，称为"清天河水"（图3—65）。

②用食、中二指指面自内劳宫穴推至肘横纹，称为"大推天河水"。

③先以运内劳宫法运之，然后屈患儿四指向上，以左手握住，再以食、中二指顶端自内关、间使循天河向上一起一落打至洪池为一次，称为"打马过天河"（图3—66）。

④以凉水滴于大横纹处，用食、中二指指面慢慢推至洪池，后以两手四指拍之，并用口吹气于天河穴透之，称为"引水上天河"。

次数：以上各法均为100～300次。

作用：清热解表，泻心火，除烦躁，润燥化痰。

主治：一切热症，如外感发热、内热、潮热、烦躁不安、口渴、弄舌、重舌、惊风、痰喘、咳嗽等病症。

5. Points on the Lower Limbs

Jimen

Location: in the medial aspect of thighs, the straigt way from the superior border of the knee to the groin.

Manipulation: Pushing from the superior border of the medial aspect of the knee up to the groin with faces of index and middle fingers is called "pushing Jimen" (Fig. 3-67).

Frequency: 100–500 times.

Function: Diuresis.

Indication: scanty dark urine, anuresis, watery diarrhea, etc.

Baichong (Xuehai Sp 10)

Location: 2 *cun* directly above the medial border of the patella.

Manipulation: Grasging the patient's left and right points with the thumbs and the middle fingers is called "grasping Baichong" (Fig. 3-68). Pushing them with the thumb is called "pushing Baichong".

Frequency: 5 times for grasping and pessing respectively, or stop soon after the patient recovers consciousness.

Function: clearing and activating the channels and collaterals, relieving spasm.

Indication: convulsion, coma, unconsciousness, paralysis of lower limbs, arthralgia-syndrome.

Zusanli (St 36)

Location: 3 *cun* below Dubi (St 35), one finger–breadth from the anterior crest of the tibia.

Manipulation: Pressing–kneading with the tip of the thumb is called "pressing–kneading Zusanli (St 36)" (Fig. 3-69). Kneading after nipping with the nail of the thumb is called "nipping-kneading Zusanli (St 36)".

Frequency: 50–100 times.

Function: strengthening the spleen and stomach, regulating

5. 下肢部穴位

箕门

位置：大腿内侧正中，膝盖上缘至腹股沟成一直线。

操作：用食、中二指指面自膝盖内侧上缘直上推至腹 股 沟，称为"推箕门"（图3—67）。

次数：100～500次。

作用：利小便。

主治：小便短赤、尿闭、水泻等。

百虫（血海）

位置：髌骨内缘直上2寸。

操作：以两手拇、中二指合拿患儿之左右两穴，称为"拿百虫"（图3—68）；用拇指按称为"按百虫"。

次数：拿、按均为5次，或醒后即止。

作用：通经活络，止抽搐。

主治：惊风抽搐、昏迷、不省人事、下肢瘫痪、痹痛等病证。

足三里

位置：犊鼻穴下3寸，胫骨前嵴外一横指处。

操作：用拇指端按揉之，称为"按揉足三里"（图3—69）；以拇指甲掐之，继而揉之，称为"掐揉足三里"。

次数：100～500次。

作用：健脾和胃，调中理气，导滞通络。

qi, removing stagnancy and obstruction of channels.

Indication: abdominal distention, abdominal pain, diarr-hea, vomiting, flaccidity of lower limbs.

Pushen (UB 61)

Location: 2 *cun* directly below Kunlun (UB 60).

Manipulation: Grasping heavily with the thumb, index and middle fingers symmetically is called "grasping Pushen", Nipping with the nail of the thumb is called "nipping Pushen" (Fig. 3–70).

Frequency: 5 times for grasping, and nipping respectively or stop soon after the patient recovers consciousness.

Function: relieving convulsion, relieving rigidity of muscles and joints.

Indication: infantile convulsion, spasm, faint, sprain of lateral malleolus.

Yongquan (K 1)

Location: at the junction between anterior 1/3 and posterior 2/3 of the sole, in the depression when the foot is in plantar flexion.

Manipulation: Kneading with the tip of the thumb is called "kneading Yongquan" (K 1) (Fig. 3–71). Pushing towards the toes with the face of the thumb is called "pushing Yongquan".

Frequency: 50–100 times kneading and pushing respectively.

Function: Pushing Yongquan (K 1) plays the roles of conducting the fire back to its origin and reducing fever of deficiency type. Kneading Yongquan (K 1) plays the role of preventing vomiting and diarrhea.

Indication: Pushing Yongquan (K 1) can be used to treat dysphoria with feverish sensation in the chest, palms and soles, restlessness at night, fever, etc. Kneading Yongquan (K 1) to the left can be used to treat vomiting, while to the right can be used to treat diarrhea.

主治：腹胀，腹痛，泄泻，呕吐，下肢痿软乏力。

仆参

位置：昆仑穴直下2寸。

操作：用拇指和食、中二指对称用力拿之，称为"拿仆参"；用拇指甲掐之，称为"掐仆参"（图3—70）。

次数：拿、掐均为5次，或醒后即止。

作用：镇惊止搐，活利关节。

主治：惊风，抽搐，昏厥，外踝关节扭挫伤。

涌泉

位置：足趾跖屈时在足掌心前正中凹陷中，相当于足掌心前1/3和后2/3之间。

操作：以拇指端揉之，称为"揉涌泉"（图3—71）；用拇指面向足趾推，称为"推涌泉"。

次数：揉、推均为50～100次。

作用：推涌泉能引火归元、退虚热。揉涌泉可止吐泻。

主治：推涌泉可用于治疗五心烦热、夜寐不安、发热等。揉涌泉主治呕吐、泄泻，左揉止吐，右揉止泻。

6. Summing-up of the Commonly-used Points

The 54 points introduced above are often used for children clinically. The points distribute all over the human body. Most of them have many kinds of effect and different indications and functions which vary with the nature of the manipulations such as intensity, speed and direction.

(1) Points and Manipulations for Relieving Superficial Syndrome by Means of Diaphoresis.

POINTS AND MANIPULATIONS

Opening Tianmen, pushing Kangong, kneading Taiyang (Extra 2), kneading Erhou Gaogu, nipping Fengchi (GB 20), kneading Yingxiang (LI 20), pushing Tianzhugu, nipping-kneading Dazhui (Du 14), grasping Jianjing (GB 21), pushing the spine, pushing Sanguan, kneading Wailaogong, nipping-kneading Yiwofeng, clearing Tianheshui, nipping-kneading Ershanmen, etc.

CLINICAL APPLICATION OF DIFFERENT MANIPULATIONS

The points and manipulations mentioned above can be used to treat various kinds of diseases caused by exogenous pathogenic factors, sush as headache, fever, stuffy nose with discharge, etc. Opening Tianmen, pushing Kangong, kneading Taiyang (Extra 2), kneading Erhou Gaogu, kneading Yingxiang (LI 20), pushing Tianzhugu, pushing the spine and grasping Janjing (GB 21) play the roles of dispelling pathogenic wind and relieving exterior syndrome, which can be used to treat various kinds of diseases caused by exogenous pathogenic factors. Squeezing-kneading Dazhui (Du 14), and clearing Tianheshui play the roles of clearing away pathogenic heat and relieving exterior syndrome, which can be used to treat cold of wind-heat type. Pushing Sanguan (three passes), kneading Wailaogong and nipping Yiwofeng play the roles of warming *yang* and dispelling cold, which can be used to treat exterior-asthenia syndrome of wind-cold type. Nipping-

6. 常用穴位小结

以上介绍的 54 个穴位均为临床小儿推拿常用穴，这些 穴 位分布于全身各部。其中，多数穴位，一穴可兼有多种功效，并且可因操作手法的轻、重、缓、急和方向顺逆的不同，其主治与作用性能亦不相同。

（1）发汗解表类

【穴位与手法】

开天门，推坎宫，揉太阳，揉耳后高骨，掐风池，揉迎 香，推天柱骨，掐揉大椎，拿肩井，推脊，推三关，揉外劳宫，掐揉一窝风，清天河水，掐揉二扇门等。

【辨证应用】

以上诸穴，能治疗各型外感及头痛、发热、鼻塞流涕等症。其中，开天门、推坎宫、揉太阳、揉耳后高骨、揉迎香、推天柱骨、推脊、拿肩井能祛风解表，可用作各型外感的常规治法；挤、揉大椎、清天河水能清热解表，可用于治疗风热型外感；推三 关、揉外劳宫、掐一窝风有温阳散寒之功，适用于治疗风寒表虚型外

kneading Ershanmen and grasping forcefully Jianjing (GB 21) and Fengchi (GB 20) play the role of diaphoresis, which can be used to treat cold of superficies of exterior–sthenia syndrome wind–cold type with fever and anhidrosis.

(2) Points and Manipulations for Clearing Heat and Purging Fire

POINTS AND MANIPULATIONS

Clearing Pijing, Ganjing, Xinjing, Feijing, Shenjing, Dachang, Xiaochang, Weijing and Tianheshui, crossing the Tianhe while beating the horse, pushing Liufu, pushing spine, nipping Shixuan (Extra 30), kneading Xiaotianxin, and Neilaogong, arc-pushing Neilaogong, kneading Erma and Yongquan (K 1), parting-pushing *yin-yang*, nipping-kneading Sihengwen, pushing Xiaohengwen, kneading Xiaohengwen of the palm, and nipping-kneading Zongjing.

CLINICAL APPLICATION OF DIFFERENT MANIPULATIONS

All the points and manipulations mentioned above play the role of clearing away pathogenic heat. Among them, the first eight points paly the roles of clearing and reducing sthenic heat-syndrome of viscera. Clearing Tianheshui mainly plays the role of clearing away pathogenic heat of *wei* and *qi* systems, pushing Liufu, Crossing the Tianhe while beating the horse plays the role of clearing away pathogenic heat of *ying* and *xue* systems. Pushing the spine plays the role of clearing away pathogenic heat and relaxing the bowels. It also can be used to clear away pathogenic heat from *wei* and *qi* systems or *ying* and *xue* systems. Nipping Shixuan (Extra 30) can be used to treat dysphoria due to heart-heat, convulsion due to hyperactivity of heat. Kneading Xiaotianxin and Neilaogong play the role of clearing away the heat from heart channel or the heat that has moved to the small intestine. It is suitable for the treatment of restlessness with frightening, infantile convulsion with spasm or scanty dark urine with burning sensation during

感；掐揉二扇门、重拿肩井、重拿风池有较明显的发汗作用，善于治疗身热、无汗的风寒表实型感冒。

（2）清热泻火类

【穴位与手法】

清脾经，清肝经，清心经，清肺经，清肾经，清大肠，清小肠，清胃经,清天河水,打马过天河，退六腑，推脊，掐十宣，揉小天心，揉内劳宫，运内劳宫，揉二马，揉涌泉，分阴阳，掐揉四横纹，推小横纹，揉掌小横纹，掐揉总筋。

【辨证应用】

以上诸穴及手法均有清热之功。其中，前八个穴位，主要能清泻所属脏腑之实热；清天河水主要用于清卫分、气分之热；退六腑、打马过天河主要用于清营分、血分之热；推脊能清热通便，并对热在卫气或热入营血诸证有治疗作用；掐十宣可用于治疗心热烦躁、热盛惊风；揉小天心、揉内劳宫能清心经有热或移热于小肠，适用于治疗惊惕不安、惊风抽搐或小便热赤等症；运内劳

urination. Arc-pushing Neilaogong, kneading Erma and kneading Yongquan (K 1) play the role of clearing away asthenic heat. They are suitable for the treatment vexation, night sweat, etc. Separating *Yinchi-Yangchi* plays the role of regulating *qi* and blood. It is suitable for the treatment of alternating episodes of chills and fever and derangement of *qi* and blood. Nipping-kneading the last four points such as Sihengwen play the role of clearing away heat, and removing obstruction. The former plays the role of regulating *qi* and blood, promoting digestion and relieving retention of food in the stomach, pushing Xiaohengwen plays the role of clearing away heat from the spleen and stomach. It can also be used to treat abdominal distention and cracked lip. Kneading Xiaohengwen of the palm plays the role of clearing away heat from the heart and lung. It can be used to treat stomatitis, accumulation of phlegm and asthma. Nipping Zongjin plays the role of clearing away the pathogenic heat in the pericardium to relieve spasm.

(3) Points and Manipulations for Reinforcing

POINTS AND MANIPULATIONS

Reinforcing Pijing, Ganjing, Xinjing, Feijing, Shenjing, Dachang, Xiaochang, kneading Feishu (UB 13), kneading the points of viscera, kneading Erma, rubbing the abdomen, kneading the umbilicus, kneading Zhongwan (Ren 12), pressing-kneading Zusanli (St 36), pushing Sanguan and pinching the spine.

CLINICAL APPLICATION OF DIFFERENT MANIPULATIONS

The first eight points and manipulations, such as reinforcing Pijing, play the role of reinforcing deficient viscera; and kneading Erma and rubbing-kneading Dantian (Elixir Field) play the role of reinforcing the kidney-*yin*. The former mainly plays the role of nourishing the kidney-*yin*, and the latter, warming and reinforcing the kidney-*yang*. The two manipulations are often used together to treat enuresis due to deficiency of the kidney-*qi* and prolapse of rectum.

宫、揉二马、揉涌泉，主要用于清虚热，适用于治疗心烦、盗汗等症；分阴阳能调和气血，适用于治疗寒热往来、气血不和之证。掐揉四横纹等后四穴，均能清热散结，前者主和气血、消食积，治疗积滞；推小横纹主清脾胃热结，治腹胀、口唇破裂；揉掌小横纹主清心、肺之热积，治口舌生疮、痰热喘咳等证；掐总筋能清心止痉。

（3）补益类

【穴位与手法】

补脾经、补肝经、补心经、补肺经、补肾经、补大肠、补小肠、揉肺俞等脏腑俞穴、揉二马、摩腹、揉脐、揉中脘、按揉足三里、推三关、捏脊等。

【辨证应用】

补脾经等前八穴及手法可补所属脏腑之虚损；揉二马、摩揉丹田均能补肾，但前者偏于滋补肾阴，后者则重在温补肾阳，二法常配合应用，用于治疗肾气不足所致的遗尿、脱肛等病证；摩

Rubbing the abdomen, kneading the umbilicus, kneading Zhong-wan (Ren 12), and pressing-kneading Zusanli (St 36) play the role of invigorating the spleen and stomach and regulating mid-dle-*jiao*. It is effective to treat asthenia of the spleen and stomach, indigestion and acquired defect. Pushing Sanguan, pinching the spine are more effective for asthenia-syndrome such as congenital defect, lack of proper care after birth, and weakness after illness, etc. Pushing Sanguan mainly plays the role of warming and invigorating *qi* and enriching blood. Pinching the spine mainly plays the role of invigorating primordial *qi* and regulating the function of the viscera.

(4) Points and Manipulations for Warming the Middle-*jiao* and Dispelling Pathogenic Cold

POINTS AND MANIPULATIONS

Nipping-kneading Yiwofeng, kneading Wailaogong, rubbing umbilicus, Zhengwan (Ren 12) and Dantian (Elixir Eield), pushing Sanguan, etc.

CLINICAL APPLICATION OF DIFFERENT MANIPULATIONS

All the points and manipulations mentioned above play the roles of warming the middle-*jiao* and dispelling pathogenic cold. Among them, nipping-kneading Yiwofeng plays the roles of warming the middle-*jiao*, activating *qi*, and relieving abdominal pain. Kneading Wailaogong also plays the role of lifting *yang qi*, which is effective for treating abdominal pain, diarrhea, prolapse of rectum and enuresis. Rubbing the umbilicus plays the role of warming *yang*, invigorating the spleen and stomach, warming the intestine. It can be used to treat borborygmus, abdominal pain, diarrhea, etc. Rubbing Zhong-wan (Ren 12) mainly plays the role of warming and reinforcing the spleen and stomach. Rubbing Dantian (Elixir Field) plays the role of warming and reinforcing primordial *qi* of the lower-*jiao*, reinforcing the kidney and strengthening body resistence. With the function of warming and heating,

腹、揉脐、揉中脘、按揉足三里四法，能健脾益胃、调和中州，

治疗脾胃功能虚弱、消化不良、后天不足等病证有良效；推三关、

捏脊善治先天不足、后天失养及病后亏损等各种体虚之证，推三

关重在温补气血，捏脊则擅于培补元气、调和脏腑。

（4）温中散寒类

【穴位与手法】

掐揉一窝风，揉外劳宫，摩脐，摩中脘，摩丹田，推三关等

【辨证应用】

以上诸法均有温中散寒之功。其中，掐揉一窝风能温中、行

气、止腹痛；揉外劳宫则兼升阳举陷，对腹痛、泄泻、脱肛、遗

尿等病证有较好的效果；摩脐可温阳健脾、益胃、暖肠，能治疗

肠鸣、腹痛、泄泻等病证；摩中脘则重在温补脾胃，以消脘腹冷

痛；摩丹田可温补下元、培肾固本；推三关其性温热，可治疗一

pushing the Sanguan can be used to treat all kinds of asthenia-cold syndromes, which, if applied in combination with the points mentioned above, will be more effective.

POINTS AND MANIPULATIONS

(5) Points and Manipulations for Promoting Digestion

Clearing-reinforcing Pijing, kneading Banmen, clearing Weijing, arc-pushing Bagua, parting-pushing Yinchi-Yangchi, kneading Zhongwan (Ren 12), parting-pushing *Fu yin-yang*, rubbing the umbilicus, foulaging-rubbing the hypochondrium, and pressing-kneading Zusanli (St 36).

CLINICAL APPLICATION OF DIFFERENT MANIPULATIONS

The manipulations mentioned above play the role of promoting digestion and removing indigested food from the stomach. Among them, clearing-reinforcing Pijing, kneading Banmen and arching-pushing Neibagua play the role of invigorating the spleen and stomach and promoting digestion and fluid transportation. Separating Yinchi-Yangchi plays the role of regulating *yin-yang* and promoting digestion. Kneading Zhongwan (Ren 12) and parting-pushing *Fu yin-yang* mainly play the role of removing indigested food from the stomach. Rubbing the umbilicus plays the role of removing retention of food from the intestine. Foulaging-rubbing the hypochondrium plays the role of relieving the depressed liver, soothing the liver and regulating the circulation of *qi*. It can be used to treat anorexia, distension and pain in the chest and hypochondrium due to stagnation of liver-*qi*. Pressing-kneading Zusanli (St 36) can strengthen the effect produced by the manipulations mentioned above.

(6) Points and Manipulations for Relieving Diarrhea

POINTS AND MANIPULATIONS

Reinforcing Pijing, Dachang, Shenjing, clearing Xiaochang, pushing from Banmen to Hengwen, rubbing the abdomen, rubbing-kneading Dantian (Elixir Field), rubbing the umbilicus, (the three points are operated counterclockwise), grasping Dujiao,

切虚寒证，与上述各穴配用有加强其温补作用的功能。

（5）消食导滞类

【穴位与手法】

清补脾经，揉板门，清胃经，顺运八卦，分阴阳，揉中脘，分推腹阴阳，摩脐，搓摩胁肋，按揉足三里。

【辨证应用】

以上诸法均有明显的助消化、导积滞的作用。其中，清补脾经、揉板门、顺运内八卦能健脾胃、助运化；分手阴阳则能调阴阳、消食积；揉中脘、分推腹阴阳重在消胃中积滞，摩脐可清理肠中积滞；搓摩胁肋有疏肝理气的作用，可用于治疗肝气郁结所致的食欲不振，胸胁胀痛等证；按揉足三里可加强上述诸法消食导滞作用。

（6）止泻类

【穴位与手法】

补脾经，补大肠，补肾经，清小肠，板门推向横纹，摩腹，摩揉丹田，摩脐(上三穴均为逆时针方向摩)，拿肚角，捏脊，推上

pinching the spine, pushing-up Qijiegu, kneading Guiwei, pressing-kneading Zusanli (St 36) and kneading Yongquan (K 1).

CLINICAL APPLICATION OF DIFFERENT MANIPULATIONS

All the above manipulations are very effective for relieving diarrhea. Among them, reinforcing Pijing, rubbing the abdomen and pinching the spine play the roles of invigorating the spleen and relieving diarrhea. Rubbing Dantian (Elixir Field) is indicated in persistent diarrhea and diseases which damage the kidney-*yang*. Clearing Xiaochang plays the role of clearing away pathogenic heat and promoting diuresis, separating the useful from the waste through the function of the small intestine. It is the most effective point to treat watery diarrhea due to pathogenic damp heat. Grasping Dujiao plays the role of relieving diarrhea and abdominal pain, which is suitable for diarrhea at the early stage when the vital-*qi* (the body's resistance) of the patient has not been damaged. Pressing-kneading Zusanli can be used to strengthen the effect produced by the above points.

(7) Points and Manipulations for Relaxing the Bowels

POINTS AND MANIPULATIONS

Clearing Dachang, pinching-kneading Boyangchi, rubbing the abdomen, kneading the umbilicus (the two points are operated clockwise), pushing down Qijiegu, kneading Guiwei, and pushing the spine.

CLINICAL APPLICATION OF DIFFERENT MANIPULATIONS

All the manipulations mentioned above have the role of relaxing the bowels. Among them, clearing Dachang and pushing the spine play the roles of clearing away pathogenic heat and relaxing bowels, which can be used to treat diarrhea due to pathogenic heat. Pinching-kneading Boyangchi i.e. Zhigou (SJ 6) of the *San-jiao* Channel of Hand-*Shaoyang* plays the roles of regulating *San-jiao* and loosening the bowels to relieve constipation. Rubbing the abdomen and kneading the umbilicus

七节骨，揉龟尾，按揉足三里，揉涌泉。

【辨证应用】

以上诸法均有明显的止泻作用。其中，补脾经、摩腹、捏脊能健脾止泻；补肾经、摩丹田主治久泻不止、损及肾阳之病证；清小肠则有清热利尿、泌别清浊的功能，是治疗湿热水泻的效穴；拿肚角适用于泄泻初期、正气未衰者，有止泻、疗腹痛的功效；其他诸法对泄泻亦有特效。按揉足三里能加强以上各穴止泻的作用。

（7）通便类

【穴位与手法】

清大肠，掐揉膊阳池，摩腹，揉脐（以上两穴均为顺时针方向摩），推下七节骨，揉龟尾，推脊。

【辨证应用】

以上诸法均能通调大便。其中，清大肠、推脊能清热通便治热泻；膊阳池即手少阳三焦经之支沟穴，掐揉之可通理三焦，润肠通便；顺时针方向摩腹、揉脐，即顺大肠行走的方向直接摩、

clockwise, in the direction of the movement of the large intestine can remove stagnation in the intestine. Kneading Guiwei and pushing down Qijiegu play the role of relaxing the bowels by promoting the peristalsis of intestinal tract and the function of the sphincter of anus.

(8) Points and Manipulations for Relieving Pain

POINTS AND MANIPULATIONS

Opening Tianmen, pushing Kangong, arc-pushing Taiyang (Extra 2) and Erhougaogu, pinching-kneading Baihui (Du 20), pinching Yintang (Extra 1), pressing-kneading Jiache (St 6), pinching Fengchi (GB 20), pressing-kneading Rugen (St 18), Rupang and Tanzhong (Ren 17), rubbing the umbilicus and Zhongwan (Ren 12), kneading Tianshu (St 25), grasping Dujiao and Jian jing (GB 21), nipping-kneading Wuzhijie, kneading Wailaogong, pinching-kneading Yiwofeng kneading Zusanli (St 36), kneading Boyangchi, pressing-kneading *Shu* points of viscera on lumbodorsal region, pressing-kneading points round the joints of extremities such as Jianyu (LI 15), Quchi (LI 11), Weizhong (UB 40) Huantiao (GB 30), etc.

CLINICAL APPLICATION OF DIFFERENT MANI- PULATIONS

All the manipulations mentioned above play the role of relieving pain to some extent in every part of the body. Among them, the manipulations of the first six points as well as pinching Fengchi and kneading Boyangchi are effective for treating headache. Pressing kneading Jiache can be used to treat toothache. The three manipulations counted from pressing-kneading Rugen (St 18) play the roles of soothing chest disorder and regulating the flow of *qi*, effective for treating stuffiness and pain in the chest. Pinching-kneading Yiwofeng is the main method of relieving pain. It can be used to treat abdominal pain and general arthralgia. The four manipulations counted from rubbing the umbilicus and pressing-kneading Zusanli (St 36) can be used to treat abdominal pain. Kneading Wailaogong

揉，能清理肠中积滞；揉龟尾、推下七节骨能促进肠道的蠕动与肛门括约肌的功能，从而起到理肠通便的作用。

（8）止痛类

【穴位与手法】

开天门，推坎宫，运太阳，**运耳后高骨**，掐揉百会，掐印堂，按揉颊车，掐风池，按揉乳根、乳旁及膻中，摩脐，摩中脘，揉天枢，拿肚角，拿肩井，掐揉五指节，**揉外劳宫**，掐揉一窝风，按揉足三里，揉膊阳池，按揉腰背部各脏腑**俞穴**，**按揉肩髃**、曲池、委中、环跳等四肢关节四周之穴位等。

【辨证应用】

以上诸法，对全身各部位的疼痛均有不同程度的治疗作用。其中，自开天门以下六法及掐风池~揉膊阳池有治头痛的功效；**按揉颊车穴能治牙痛**，自按揉乳根以下三法，能宽胸理气，善治胸部闷痛；掐揉一窝风为止痛要法，能治腹痛及周身痹痛；自摩脐以下四法及按揉足三里，可治腹痛，揉外劳宫善治虚寒性腹痛；**按揉腰背部各脏腑俞穴**，除能消除局部肌肉疼痛外，还能对相应脏腑

· 511 ·

is more effective for abdominal pain of asthenia-cold type. Pressing-kneading the *Shu* points of viscera on the lumbodorsal region can be used to relieve radiating pain on the lumbodorsal region due to visceral disorder and pain in internal organs apart from relieving local muscular pain. Pressing-kneading the points round the joints of the extremities can be used to treat arthralgia of corresponding joints. If it is used together with nipping-kneading Yiwofeng, it will be more effective.

(9) Points and Manipulations for Inducing Diuresis

POINTS AND MANIPULATIONS

Clearing Xiaochang, kneading Boyangchi, clearing Shenjing, kneading Erma, kneading Xiaotianxin, palm-rubbing or pushing-pressing Dantian (Elixir field) and pushing Jimen.

CLINICAL APPLICATION OF DIFFERENT MANIPULATIONS

All the manipulations mentioned above play the role of inducing diuresis. Among them, kneading Erma and palm-rubbing Dantian (Elixir Field) play the roles of nourishing the kidney-*yin*, inducing diuresis for treating stranguria and are used to treat the symptoms of scanty dark urine and stranguria. Clearing Shenjing, Xiaochang and nipping-kneading Boyangchi play the roles of clearing away damp-heat from the lower-*jiao*, separating the useful from the waste (through the function of the small intestine). They are often used to treat scanty dark urine due to heat in the bladder. Clearing Xiaochang is used with kneading Xiaotianxin to treat scanty dark urine, anuresis due to heat having moved into the small intestine from the Heart Channel. Pushing Jimen and pushing-pressing Dantian (Elixir Field) are most effective for treating uroschesis.

(10) Points and Manipulations for Relieving Vomiting

Clearing Weijing, pushing from Hengwen to Banmen, arc-pushing Bagua counter clockwise, separating abdominal

疾病所引起的腰背部牵涉痛及内脏疼痛有治疗作用；**按揉肢节周围的穴位能治疗相应关节的痹痛，如与掐揉一窝风配合使用，则疗效更佳。**

（9）利小便类

【穴位与手法】

清小肠，揉膊阳池，清肾经，揉二马，揉小天心，摩或推按丹田，推箕门。

【辨证应用】

以上诸法均有利尿作用。其中，揉二马、摩丹田能滋补肾阴、利水通淋，主治小便短赤淋沥不畅之证；清肾经、清小肠、掐揉膊阳池能清利下焦湿热、泌别清浊，多用于治疗膀胱蕴热之小便短赤之证；清小肠与揉小天心配用能治心经有热，移热于小肠所致的小便短赤、尿闭等证；推箕门，推按丹田对尿潴留疗效显著。

（10）止呕吐类

清胃经，横纹推向板门，逆运八卦，分腹阴阳，按弦走搓摩，推天柱骨，按揉天突，揉涌泉。

Yin-Yang, foulaging-rubbing just in the the same way as touching the string, pushing Tianzhugu, pressing-kneading Tiantu (Ren 22), and kneading Yongquan (K 1).

CLINICAL APPLICATION OF DIFFERENT MANIPULATIONS

All the manipulations mentioned above play the role of relieving vomiting. Among them, clearing Weijing plays the role of clearing away pathogenic heat from the stomach, so it can be used to treat vomiting due to pathogenic heat. Pushing Tianzhugu and pressing-kneading Tiantu (Ren 22) play the role of keeping the adverse *qi* downwards and relieving vomiting, being effective for vomiting due to wind-cold or wind-heat. Separating abdominal Yin-Yang, foulaging-rubbing just in the same way as touching strings play the roles of promoting digestion and removing retention of food in the stomach. So they can be used to treat vomiting due to improper diet. Pushing from Hengwen to Banmen is more effective for treating vomiting due to various causes. Arc-pushing Neibagua counterclockwise plays the roles of keeping the adverse *qi* downwards and promoting digestion. It is more effective for vomiting due to improper diet. Kneading Yongquan (K 1) plays the role of withdrawing the fire to its origin. It is often used to treat vomiting due to asthenia-heat.

(11) Points and Manipulations for Soothing Chest Oppression, Regulating the Flow of *Qi*, Eliminating Phlegm and Relieving Cough and Asthma

POINTS AND MANIPULATIONS

Kneading or squeezing-pinching Tiantu, pushing-kneading Tanzhong (Ren 17), kneading Rugen (St 18) and Rupang, kneading Feishu (UB 13), lifting-pinching or squeezing-pressing Dazhui (Du 14), foulaging-rubbing the hypochondrium, reinforcing Feijing, clearing Feijing, reinforcing Shenjing, arc-pushing Neibagua clockwise, and kneading Xiaohengwen of the palm.

【辨证应用】

以上诸法均有止呕之功。其中，清胃经能清胃府积热而治热
所致呕吐；推天柱骨、按揉天突可降逆止呕，善治感受风寒或风热所致
的呕吐；分腹阴阳、按弦走搓摩有明显的消食导滞作用，故可用
于治疗伤食呕吐；横纹推向板门是治呕吐的效穴，各种原因所致
的呕吐均可应用；逆运内八卦能降气消食，善治伤食吐；揉涌泉
能引火归元，常用于治疗虚热呕吐。

(11)宽胸理气、化痰、止咳、平喘类

【穴位与手法】

揉天突或挤捏天突，推揉膻中，揉乳根、乳旁，揉肺俞，提
捏或挤压大椎，搓摩胁肋，补肺经，清肺经，补肾经，顺运内八
卦，揉掌小横纹。

CLINICAL APPLICATION OF DIFFERENT MANI-PULATIONS

All the manipulations mentioned above are important methods of regulating the flow of *qi*, relieving cough and asthma and eliminating phlegm. Among them, the first five manipulations play the roles of relieving cough, eliminating phlegm, normalizing the lung and relieving asthma. Kneading Tiantu mainly plays the role of relieving asthma and is effective for asthma with rale. The other four manipulations and arc-pushing Neibagua clockwise play the role of relieving chest fullness and promoting the circulation of *qi*, which can be used to treat stuffiness in the chest, cough, rale, etc. Kneading Feishu (UB 13) and reinforcing Feijing play the roles of replenishing and restoring the lung-*qi*, which can be used to treat persistent cough due to deficiency of the lung. Reinforcing Shenjing plays the roles of nourishing the kideny and strengthening *yang*, which can be used to treat dyspnea due to deficiency of the kidney. Foulaging-rubbing the hypochondrium plays the role of soothing the liver and clearing away phlegm. Clearing Feijing, lifting-pinching or squeezing-pressing Dazhui and kneadnig Xiaohengwen of the palm play the role of clearing away lung-heat, relieving cough and eliminating phlegm, which are mainly used to treat dyspnea of wind-heat type, rale, whooping cough, etc.

(12) Points and Manipulations for Relieving Convulsion and Allaying Excitement

POINTS AND MANIPULATIONS

Opening Tianmen, pushing Kangong, kneading Taiyang (Extra 2), pressing-kneading Baihui (Du 20), nipping Yintang (Extra) clearing Ganjing, reinforcing Xinjing, clearing Xinjing, and nipping-kneading Xiaotianxin and Wuzhijie.

CLINICAL APPLICATION OF DIFFERENT MANI-PULATIONS

All the manipulations mentioned above play the roles of relieving convulsion and tranquilizing the mind. Among

【辨证应用】

以上诸法均为理气、止咳、化痰、平喘之要法。其中，前五法均有止咳化痰，利肺平喘之功效，揉天突偏重于降逆平喘，善治哮喘痰鸣；其他四法及顺运内八卦有开胸利气的作用，可用于治疗胸闷、咳嗽、痰鸣等病证；揉肺俞与补肺经能补益肺气，适用于肺虚久咳之证；补肾经能滋肾壮阳，可治肾虚喘咳；搓摩胁肋能疏肝气、消积痰；清肺经、提捏或挤压大椎穴、揉掌小横纹能清宣肺热、止咳化痰，主治风热型喘咳、痰鸣、百日咳等病证。

(12) 镇惊安神类

【穴位与手法】

开天门，推坎宫，揉太阳，按揉百会，掐印堂，清肝经，补心经，清心经，掐揉小天心，掐揉五指节。

【辨证应用】

以上诸法都有明显的镇惊安神的作用。其中，自开天门以下五法，能醒脑安神、镇静除烦、明目益智；清肝经能平肝泻火、

them, the first five manipulations play the roles of restoring consciousness and allaying excitement, tranquilizing and relieving restlessness, improving vision and promoting intelligence. Clearing the liver channel plays the roles of calming the liver, removing fire from the liver and relieving depressed liver and restlessness, which is used to treat convulsion and dysphoria with feverish sensation in the chest, palms and soles. Clearing Xinjing, nipping-kneading Xiaotianxin play the role of clearing away heat from the heart channel, which is mainly used to treat infantile convulsion, morbid night crying of babies, restlessness due to flaring heart-fire. Reinforcing Xinjing plays the role of nourishing the heart to calm the mind, which is mainly used to treat restlessness due to deficiency of *qi* and blood. Nipping-kneading Wuzhijie plays the roles of allaying excitement, relieving convulsion and expelling wind-phlegm, which can be used to treat convulsion and restlessness due to heat-transmission from obstruction of windphlegm.

(13) Points and Manipulations for Restoring Consciousness and Relieving Spasm

POINTS AND MANIPULATIONS

Opening Tianmen, pushing Kangong, pinching Renzhong (Du 26), pinching Shixuan, grasping Baichong and Pushen (UB 61), pressing Jiache (St 6) and grasping Weizhong (UB 40), Chengshan (UB 57), Quchi (LI 11) and Hegu (LI 4).

CLINICAL APPLICATION OF DIFFERENT MANIPULATIONS

The first four manipulations play the roles of restoring consciousness and causing resuscitation, which can be used to treat infantile convulsion and fainting spell. Pressing Jiache (St 6) can be used to treat trismus. Pinching, kneading, pressing, grasping forcefully on the points distributed on the extremities play the roles of relieving convulsion, calming the endogenous wind and stopping twitch.

解郁除烦，主治惊风躁动、五心烦热；清心经、掐揉小天心能清

心经之热，主治心火炽盛所致的惊风、夜啼、烦躁不安等证；补

心经可养心安神，主治气血虚弱之心烦不安等证；掐揉五指节能

安神镇惊、祛风痰，治疗风痰内结，郁久化热所引起的惊风、惊

惕不安之证。

　　(13) 醒神开窍、止抽搐类

【穴位与手法】

　　开天门，推坎宫，掐人中，掐十宣，拿百虫，拿仆参，按颊

车，拿委中，拿承山，拿曲池，拿合谷。

【辨证应用】

　　前四法能醒神开窍，主治惊风、昏厥等病证；按颊车能治牙

关紧闭；其他肢节四周各穴，若用较重的手法掐揉、按拿之，则

有镇惊、熄风、止抽搐的功用。

Section 3

Points for Attention in Performing Child Massage

1. Suitable Age and Massage Area

(1) Suitable Age

Child massage operated mainly on points of the hands is suitable for children under 12, with the effect of treatment most prominent in children under 6. Clinical experience shows that the younger the age the more effective it will be. For elder children the treatment can be done in combination with adult massage which is operated mainly on the points on the body.

(2) Massage Area

Massage areas vary with the points used in clinical treatment. When the points on the fourteen regular channels, extra-points and the special points on the trunk and the lower limbs for children are selected, the symmetrical points on both right and left sides are generally operated on at the same time, except a few points, for instance, Jimen (SP 11), which is usually operated on one side, but in serious cases, on both sides. When the special points on the upper limbs are selected, the manipulation is often unilateral. In ancient times, the doctor only operated on boy's left hand and on girl's right hand. But nowadays there is no difference in sex. The doctor operates on points of the left hand in both sexes. If there is a abrasion or other injury which prevents the left hand from being operated, the right hand can be manipulated instead.

2. Irritating Extent and Reinforcing and Reducing Effect of Child Massage

The irritating extent of the manipulations includes the

第三节 小儿推拿临床须知

1. 小儿推拿的适宜年龄与操作部位

（1）适宜年龄：以运用手穴为主的小儿推拿疗法，适用于12周岁以下的儿童。其中，以6周岁以下的儿童疗效为佳。临床经验表明，年龄越小，其治疗效果越好。对年龄较大的儿童，可配合应用以体穴为主的成人推拿手法进行治疗。

（2）操作部位：在小儿推拿临床中，由于采用的穴位不同，其操作部位也各异。当取用十四经穴、奇穴与躯干部及下肢部的小儿推拿特定穴时，一般采用双侧穴位同时操作，即在推拿上述部位的穴位时，左右对称的同名穴都要同时进行推拿，但也有个别穴位例外，如箕门穴，通常情况下推单侧，病情较重时推双侧。当取用上肢的小儿推拿特定穴时，则仅用单侧穴位。在古代，对男孩只推拿左手，而对女孩则只推拿右手；现代的小儿推拿医生多不分病儿的男女，均取左手的穴位操作。如左手有擦伤或其他情况不便于操作时，也可推拿右手。

2. 小儿推拿手法的刺激量与补泻作用

手法刺激量的强度包括手法作用力的大小、频率的快慢和持

pushing strength, the frequency and the duration. Generally pushing-forcefully with quick frequency and long duration can result in heavy irritation, otherwise it can result in weak irritation. Irritating extent of the manipulation is decided according to the child's age, his health status, the severity of his illness and the points selected (main points or supplementary points). Take the most commonly-used straight-pushing for example. If the frequency of manipulation is 200—300 times a minute, the duration of manipulation in different age groups can be found in the following table.

Duration of Irritation Required for Straight-pushing Manipulation

Age	Point	
	Main Point	Supplementary point
within 6 months	1–1.5 minutes	30 seconds
6 months–1 year	1.5–3 minutes	30 seconds– 1 minute
1–3 years	3–4 minutes	1–1.5 minutes
3–6 years	4–5 minutes	1.5–2 minutes
above 6 years	5–7 minutes	2–3 minutes

Apart from irritating extent, reinforcing or reducing manipulation can be selected according to the patient's condition. The effect of reinforcing and reducing manipulations depends on the irritating extent and the direction of strength. Traditionally, the operation with great strength, quick frequency, short duration and in opposite direction of the course of the channel is called reducing manipulation. The operation with a little strength, low frequency, long duration and in the same direction of the course of the channel is called reinforcing manipulation.

It is a complicated and difficult clinical problem to use reinforcing and reducing manipulation properly because the patients

续时间的长短等因素。一般说来，用力重、频率快、持续时间长的手法为强刺激；反之则为弱刺激。治疗时对患儿采取多大的刺激量，需根据患儿的年龄、体质、病情及具体穴位（主穴或配穴）而定。以临床最常用的直推法为例，如果按每分钟200—300次的频率来计算，则不同年龄刺激时间的掌握可参考下表：

小儿直推法刺激时间表

穴位 年龄	主 穴	配 位
6个月以内	1～1.5分钟	30秒
6个月～1周岁	1.5～3分钟	30秒～1分钟
1周岁～3周岁	3～4分钟	1～1.5分钟
3周岁～6周岁	4～5分钟	1.5～2分钟
6周岁以上	5～7分钟	2～3分钟

临床除注意刺激量外，还应根据病情的虚实，采用或补或泻的操作方法。而手法的补泻作用是由一定的刺激量与作用力的方向来决定的。传统推拿学认为，凡手法作用力大、频率快、操作时间短或相对较短、逆经方向操作（在腹部则顺时针方向操作）者，称为泻法；若作用力较轻柔、频率稍慢、操作时间长、顺经方向操作（在腹部则逆时针方向操作）则为补法。

临床上，要恰当掌握刺激量与手法补泻的操作，是一个比较

are usually different in age and health status, the severity of their illness is ever changing, and the onset of the children's diseases is abrupt and can progress quickly. So we should never stay in rut. Based on general rules, we must sum up the experience in practice. Only in this way can we use reinforcing and reducing manipulations accurately according to the patient's condition.

3. Commonly-used Medium for Child Massage

All the doctors in history have attached great importance to the combination of manipulation with the application of medium. We can find the earliest child massage method which called "paste massage" from the documents written in Han and Tang Dynasties. Since Ming and Qing Dynasties, pediatric massagist have also stressed that "pushing must be done with juice". "Juice" here means liquid medium. The use of medium is not only helpful to the operation, but also protects the skin from damage. It can also improve the curative effect, and widen the treatment scope of pediatric masso-therapy. Apart from talc powder, Chinese ilex oil, sesame oil, wintergreen oil, massage lotion used in massage for adults, other mediums are often used as follows:

1) Ginger Juice: Smash cleaned fresh ginger, filter it and then add some water to the juice. It can be used in spring and winter. It plays the roles of smoothing skin, dispelling cold, warming yang, and relieving superficial syndrome by means of diaphoresis.

2) Chinese Onion Juice: Cut Chinese onion into small pieces. Steep them in a certain amount of alcohol for 24 hours. It can be used after filtrition in winter and spring. It plays the roles of smoothing the skin, dredging the channel, activating the blood circulation, dispelling cold, relieving superficial syndrome.

3) Peppermint Juice (*Aqua Menthae*): Take some peppermint leaves, steep and filter them. Then it can be used in summer. It plays the roles of smoothing the skin, clearing away pathogenic heat and relieving superficial syndrome, removing

复杂且难以掌握的问题。这是因为患儿年龄、素质各不相同，病情千变万化，并且小儿的发病特点是发病急骤，传变迅速，因此，决不能墨守成规，必须在掌握上述一般规律的基础上，不断积累实践经验，才能根据病人的具体情况，准确把握刺激量及补泻手法的应用。

3. 小儿推拿常用介质

对于小儿推拿，历代医家都十分重视手法与介质结合运用。从汉唐时期的推拿文献中，我们就可看到，中国小儿推拿最早的治疗形式就是"膏摩"。明、清以来，小儿推拿医家也都十分强调"推必用汤"。这里所说的"汤"，即液体介质之意。介质的正确使用，不但方便操作，保护患儿皮肤，且能明显地提高疗效，扩大小儿推拿的治疗范围。目前临床常用的小儿推拿介质，除成人推拿常用的滑石粉、冬青油、麻油、冬绿油、按摩乳外，还有以下几种：

1）姜汁：把生姜洗净捣烂，滤汁去渣，然后加入适量的水，便可应用。多用于冬、春季节，有滑润皮肤、温阳散寒、发汗解表的作用。

2）葱水：取葱白切碎，用适量的酒精浸泡24小时后，滤汁去渣，即可应用。亦多用于冬、春季节，有滑润皮肤、通经活血、散寒解表的作用。

3）薄荷水：取少量薄荷叶，用水浸泡后滤汁去渣，即可应

summer-heat, reducing fever.

4) Chinese Ilex Oil: It is a kind of mixed liquid or medicinal ointment which is prepared with Chinese ilex oil, vaseline, peppermint oil or glycerin. The dispensing is as follows:

Name	Winter	Summer
Chinese Ilex oil	17%	15%
peppermint oil	3%	5%
vaseline	80%	80%

5) Egg White: Take one egg and remove the egg yolk. The egg white can then be used. It plays the roles of smoothing the skin, clearing away pathogenic heat and moistening the lung.

4. The Principle of Formulation and Prescription Writing

The prescription is made up according to the rule of compatibility, based on clinical diagnosis of diseases and differentiation of sysdromes, the function of points, the effect of manipulations and their relationship. There are three parts that need attention — selecting points, choosing manipulations and determining the extent of irritation.

"Points selecting" means that the points selected are divided into principal points and coordinating points according to their therapeutic effect. Coordinating point includes supplementary and adjuvant points. A principal point is a point which plays the main role in treating the cause of the disease and its main symptoms. A supplementary point is a point which coordinates with the principal point to treat diseases. It can enhance the curative effect. An adjuvant point is a point which supports the principal point in treating diseases. It can also decrease the side effect produced by the main point. There

用。多在夏季应用，有滑润皮肤、清热解表、消暑退热的作用。

4）冬绿油：是用冬青油与凡士林、薄荷油或甘油等配成的混合液或膏剂，常用比例如下：

名　　　称	冬　　天	夏　　天
冬 青 油	17%	15%
薄荷脑(油)	3%	5%
凡 士 林	80%	80%

5）鸡蛋清：取鸡蛋一个，去其蛋黄，所剩的蛋清即可使用。有滑润皮肤、清热滑润肺的作用。

4．小儿推拿的组方原则与处方书写

小儿推拿治疗处方是在临诊辨证、立法的基础上，根据穴位的性能、手法的功效及其相互关系，按照一定的配伍规律组合而成的。在组方时，应注意选穴、定法、定量三个方面的问题。

"选穴"是指将所选的穴位，按其治疗作用的大小，分为主穴与配穴两种。其中，配穴又有辅穴与佐穴之别。主穴是在治疗病因与主证中起主要治疗作用的穴位；辅穴是辅助主穴治疗病因与主证的穴位，与主穴能产生直接的协同作用，并可加强其疗效；佐穴是协助主穴治疗兼证或制约主穴副作用的穴位。在一个处方中，一般主穴较少，一至三个；辅穴与佐穴常根据具体情况而

are only a few principal points, usually 1—3, in one prescription. The supplementary and adjuvant points are selected on the basis of the patient's condition. Generally, the principal points and supplementary points prescribed in a prescription must be clearly pointed out and coordinate to each other, as ancient doctors held that "a massage prescription had to be done in the way as the task allotment among the officials of different ranks, the monarch, minister, assistant and guide."

"Determining manipulations" means that the manipulations on each point which play the roles of reinforcing, reducing, heat-clearing, warming, sweating, activating, regulating, scattering must be clearly determined respectively. For instance, when the doctor treats the patient with cough due to lung-heat he must prescribe "clearing Feijing" instead of "pushing Feijing", because the former means that the doctor uses pushing manipulation centrifugally on the point of Feijing on child's end part of the ring finger while the latter includes needs pushing in two directions called centrifugation and centripetalness.

"Determining the extent of irritation" means that the doctor must determine the irritating extent to each point, according to the patient's condition and the main points and the auxiliary points prescribed, including the frequency and duration. Generally, the duration of irritation to the main point lasts longer, to the supplementary points, shorter and to the supporting points, the shortest.

When the doctor writes a precription, he usually writes the main words which refers to the point in the middle. Before this, the technique which expresses manipulations must be clearly written down along with the irritating extent and duration on the right corner of the paper. For the whole prescription the point prescribed must be in the order of the main points, supplementary points and adjuvant points. It also can be arranged in the order of the points on the head and face first and then the points on upper limbs, chest, stomach, back and

定，可多可少。总之，从总体上来说，整个处方的用穴，要主次分明，协调统一。正如古代医家所说的推拿用穴"即如用药者之必有君、臣、佐、使也。"

"定法"即是根据治则明确每个穴位的操作手法，或补、或泻、或清、或温、或汗、或通、或和、或散，都要一一确定，不可模棱两可。例如在治疗肺热咳嗽时，应注明"清肺经"，而不可只写"推肺经"。这是因为前者要求医者在患儿无名指末节的肺经穴上做离心方向直推；而后者则包括离心与向心两个方向的直推动作，是相反的两种操作方法的统称。

"定量"是要求医者根据病人的情况与处方中穴位的主次，确定对每个穴位的刺激量，包括推拿的次数或时间。一般说来，对主穴的刺激时间较长，辅穴次之，佐穴较少。

在具体书写小儿推拿处方时，就每个穴位而言，一般以穴位名称为主干词写在中间，在其前方要写清表示操作方法的手法动作名称，而在其右下角则标明作为刺激量的操作次数与时间，而对于整个处方的书写，则应按先主穴，再辅穴，后佐穴的顺序书写。也可前先头面部穴位，再上肢，后胸腹、腰背与下肢部穴位的顺序，但一般应尽量要求二者的统一。临床实际操作时，一

lower limbs. The doctor must operate according to the order prescribed.

For example, if the child has as his symptoms watery stool with foam, light colour and no stink, borborygmus with stomachache, pale face, no thirst, prolonged urine, smooth and white fur on the tongue, soft and floating pulse, red superficial venule of the index finger, then the disease is diagnosed as diarrhea due to pathogenic cold-dampness. The principle of treatment is dispelling pathogenic cold by warming the middle-*jiao*, eliminating the dampness and stopping diarrhea. The prescription of massage is as follows: reinforcing Pijing and Dachang for 500 times, pushing Sanguan for 300 times, kneading Wailaogong 100 times, kneading Yiwofeng 50 times, pushing Liufu 50 times, rubbing the abdomen and kneading the umbilicus 500 times, pushing-up Qijiegu 100 times, kneading Guiwei 50 times, and pressing-kneading Zusanli (St 36) 30 times. Among them, the first three points are principal points, while kneading Wailaogong, rubbing abdomen and kneading umbilicus, pushing-up Qijiegu, kneading Guiwei are supplementary. Kneading Yiwofeng and pressing-kneading Zusanli are supporting points to treat abdominal pain. Pushing Liufu plays the role of preventing heat side effect due to the manipulation of pushing Sanguan. The arrangement of the points prescribed above is basically decided according to the principle that the main points must be arranged before the supplementary points, along with the arrangement of points on the part of the body. Additionally, if there is a point which needs strong irritation, it will be the last one to be operated. If this point receives manipulations at first, it may cause the child to cry, and interrupts the treatment.

5. Indications and Contraindications of Child Massage

Child massage is widely used. It is indicated in treating various diseases including internal disorders, trauma and diseases

般是按照处方的先后次序进行操作。

例如，若患儿表现为：大便清稀多沫，色淡不臭，肠鸣腹痛，面色淡白，口不渴，小便清长，苔白腻，脉濡，指纹色红。辨证为寒湿泻。治法为温中散寒、化湿止泻。据此则拟推拿处方如下：补脾经 500 次，补大肠 500 次，推三关 300 次，揉外劳宫 100 次，揉一窝风 50 次，退六腑 50 次，摩腹揉脐 500 次，推上七节骨 100 次，揉龟尾 50 次，按揉足三里 30 次。其中，前三穴为主穴；揉外劳宫、摩腹揉脐、推上七节骨、揉龟尾四穴为辅穴；揉一窝风与按揉足三里为治疗腹痛等兼症的佐穴，退六腑则是为防止推三关的温热作用太过而设的起反佐作用的穴位。以上处方的穴位排列次序基本上是按主穴在先，配穴在后的原则，并兼顾了以穴位所在部位为先后的要求。此外，如在某一处方中有需要用强刺激手法的穴位，则应放在最后进行操作。因为如果此类穴位在一开始就操作，则会引起患儿哭闹以致治疗无法进行。

5．小儿推拿的适应症与禁忌症

小儿推拿的适应症相当广泛，凡小儿内、伤、五官科的各种病

of the eyes, nose, mouth and ears, with good effect, especially for children with the symptoms in digestive and respiratory systems. The usage is being widened along with the development of pediamassage. It can also stimulate the appetite, promote health, enhance the immunity of the body against diseases and foster growth. It is convenient, effective in contrast with drugs and acceptable by the children and their parents.

It is not suitable for skin and external diseases, such as carbuncle and ulcers, fracture, dislocation of joint, and acute infectious diseases.

6. Other Points for Attention

1) Keep appropriate temperature in the treating room, avoid overwarm and overcold and catching cold.

2) When the doctor treats the patient, he must be amicable and exerts light strength carefully and gently. The doctor's finger nail has to be cut round with appropriate length and smooth edge before operating. The cold hands which touch the child suddenly may cause the baby patient to cry so the doctor has to warm his hands before operating.

3) In the treatment the doctor must pay attention to the child's position which should be convenient for him to operate and comfortable. The child can be seated, lie in bed or be carried by his mother.

4) Generally, the doctor's left hand is the fixing hand, the right hand is the operating hand. The doctor uses his left hand to fix the child's limbs and also let the points expose in order that the right hand can operate successfully But he should not grasp the child too tightly or keep the child's limbs in a certain position for a long time lest the child feel uncomfortable, painful and frightened. So the two hands must cooperate with each other in the movement with the child's limbs in different positions without interrupting the operation.

5) For other matters that call for attention, refer to the

证皆可应用，并有良好的疗效。特别是对小儿消化、呼吸系统病症的疗效尤为显著。随着小儿推拿学的不断发展，其适应范围还在继续扩大。另外，小儿推拿对健康儿童又有增进饮食、强壮身体、提高机体的免疫力与抗病能力、助长发育等作用，且较药物更方便、更有效，更乐于被家长和小儿接受。

凡疮疡、骨折、脱位、急性传染病等均不宜于推拿治疗。

6．其他注意事项

1）治疗室内应保持适宜的温度，避免过冷、过热及受风着凉。

2）医者应态度和蔼可亲，操作时动作宜轻柔，细心耐心。操作前，术者必须将指甲修剪圆整，长短适宜，边缘光滑；天冷时，应先将双手温暖后再进行操作，以免凉手突然刺激患儿，引起患儿哭闹。

3）治疗时，要注意患儿的体位，或坐或卧，或由母亲怀抱，既要方便操作，又要力求舒适自然。

4）操作时，一般术者的左手为固定手，右手为操作手。固定手既要握持固定好患儿的肢体，又要将穴位充分暴露，以保证右手顺利地操作。但又不可握捏太紧，强制性地将患儿的肢体长时间地固定在某一位置，以免引起患儿不适、疼痛与恐惧。所以，操作时术者的双手要配合默契、协调一致，在不妨碍操作的前提下，术者双手可边操作、边随患儿的肢体作前后或上下移动。

5）其他注意事项基本同成人推拿。

chapter concerning the massage for adults.

Section 4

Treatment of Common Diseases

Infantile Diarrhea

Infantile diarrhea, also called indigestion, refers to increased frequency of defecation with thin or even watery stool.
Though it can occur in four seasons, it occurs more often in
summer and autumn. Children under 2 years are most frequently affectd. Traditional Chinese medicine holds that the
main causes of the disease are exogenous pathogenic factors
(including pathogenic cold, dampness, summer-heat and heat),
improper diet or deficiency of the spleen and stomach. Now
the causes of the disease are considered to be associated with
infection by pathogenic colibacillus, viruses, mycetes and other
infections apart from the factors of diet and climate.

MAIN SYMPTOMS

1. Diarrhea due to Cold-dampness

The main symptoms are thin stool with foam or watery
stool light in colour with no stink, borborygmus with
stomachache, pale face, no thirst, cold extremities, prolonged
urine, smooth and white fur on the tongue, slow pulse and
reddish superficial venule of the index finger.

2. Diarrhea due to Dampness-heat

The child passes loose stool the moment he feels abdominal
pain. The onset is abrupt with yellowish-brown and stinking
stool. The child has a slight fever, feels thirsty with less
yellow-coloured urine, red anus with burning sensation, red
tongue, yellowish and greasy fur, smooth pulse and purple
superficial venule of the index finger.

3. Diarrhea due to Indigestion

第四节　常见病的治疗

婴幼儿腹泻

婴幼儿腹泻，亦名消化不良，临床以大便次数增多、粪便稀薄甚至如水样为主症。本病一年四季均可发病，但以夏、秋两季为多。患儿多为2岁以下的婴幼儿。中医认为，本病多因感受外邪(包括寒、湿、暑、热之邪)、内伤乳食或脾胃虚弱所致。现代医学认为婴幼儿腹泻除与饮食、气候等因素有关外，尚与致病性大肠杆菌、病毒、霉菌及其他感染有关。

【主证】

1. 寒湿泻

大便清稀多沫或呈水泻，色淡不臭，肠鸣腹痛，面色淡白，口不渴，四肢欠温，小便清长，舌苔白滑，脉迟，指纹淡红。

2. 湿热泻

腹痛即泻，急迫暴注，粪便稀薄，色黄褐热臭，身有微热，口渴，尿少色黄，肛门色红灼热，舌质红，苔黄腻，脉滑数，指纹紫红。

3. 伤食泻

The child cries before passing stool and feels abdominal distention and pain, which may be allayed after defecation. The child patient passes more sour and stinking stool accompanied with halitosis and anorexia. The child suffering from diarrhea due to indigestion passes stool green in colour with lumps of milk, accompanied with eructation with fetid odour, nausea, vomiting, thick fur, smooth pulse and purple superficial venule of the index finger.

4. Diarrhea due to Hypofunction of the Spleen

The symptoms and signs are repeated attacks of diarrhea with long duration, abdominal frequent passage of loose stools with light white colour lumps of milk and residue of food. It occurs more often after meals. The patient has emaciation with sallow complexion, anorexia, pale tongue with thin fur, floating pulse and reddish superficial venule of the index finger.

If the diarrhea lasts long, it can damage the kidney-*yang*, manifested as pale complexion, watery stools with more frequency, cold limbs, pale tongue with white fur, feeble pulse, or even persistent diarrhea with undigested food in the stool, cold extremities, faint pulse and mental confusion due to the exhaustion of the body fruid and *yang*.

TREATMENT

1. Essential Prescription

Pushing Pijing and Dachang, arc-pushing Neibagua, rubbing the abdomen, pushing-up Qijiegu, kneading Guiwei and pressing Zusanli (St 36).

2. Modification of Prescription according to Different Syndromes

Diarrhea due to Cold-dampness: Reinforcing Pijing and Dachang, rubbing the abdomen (reinforcing method) as well as pushing Sanguan and kneading Wailaogong

Diarrhea due to Dampness-heat: Reinforcing Pijing, clearing Dachang, rubbing the abdomen (reducing method or uniform reinforcing-reducing method); clearing Xiaochang

腹部胀痛，泻前哭闹，泻后痛减，大便酸臭量多，口臭纳呆。伤于乳者，可见有绿色大便及乳块，并伴有嗳腐、恶心、呕吐。舌苔厚或腻，脉滑，指纹紫滞。

4. 脾虚泻

久泻不止，经常反复发作，大便稀薄，水谷不化，其色淡白，夹有奶块及食物残渣，多在食后作泻，面黄体瘦，食欲不振，舌质淡，苔薄白，脉濡，指纹淡红。

若腹泻日久不愈，进而可损及肾阳，症见面色㿠白、大便水样、次数频多、四肢厥冷、舌质淡、苔白、脉细弱无力，甚至出现腹泻不止、完谷不化、四肢逆冷、脉微欲绝、昏不识人等津竭阳脱之证。

【治疗】

1. 基本处方

推脾经，推大肠，运内八卦，摩腹，推上七节骨，揉龟尾，按揉足三里。

2. 随证加减

寒湿泻：用补脾经、补大肠、摩腹（补法），加推三关、揉外劳宫。

湿热泻：用清补脾经、清大肠、摩腹（泻法或平补平泻），加清小肠、清天河水。

and Tianheshui should also be added.

Diarrhea due to Indigestion: Reinforcing Pijing, clearing Dachang, rubbing the abdomen (reducing method or uniform reinforcing-reducing method), can be used. Kneading Banmen and parting-pushing abdominal *Yin-Yang* should be added.

Diarrhea due to Hypofunction of the Spleen: Reinforcing Pijing and Dachang, rubbing the abdomen (reinforcing manipulation) and pinching the spine. Based on the prescription, reinforcing Shenjing, kneading Wailao, kneading Shenshu (UB 23) can be added for the patient with deficiency of spleen and kidney-*yang*. Severe cases should be treated by combining traditional Chinese medicince with Western medicine.

All the manipulations mentioned above can be increased or decreased according to the symptoms and signs. Parting-pushing abdominal *Yin-Yang* can be added for the patient with abdominal distention, rubbing Yiwofeng and grasping Dujiao for the patient with abdominal pain, pushing Tianzhugu for the patient with vomiting, kneading Baihui and pushing-pressing Houchengshan (see Notes below) for the patient with persistent diarrhea.

3. Points for Attention

Massage can be performed once a day. If the patient is in severe condition, it can be done twice a day. Each course of treatment covers 3 days. The patient can recover after 1—3 days' treatment. If the treatment shows no effect, additional 1—2 courses of treatment are needed.

Notes:

Baihui (Du 20): This point is located at the midpoint on a line connecting the apices of both ears. Pressing-kneading manipulation can be used with pressing 3—5 times and kneading 100—300 times. It has the functions of lifting *yang* and treating collapse, indicating to chronic diarrhea, enuresis, prolapse of the rectum, etc.

Houchengshan point: This point is located at the top of

伤食泻：用补脾经、清大肠、摩腹(平补平泻)，加揉板门、分推腹阴阳。

脾虚泻：用补脾经、补大肠、摩腹(补法)，加捏脊。

脾肾阳虚者，可在脾虚泻处方的基础上，加用补肾经、揉外劳宫、揉肾俞。

病情危重者，应中西医结合治疗。

以上诸法，如遇其他兼症，还可随症加减。若腹胀者，加分推腹阴阳；腹痛者，加揉一窝风、拿肚角；呕吐者，加推天柱骨；久泻不止者，加按揉百会、推按后承山(见后注)。

3．注意事项

推拿为每日1次，重者可每日2次，3日为1疗程。一般治疗1～3日即可痊愈。若一个疗程不愈者，可继续治疗1～2个疗程。

注：

百会穴：位于两耳尖直上头顶正中。操作时用按揉法，按3—5次，揉100—300次。有升阳举陷的作用。主治久泻、遗尿、脱肛等。

后承山穴：位于小腿腓肠肌两肌腹之间凹陷中的顶端。操作

the depression, between the two bellies of gastrocnemius muscle.

Manipulation; Pushing-pressing manipulations can be used. Pressing 3—5 times first, then pushing 100—300 times or till heat sensation occurs. Pushing-pressing in the direction to popliteal fossa can be used to treat chronic diarrhea, while pushing-pressing in the opposite direction to the heel can be used to treat constipation.

Vomiting

Vomiting is a symptom, manifested as the adverse rising of food from the stomach by the mouth and nose. In the antient literature of TCM, it is devided into three types, namely "ou" (vomiting with food and sound), "tu" (vomiting with food but without sound), "ganou" (vomiting with sound but without food). Vomiting is a common symptom in clinical pediatrics. It may occur as a single disorder or as a symptom of many other diseases. Children at any age can be affected. It occurs mostly in children under the age of 1 year. TCM holds that vomiting is often caused by exogenous pathogenic factors (such as pathogenic cold, dampness, summer-heat and heat) and improper diet or dirty food. Modern medicine believes that it is due to adverse peristalsis of the esophagus, the stomach or the intestinal tract accompanied by spasmodic contraction of abdominal muscles, which forces food and other contents to cast up from the stomach by way of the esophagus, mouth and nose. Additionally, because of the delicate stomach, relaxation of cardia, if the infant is fed improperly, intakes extra air or overfed, the milk can adversely flow to the mouth, then overflow from the mouth. This, in TCM, is called "milk eructation" which should not be considered as a disease.

MAIN SYMPTOMS

1. Vomiting due to Pathogenic Cold

It often occurs at a certain time after meals. The food vomited is not sour and odorous. The symptoms and signs

时用推按法，先按后推，按 3～5 次，推100～300 次或以 热 为度。向腘窝的方向推按治疗久泻，反之向足跟方向推 按 治 疗 便秘。

呕 吐

呕吐是以胃内容物逆行而上，从口腔或鼻腔涌出为主要表现的病症。对于这一症状的描述，古人又有有物有声谓之呕，有物无声谓之吐，有声无物谓之干呕之说。呕吐是儿科临床常见的症状，既可单独出现，也可见于多种疾病中。本症可见于各种年龄的儿童，但以周岁内婴儿为多见。中医认为，呕吐多 因 感 受 外邪(如寒、湿、暑、热之邪)、饮食不节或不洁所引起。现代医学认为是由于食管、胃或肠道呈逆蠕动并伴有腹肌强力 痉 挛 性 收缩，迫使食物或胃内容物从口、鼻腔涌出。另外，由于婴儿胃脏娇嫩、贲门松弛，如果喂养不当或吸入空气过多，或喂乳 过 多，可在乳后有少量乳汁倒流口腔，并从口角溢出，称之为"溢 乳"，不属病态。

【主证】

1. 寒吐

呕吐乳食多在食后经过一段时间发生。吐物味不酸臭，面色

may include pale complexion, fatigue, cold extremities, abdominal pain that may be relieved by warmth, loose stools, pale tongue with thin and white fur, sunken and slow pulse, and reddish superficial venule of the index finger.

2. Vomiting due to Pathogenic Heat

It occurs soon after meal. The food vomited is sour and offensive. The patient often has fever, restlessness, thirst, red coloured lip, thin stools with offensive smell or constipation, dark urine, reddened tongue, yellow and greasy fur on the tongue, rapid pulse, and purple superficial venule of the index finger.

3. Milk Vomiting

It is manifested as frequent vomiting with sour and offensive milky fragments and indigestive food, halitosis, slight fever or no fever, stuffiness in the chest and anorexia, abdominal pain and distention, constipation or sour and stink stools, white and greasy tongue fur, smooth and full pulse, dark and superficial venule of the index finger.

TREATMENT

1. Essential Prescription

Pushing Pijing, pushing from Hengwen to Banmen, arc-pushing Neibagua, kneading Zhongwan (Ren 12), pressing-kneading Zusanli (St 36), and pushing Tianzhugu.

2. Modification of Prescription according to Syndromes

Cold type vomiting: In addition to reinforcing Pijing, kneading Wailaogong and pushing Sanguan can be prescribed.

Heat type vomiting: Reinforcing-clearing Pijing as well as clearing Weijing, Dachang and Tianheshui and pushing-down Qijiegu can be prescribed.

Vomiting due to improper diet: Reinforcing-clearing Pijing can be prescribed, with kneading Banmen, and separating abdominal *yin-yang* as additional manipulations.

3. Points for Attention

The massage is conducted once a day or in severe cases, twice a day. One course of treatment consists of 3 days.

苍白，精神疲惫，四肢欠温，腹痛喜暖，大便溏薄，舌质淡，苔薄白，脉沉迟，指纹淡红。

2. 热吐

食入即吐，呕吐物酸臭，身热烦躁，口渴唇红，大便稀溏臭秽或秘结，小便黄，舌质红，苔黄腻，脉数，指纹紫红。

3. 伤乳食吐

呕吐频繁，吐出酸臭乳块和未消化的食物，口气臭秽，身发微热或不发热，胸闷厌食，肚腹胀痛，大便秘结或泻下酸臭，苔白厚腻，脉滑实，指纹暗滞。

【治疗】

1. 基本处方

推脾经、横纹推向板门、运内八卦、揉中脘、按揉足三里、推天柱骨。

2. 随证加减

寒吐：用补脾经，加揉外劳宫、推三关。

热吐：用清补脾经，加清胃经、清大肠、清天河水、推下七节骨。

伤食吐：用清补脾经，加揉板门、分腹阴阳。

3. 注意事项

推拿为每日1次，重者每日2次，3日为1个疗程。一般治

Generally, the patient will recover from his illness after three days' treatment. If it shows no effect after 1 course, 1 or 2 more courses should be continued.

Abdominal Pain

Abdominal pain which can occur in many diseases is one of common clinical symptoms in pediatrics. TCM believes that many factors can lead to abdominal pain. It is mainly caused by retention of pathogenic cold-heat in the intestine, stagnation of milk and food, parasitic infestation, and hypofunction of the spleen and stomach. Abdominal pain caused by organic pathologic changes must be diagnosed and treated early in order to avoid deterioration of the disease.

MAIN SYMPTOMS

1. Abdominal Pain due to Pathogenic Cold

The disease is manifested as abrupt abdominal pain with dysphoric crying. It occurs mostly after catching cold or eating raw and cold food. It may be aggravated by cold and relieved by warmth. The other symptoms are black and pale complexion, desire for heat and aversion to cold, watery stool, light-coloured urine, pale tongue with moist and white fur, and reddish superficial venule of the index finger.

2. Abdominal Pain due to Pathogenic Heat

The disease is manifested as paroxysmal abdominal pain and tenderness, burning abdominal wall, flushed cheeks, warm breath, red lips, extreme thirst, constipation, dark urine, red tongue with yellowish and greasy fur, and purplish superficial venule of the index finger.

3. Abdominal Pain due to Improper Diet

The disease is manifested as abdominal distention and pain, tenderness, anorexia, acid regurgitation and eructation with fetid odor, nausea, vomiting, frequent break of wind from bowels, diarrhea or constipation, less pain after fecal discharge, thin and greasy fur on the tongue, smooth pulse and purple superficial venule of the index finger.

疗1～3日即可痊愈，若治疗1个疗程不愈，可继续推拿1～2个疗程。

腹　痛

腹痛是小儿临床常见的症状，可见于多种疾病中。中医认为，导致腹痛的原因很多，主要是由于寒热之邪结于肠间，或乳食积滞、或蛔虫内扰，以及脾胃虚寒等原因所致。对某些器质性病变引起的腹痛，应早诊断，早处理，以免贻误病情。

【主证】

1. 寒痛

腹痛骤发，哭叫不安，多在受凉或饮食生冷后发生，遇冷更剧，得热较舒，面色青白，喜热恶寒，大便清稀，小便清长，舌质淡，苔白滑，指纹淡红。

2. 热痛

腹痛时作时止，痛时拒按，肚皮发烫，面赤，口气热，唇红，烦渴，便秘尿赤，舌质红，苔黄腻，指纹紫红。

3. 伤食痛

腹部胀痛、拒按，厌食，嗳腐吞酸，恶心，呕吐，矢气频作，腹泻或便秘，便后痛减，苔厚腻，脉滑，指纹紫滞。

4. Abdominal Pain due to Helminths

The disease is manifested as abrupt abdominal pain which is more severe round the umbilicus, peristaltic mass in the abdomen which is palpable now and then, the history of fecal discharge with worms in most cases, emaciation, anorexia or paroxia. If the ascaris enter the biliary tract, paroxysmal colicky pain can occur in the right upper abdomen which may be accompanied with vomiting, thick fur on the tongue and wiry pulse.

5. Abdominal Pain due to Asthenia-cold

The disease is manifested as dull abdominal pain, inclination for local pressure and warmth, sallow complexion, emaciation, anorexia, diarrhea, pale tongue with thin and whitish fur, reddish superficial venule of the index finger.

TREATMENT

1. Essential Prescription

Kneading Yiwofeng, palm-rubbing the abdomen, kneading the umbilicus, grasping Dujiao, pressing the corresponding points of the Bladder Channel such as Ganshu (UB 18), Danshu (UB 19), Pishu (UB 20), Weishu (UB 21) and Shenshu (UB 23) and pressing-kneading Zusanli (St 36).

2. Modification of Prescription according to Different Syndromes

Abdominal Pain due to Pathogenic Cold: Adding reinforcing Pijing, kneading Wailaogong and pushing Sanguan.

Abdominal Pain due to Pathogenic Heat: Adding reinforcing-clearing Pijing, clearing Weijing and clearing Tianheshui.

Abdominal Pain due to Improper Diet: Adding reinforcing Pijing, clearing Dachang, kneading Banmen, arc-pushing Neibagua, and separating abdominal *Yin* and *Yang*.

Abdominal Pain due to Ascariasis: Adding kneading Wailaogong, pushing Sanguan and kneading Tianshu (St 25).

Abdominal Pain due to Asthenia-cold: Adding reinforcing Pijing, reinforcing Shenjing, kneading Wailaogong.

3. Points for Attention

4. 虫痛

腹痛突然发作，以脐周为甚，有时可在腹部摸到蠕动之块状物，时隐时现，患儿多有便虫病史，形体消瘦，食欲不振，或嗜食异物。如蛔虫钻入胆道，则可出现右上腹阵发性绞痛，时作时止，或伴有呕吐，舌苔厚，脉弦。

5. 虚寒腹痛

腹痛隐隐，喜暖喜按，面色萎黄，形体消瘦，食欲不振，易发腹泻，舌质淡，苔薄白，指纹淡红。

【治疗】

1. 基本处方

揉一窝风，摩腹，揉脐，拿肚角，按膀胱经相应俞穴，如肝俞、胆俞、脾俞、胃俞、肾俞等，按揉足三里。

2. 随证加减

寒痛：加补脾经，揉外劳宫、推三关。

热痛：加清补脾经、清胃经、清天河水。。

伤食痛：加补脾经、清大肠、揉板门、运内八卦、分腹阴阳。

虫痛：加揉外劳宫、推三关、揉天枢。

虚寒痛：加补脾经、补肾经、揉外劳宫。

3. 注意事项

Once a day or twice a day in severe cases. One course of treatment includes three days. Generally the patient can recover from his illness after 1–3 days' treatment. If it shows no effect after one course, 1 or 2 more courses should be added.

Malnutrition and Food Stagnation of Children

This disease includes malnutrition of children and stagnation of food in the stomach. Stagnation of food in the stomach is a syndrome of chronic digestive disorder due to retention of milk and food in the stomach, manifested as anorexia, indigestion, emaciation and irregular bowel movement. Malnutrition of children refers to deficiency of body fluid and qi, manifested as emaciation, dry skin, brittle hairs, listlessness, and abdominal distention with visible superficial veins. The two syndromes are usually differentiated from each other according to their severity. The symptom of stagnated food in the stomach can develop malnutrition as it was said in ancient time that "most cases with malnutrition result from stagnated food in the stomach." Parasitic infection can also develop malnutrition. The disease occurs more often in infants under the age of 3. TCM holds that stagnation of food is due to improper feeding to the infant, which damages the spleen and stomach resulting in disorder of transportation of the spleen and stomach; malnutrition of children is due to stagnated food in the stomach or other factors, resulting in weakness of the spleen and stomach leading to nutritional disorder, and deficiency of qi and blood.

The disease is almost as the same as "infantile malnutrition" in Western medicine. Complications such as hypochromemia and, vitamin (A. B. C. D) difficiency may occur in severe patients due to low resistance against diseases, which may affect the infant's normal growth.

推拿每日1次，重者可1日2次，3日为1个疗程。一般治疗1～3日即可痊愈。若1个疗程不愈，可续续治疗1～2个疗程。

疳　积

疳积是疳证和积滞的总称。积滞是指乳食积聚留滞于中焦所引起的一种慢性消化功能紊乱的综合征，临床以不思饮食、食而不化、形体消瘦、大便不调为特征。疳证则是指气液干涸，临床以身体羸瘦、毛发枯焦、神疲乏力、腹大筋暴为特征。积滞与疳证有轻重程度之不同，疳证往往是积滞的进一步发展，故古人有"无积不成疳"的说法。小儿感染诸虫，亦可转变为疳证。本病多见于3岁以下的婴儿。中医认为，积滞是由于乳食不节，伤及脾胃，以致脾胃运化失司引起；疳证是因积滞或其他原因导致脾胃虚弱，以致营养失调、气血亏虚所致。

本病大致相当于西医之"小儿营养不良"。重者可因抵抗力极度低下，产生各种并发症，临床以低血色素性贫血、各种维生素（A、B、C、D）缺乏等为多见，久之可影响患儿正常发育。

MAIN SYMPTOMS

1. Damage of the Spleen due to Stagnation of Food

Manifested as emaciation, fullness of the abdomen, loss of appetite, indigestion, irregular bowel movement with fetid odor or slight fever, listlessness, restlessness in sleep, thick and greasy fur on the tongue and purple and stagnated superficial venule of the index finger.

2. Deficiency of both *Qi* and **Blood**

Manifested as sallow or pale complexion, brittle hair with hepotrichosis, emaciation, big head with thin neck, big and rigid abdomen, visible superficial veins, loss of appetite, diarrhea with loose stools, cloudy urine, listlessness or irritability, restlessness in sleep, weak cry, cold extremities, maldevelopment, pale tongue with white and thin fur, and light-coloured superficial venule of the index finger.

TREATMENT

1. Essential Prescription

Reinforcing Pijing, arc-pushing Bagua, kneading Zhongwan (Ren 12), pressing-kneading Zusanli (St 36) and pinching the spine.

2. Modification of Prescription according to Syndromes

Damage of the Spleen due to Stagnation of Food: Kneading Banmen, pushing Sihengwen and separating abdominal Yin and Yang can be added.

Deficiency of both Qi and Blood: Pinching and kneading Sihengwen, reinforcing Shenjing, kneading Wailaogong and pushing Sanguan can be added.

In the above two types, if constipation occurs, kneading Wailaogong and pushing Sanguan can be cancelled while clearing Dachang and pushing down Qijiegu can be added. For patients with diarrhea and loose stools, reinforcing Dachang and pushing-down Qijiegu can be added. For patients with hyperhidrosis, kneading Shending can be added. For patients with deficiency of *yin* fluid manifested as feverish sensation in the

【主证】

1. 积滞伤脾

形体消瘦，腹部胀满，不思乳食，食而不化，大便不调，常有恶臭，或有低热，精神萎靡，夜眠不安，舌苔厚腻，指纹紫滞。

2. 气血两亏

面色萎黄或㿠白，毛发枯黄稀疏，骨瘦如柴，头大颈细，肚大坚硬，青筋暴露，懒进饮食，大便溏泻，小便混浊，精神萎靡或烦躁，睡卧不宁，啼声低弱，四肢不温，发育障碍，舌质淡，苔薄白，指纹色淡。

【治疗】

1. 基本处方

补脾经，运八卦，揉中脘，按揉足三里，捏脊。

2. 随证加减

积滞伤脾型：加揉板门、推四横纹、分腹阴阳。

气血两亏型：加掐揉四横纹、补肾经、揉外劳宫、推三关。

以上两型，若大便秘结者，去揉外劳宫、推三关，加清大肠、推下七节骨；便溏者，加补大肠，推上七节骨；汗多者，加揉肾

heart and the centres of the palms and soles, night sweat and reddish bright tongue, pushing Sanguan and kneading Wailaogong can be cancelled while clearing Ganjing, pinching-kneading Xiaotianxin and Wuzhijie can be added. For patients with aphtha and tongue sore, pinching-kneading Xiaohengwen and kneading Zongjin can be added. For patients with conjunctival congestion accompanied with photophobia, tearing, dryness and pain, clearing Ganjing and kneading Shenjing can be added. For patients with cough and asthma, clearing Feijing, pushing-kneading Tanzhong (Ren 17) and kneading Feishu (UB 13) can be added. Pinching the spine can be used in cooperation with acupuncture treatment of Sihengwen to treat the disease, once every other day or twice a week with good result.

3. Points for Attention

The massage is done once a day. One treatment course includes 6 times. Generally, the patient with stagnation of food in the stomach can be cured after 1 course of treatment. The patient with malnutrition can be cured after 1-3 courses of treatment. If the patient is not cured, one more course should be continued 1 or 2 days later.

Constipartion

It refers to a condition of difficulty in defecation, including disposia or with desire to defecate, long intervals as well as reduced amount of feces. TCM holds that constipation results mainly from retention of sthenia heat in the stomach and the intestines, and the deficiency of *qi* and blood.

MAIN SYMPTOMS

1. Sthenia-type Constipation

The condition is manifested as disposia, long intervals, flushed face, fever, saburra, red lips, excessive thirst, desire for cold drink, scanty dark urine, feeling of fullness and stuffiness in the chest and hypochondrium, poor appetite, abdominal

顶；阴液不足，症见五心烦热、盗汗、舌红苔光剥者，去推三关、揉外劳宫，加清肝经、掐揉小天心、掐揉五指节；口舌生疮者，加掐揉小横纹、揉总筋；目赤多眵、艰涩难睁者，加清肝经、揉肾纹；咳嗽痰喘者，加清肺经、推揉膻中、揉肺俞。

本病单用捏脊配合针刺四横纹治疗，隔日或每周两次，效果亦佳。

3. 注意事项

推拿每日 1 次，6 次为 1 个疗程。一般积滞治疗 1 个疗程、疳证治疗 1～3 个疗程即可痊愈。若不愈者，可停止 1～2 天，然后再进行下一个疗程。

便　秘

便秘是指粪便排泄不畅，包括秘结不通、排便间隔时间延长或虽有便意而排出困难以及粪量减少等。中医认为，肠胃积热、气血虚弱为本证的主要原因。

【主证】

1. 实秘

大便干结不通，或排便间隔延长，面赤身热，口臭唇赤，烦

distention and pain, dry, rough and yellowish fur and purple superficial venule of the index finger.

2. Asthenia-type Constipation

Defecation is difficult although stools are not hard. The patient has pale face, light coloured fingernails, emaciation, lassitude, pale tongue with thin whitish fur and light coloured superficial venule of the index finger.

TREATMENT

1. Essential Prescription: Clearing Dachang, arc-pushing Neibagua, pressing-kneading Boyangchi, rubbing the abdomen (reducing manipulation), pressing-kneading Zusanli (St 36), and pushing down Qijiegu.

2. Modification of Prescription according to Syndromes

Sthenia-type constipation: Clearing Tianheshui, pushing Liu Fu and foulaging-rubbing hypochondrium can be added.

Asthenia-type constipation: Reinforcing Pijing, pushing Sanguan and kneading Erma can be added.

3. Notes

The massage is performed once a day. One treatment course includes three times. Generally, the patient will recover after 1—3 times of treatment. If there is no effect, 1 or 2 more courses of treatment should be continued.

Common Cold

Cold, which is generally called "attack of pathogenic wind", refers to diseases due to exogenous pathogenic factors, manifested as fever, chillness, stuffy nose, nasal discharge, cough, headache and general aching. It can occur in any seasons of the year. The incidence is highest in winter and spring. Its cause is affection of wind-cold or wind-heat pathogen. Complications may occur along with the disease such as sputum, stagnated food in the stomach and convulsion, because infants have delicate lung, deficiency of the spleen-*qi* and aplasia of nervous system.

渴喜冷饮，小便短赤，胸胁痞满，纳食减少，腹部胀痛，苔黄燥，指纹色紫。

2．虚秘

大便努挣难下，便不坚硬，面色㿠白无华，爪甲色淡，形体消瘦，神疲乏力，舌质淡，苔薄白，指纹色淡。

【治疗】

1．基本处方

清大肠，运内八卦，按揉膊阳池，摩腹（泻法），按揉足三里，推下七节骨。

2．随证加减

实秘：加清天河水、退六腑、搓摩胁肋。

虚秘：加补脾经、推三关、揉二马。

3．注意事项

推拿每日1次，3次为1个疗程。一般治疗1～3次即可痊愈。若不愈，可继续治疗1～2个疗程。

感　冒

感冒即外感，俗称"伤风"，临床以发热、恶寒、鼻塞、流涕、咳嗽、头痛、身痛为主症。本病一年四季均可发病，但以冬春二季发病率为高。其发病原因主要是外感风寒或风热时邪。由于小儿肺脏娇嫩，脾常不足，神志怯弱，感邪之后，常可出现夹痰、夹滞、夹惊等兼证。

MAIN SYMPTOMS

1. Common Cold of Wind-cold Type

Severe chillness, slight fever, anhidrosis, stuffy nose with watery discharge, sneezing, cough with watery sputum, headache, itching of the throat, thin and whitish fur on the tongue, floating and tense pulse, and floating red coloured superficial venule of the index finger.

2. Common Cold of Wind-heat Type.

High fever, slight chillness, perspiration, stuffy nose with turbid discharge, sneezing, cough with yellowish and thick sputum, headache, swelling and sore throat, dry mouth and thirst, red tongue with thin and yellowish fur, floating and rapid pulse, and floating red coloured superficial venule of the index finger.

3. Complications

(1) Cough with Sputum: Severe cough with dull voice, rale, greasy and thick fur on the tongue, floating smooth and rapid pulse, purple and stagnated superficial venule of the index finger.

(2) Common Cold with Stagnated Food: Abdominal distention and fullness, loss of appetite, vomiting with fetid odor, eructation with fetid odor, soure and odor stools, abdominal pain with diarrhea or constipation, scanty dark urine, greasy and thick fur on the tongue, full and smooth pulse, and purple and stagnated superficial venule of the index finger.

(3) Common Cold with Fear: Night cry due to fright, restlessness in sleep, reddish tip of the tongue, wiry and rapid pulse, and black-purple superficial venule of the index finger.

TREATMENT

1. Essential Prescription

Opening Tianmen, parting-pushing Kangong, kneading Taiyang (Extra 2), kneading Erhou Gaogu and conducting Huangfeng Rudong.

【主证】

1. 风寒型

恶寒重，发热轻，无汗，鼻塞，流清涕，喷嚏，咳嗽，吐痰清稀，头痛，喉痒，舌苔薄白，脉浮紧，指纹浮红。

2. 风热型

发热重，恶寒轻，有汗，鼻塞，流浊涕，喷嚏，咳嗽，吐痰黄稠，头痛，咽部红肿疼痛，口干而渴，舌质红，苔薄黄，脉浮数，指纹浮露，色较红赤。

3. 兼症

(1) 夹痰：兼见咳嗽较剧、咳声重浊、喉中痰鸣，舌苔厚腻、脉象浮滑而数，指纹紫滞。

(2) 夹食滞：兼见脘腹胀满、不思乳食、呕吐酸腐、口气秽浊、大便酸臭、或腹痛泄泻、或大便秘结、小便短赤、舌苔厚腻、脉滑实，指纹紫滞。

(3) 夹惊：兼见惊惕啼叫、睡卧不宁、舌尖红赤、脉弦数、指纹青紫。

【治疗】

1. 基本处方

开天门，分推坎宫，揉太阳，揉耳后高骨，黄蜂入洞。

2. Modification of Prescription according to Syndromes

Common Cold of Wind-cold Type: Kneading Ershanmen and pushing Sanguan can be added.

Common Cold of Wind-heat Tpye: Clearing Feijing and Tianheshui and pushing Tianzhugu can be added.

Common Cold with Sputum: Kneading Rupang and Rugen (St 18) and foulaging-rubbing Xielei can be added.

Common Cold with Stagnated Food: Reinforcing Pijing, kneading Banmen, arc-pushing Bagua and rubbing the abdomen can be added.

Common Cold with Fear: Clearing Ganjing and pinching-kneading Xiaotianxin and Wuzhijie can be added.

Common Cold with Cough: Pushing-kneading Tanzhong (Ren 17) and kneading Feishu (UB 13) can be added.

3. Notes

Once a day, two times for severe patient. One course of treatment includes 3 days. Generally the patient will recover after 1—3 day's treatment. If there is no effect, another course should be continued.

Fever

It is a common symptom with the body temperature above the normal standard, which is commonly seen in pediatric department. Fever is usually caused by exogenous pathogenic factors, stagnated heat in the lung and stomach, and deficiency of *yin*-liquid.

MAIN SYMPTOMS

1. Fever due to Exogenous Pathogenic Factors

Wind-cold type: Manifested as slight fever, severe chillness, anhidrosis, headache, stuffy nose with watery discharge, thin and whitish fur on the tongue, floating pulse and floating red superficial venule of the index finger.

Wind-heat type: Manifested as higher fever, slight chillness,

2. 随证加减

风寒型：加揉二扇门、推三关。

风热型：加清肺经、清天河水、推天柱骨。

夹痰者：加揉乳旁、揉乳根、搓摩胁肋。

夹食滞者：加补脾经、揉板门、运八卦、摩腹。

夹惊者：加清肝经、掐揉小天心、掐揉五指节。

兼咳嗽者：加推揉膻中、揉肺俞。

3. 注意事项

推拿为每日1次，重者每日2次，3日为1疗程。一般治疗
1～3日即可痊愈。如不愈，可继续进行下一个疗程的治疗。

发　热

发热是指体温异常升高，是儿科常见的一个症状，多由感受
外邪、肺胃郁热、阴液亏损等原因引起。

【主证】

1. 外感发热

外感风寒：证见发热轻，恶寒重，无汗，头痛，鼻塞，流清
涕，舌苔薄白，脉浮，指纹浮红。

外感风热：证见发热重，恶寒轻，头痛，微汗出，鼻塞，流

headache, slight perspiration, stuffy nose with yellowish discharge, sore throat, dry mouth and thirst, reddish tongue with thin and yellowish fur, floating and rapid pulse, and red-purple superficial venule of the index finger.

2. Sthenia-heat of the Lung and Stomach: Mainfested as high fever, flushed cheeks with red lip, thirst with a desire for drink, feeling dry in the mouth and nose, shortness of breath, loss of appetite, fidgets, constipation, yellowish urine, red tongue with dry, rough and yellowish fur, fullness and rapid pulse, and dark-purple superficial venule of the index finger.

3. Fever due to *Yin*-deficiency: Manifested as fever in the afternoon, feverish sensation in the chest, palms and soles, spontaneous perspiration or night sweat, emaciation, poor appetite, reddish tongue with a little fur or exfoliated fur, thready and rapid pulse, and light purple superficial venule of the index finger.

TREATMENT

1. Fever due to Exogenous Pathogenic Factors:

(1) Essential Prescription: Opening Tianmen, pushing Kangong, kneading Taiyang (Extra 2) and Erhou Gaogu, clearing Tianheshui.

(2) Modification of Prescription According to Different Syndromes

Wind-cold Type: Pinching-kneading Ershanmen and grasping Fengchi can be added.

Wind-heat Type: Pushing Tianzhugu and the spine should be added

Huangfeng Rudong can be added for patients suffer from stuffy nose with watery discharge. Clearing Feijing, arc-pushing Bagua, pushing-kneading Tanzhong (Ren 17) can be added for patients with cough. Reinforcing-clearing Pijing, kneading Banmen, arc-pushing Bagua and kneading Zhongwan (Ren 12) can be added for patients with retention of food. Pushing Tianzhugu and pushing from Hengwen to Banmen can be added for patients with vomiting. Clearing Ganjing and pin-

黄涕，咽部红肿疼痛，口干而渴，舌质红，苔薄黄，脉浮数，指纹红紫。

2. 肺胃实热

高热，面赤唇红，渴而引饮，口干鼻燥，气促，不思乳食，烦燥，便秘尿黄，舌质红，苔黄燥，脉数实，指纹深紫。

3. 阴虚发热

午后发热，五心烦热，自汗或盗汗，形体消瘦，食欲减退，舌红少苔或花剥苔，脉细数，指纹淡紫。

【治疗】

1. 外感发热

基本处方

开天门，推坎宫，揉太阳，揉耳后高骨，清天河水。

随证加减

外感风寒：加掐揉二扇门、拿风池。

外感风热：加推天柱骨、推脊。

此外，若鼻塞流涕者，加黄蜂入洞；咳嗽者，加清肺经、运八卦、推揉膻中；夹食滞者，加清补脾经、揉板门、运八卦、揉中脘；呕吐者，加推天柱骨、横纹推向板门；夹惊者,加清肝经、

ching-kneading Xiaotianxin and Wuzhijie can be added for patients with fear.

2. Sthenia-heat of Lung and Stomach

Essential Prescription

Clearing Feijing, Weijing and Dachang, kneading Banmen, motioning Bagua, clearing Tianheshui, Reducing Liu Fu, kneading Tianshu, and pushing the spine.

3. Fever due to *yin*-deficiency:

Essential Prescription

Reinforcing Pijing, Feijing and Shenjing, kneading Erma, motioning Neilaogong, clearing Tianheshui, pressing-kneading Zusanli (St 36), and pushing Yongquan (K 1).

4. Points for Attention

Once a day, 2 or 3 times for severe patient. One course of treatment includes 3 times. Generally the patient can recover after 1—3 day's treatment. If there is no effect, another course should be continued.

Cough

Cough is the most common symptom among the diseases of the respiratory system. It can be caused by many diseases such as common cold, asthma, pneumonia, etc. The cough mentioned here is caused by acute and chronic bronchitis. TCM considers that the main cause of the disease is catching exogenous pathogenic factors (such as wind-cold, wind-heat and dryness) and internal damage of *Zang*-organs and *Fu*-organs.

MAIN SYMPTOMS

1. Cough due to Exogenous Pathogenic Factors: Manifested as cough with sputum, stuffy nose, nasal discharge, chillness, fever, headache, thin fur of the tongue and floating pulse. If the disease is caused by wind-cold, the patient may have cough with sputum and watery nasal discharge with white colour, severe chillness, slight fever, anhidrosis, and thin and whitish tongue fur. If it is due to wind-heat, the patient may have cough with

掐揉小天心、掐揉五指节。

2．肺胃实热

基本处方：

清肺经，清胃经，**清大肠**，揉板门，运内八卦，清天河水，退六腑，揉天枢，推脊。

3．阴虚发热

基本处方：

补脾经，补肺经，补肾经，揉二马，运内劳宫，清天河水，按揉足三里，推涌泉。

4．注意事项

推拿每日1次，重者每日2～3次，3日为1个疗程。一般治疗1～3日均可痊愈，若不愈，可继续进行下一个疗程。

咳　嗽

咳嗽是呼吸系统疾病最常见的一个症状，可由多种疾病如感冒、哮喘、肺炎等引起。本文主要讨论急、慢性支气管炎所致的咳嗽。中医认为，本证多因感受外邪(如风寒、风热、燥邪)、内伤脏腑所致。

【主证】

1．外感咳嗽

咳嗽有痰，鼻塞，流涕，恶寒，发热，头痛，苔薄，脉浮。

若为外感风寒，可兼见痰、涕清稀色白，恶寒重、发热轻,无汗,

sputum and thick yellowish nasal discharge, slight chillness, high fever, slight perspiration, thirst, sore throat, thin and yellowish fur and floating and rapid pulse.

2. Cough due to Internal Injury: manifested as protracted cough, slight fever, unproductive cough with little sputum or productive cough with much sputum, pale face, spontaneous perspiration or night sweat, poor appetite, lassitude, emaciation, pale tongue with whitish fur or reddish tongue with little fur, and thready and rapid pulse.

TREATMENT

1. Essential Prescription

Clearing Feijing, arc-pushing Neibagua, pressing-kneading Tiantu (Ren 22), pushing-kneading Tanzhong (Ren 17), kneading Rupang and Rugen (St 18), and kneading Feishu (UB 13).

2. Modification of Prescription According to Different Syndromes

Cough due to Exogenous Pathogenic Factors

Wind-cold Type: The major four manipulations (pushing Zanzhu and Kangong, kneading Taiyang (Extra 2) and Erhou Gaogu), pushing Sanguan and pinching-kneading Ershanmen can be added. For treatment of cough of wind-heat type, the major four manipulations and clearing Tianheshui can be added.

Cough Caused by Internal Injury: Reinforcing Pijing, Shenjing and Feijing can be added. For weak patients with protracted cough, pushing Sanguan and pinching the spine can be added. For patients with cough due to *yin*-deficiency, kneading Erma can be added. Foulaging-rubbing the hypochondria and kneading Fenglong (St 40) can be added for patients with difficulty to cough up sputum.

3. Points for Attention

Once a day, 2 times for severe patient. One course of treatment includes 3 days. Generally, the patient can recover

苔薄白。若为外感风热，可兼见痰、涕黄稠，恶寒轻，发热重，微汗出，口渴，咽痛，苔薄黄，脉浮数。

2．内伤咳嗽

久咳不已，身有微热，或干咳少痰，或咳嗽痰多，面色㿠白，自汗或盗汗，食欲不振，神疲乏力，形体消瘦，舌质淡，苔白或舌红少苔，脉细数。

【治疗】

1．基本处方

清肺经，运内八卦，按揉天突，推揉膻中，揉乳旁，揉乳根，揉肺俞。

2．随证加减

外感咳嗽：外感风寒，加四大手法、推三关、掐揉二扇门；外感风热，加四大手法、清天河水。

内伤咳嗽：加补脾经、补肺经、补肾经。久咳体虚者，加推三关、捏脊。阴虚咳嗽，加揉二马。痰吐不利，加搓摩胁肋、揉丰隆。

3．注意事项

推拿每日1次，重者每日2次，3日为1个疗程。一般治

after 1 course of treatment. If there is no effect, another course should be continued.

Asthma

Asthma is one of the allergic diseases manifested by shortness of breath and audible wheezing which may be so severe as to cause the patient to open his mouth and raise his shoulders to gasp for breath, with difficulty in falling asleep. Asthma hereof may mean "bronchial asthma" and "asthmatic bronchitis" named in Western medicine. TCM considers that the cause of the disease is due to weakness, stagnation of phlegm-dampness resulting from exogenous pathogenic factors (including wind-cold, wind-heat orcontact with allergens or eating allegenic food by mistake) or excitement

MAIN SYMPTOMS

Before the onset, some of the patients may have prodromata of sneezing and discomfort. It can also occur suddenly. The major symptoms of the disease are stuffiness in the chest and rapid respiration with bronchial wheezing. The infant suffering from the disease has to sit up. Generally, the onset may last from several minutes to several hours, even several days for severe patients, accompanied by cyanosis, sweating, rugular varicosity named "continuous state of asthma". When the attack is relieved, the patient will cough up some frothy mucoid sputum first. The disease can occur repeatedly with the complications of pulmonary emphysema, pulmonary heart disease, etc.

1. Heat-type Asthma

It occurs with thick and yellowish sputum, restlessness, thirst and desire to drink, reddish tongue with thin yellowish fur and purple superficial venule of the index finger. It occurs mostly during hot seasons.

2. Cold-type Asthma

It occurs with watery sputum which is white and frothy, pale tongue with whitish thin fur, and reddish superficial venule

疗一个疗程即可痊愈，若不愈，可继续下一个疗程。

哮　喘

哮喘是一种过敏性疾患，临床以呼吸急促、喘鸣有声，甚者张口抬肩，难以平卧为主症。可包括西医所称的"支气管哮喘"和"喘息型支气管炎"。中医认为，本证多因素体虚弱，内有痰湿，当感受外邪（包括感受风寒、风热或接触过敏原，或误食致敏食物等）或情绪激动时而诱发。

【主证】

在哮喘发作前，某些患者可有打喷嚏、全身不适等前驱症状，但亦可突然发作。主要症状为胸闷、呼吸急促，并伴有哮鸣音，患儿常被迫坐起。每次发作一般持续几分钟，甚者几小时不等，严重者可达几天，并可出现紫绀、汗出、颈静脉怒张，称为"哮喘持续状态"。哮喘发作缓解时，先咯出大量泡沫性粘稠痰液，然后停止。本病反复发作，迁延日久，可并发肺气肿、肺心病等。

1. 热哮

哮喘发作，吐痰黄稠，心烦不安，口渴喜饮，多发于炎热季节，舌质红，苔薄黄，指纹紫。

2. 冷哮

哮喘发作，吐痰清后，色白多沫，多发于寒冷季节，舌质淡，

of the index finger. It occurs mostly during cold seasons.

TREATMENT

1. Essential Prescription

Pushing Feijing, arc-pushing Neibagua, kneading Tiantu (Ren 22), pushing-kneading Tanzhong (Ren 17), kneading Feishu (UB 13), and foulaging-rubbing the hypochondria.

2. Modification of Prescription according to Syndromes

Heat-type: Clearing Feijing and Tianheshui can be added.

Cold-type: Reinforcing Feijing, pushing Sanguan and kneading Wailaogong can be added. Pushing Sanguan, reinforcing Pijing and Shenjing and kneading Erma can be added for weak patients due to protracted illness and failure of the kidney in preserving *qi*.

3. Points for Attention

Once a day, or twice for severe patients. One course of treatment includes 6 days. Generally the symptoms can be relieved or disappear after 1—5 courses of treatment. Treatment can be carried out continuously without intervals between courses, or with an interval of 1 or 2 days.

Enuresis

It refers to involuntary passage of urine in children over 3, occurring especially during sleeping at night. So it is also called "bed-wetting". It may occur in children under 3, resulting from insufficiency of the cerebrospinal cord and unforming of regular passage of urine. This is not considered as illness. TCM holds that the major causes of the disease are deficiency of kidney-*qi*, insufficiency of both the spleen and lung after illness, and loss of retaining power due to deficiency of *qi*.

MAIN SYMPTOMS

The child passes urine involuntarily during sleeping. It occurs more often during day time when the patient feels tired or in cloudy and raining days, once every several nights but

苔薄白，指纹淡红。

【治疗】

1. 基本处方：

推肺经，运内八卦，揉天突，推揉膻中，揉肺俞，搓摩胁肋。

2. 随证加减

热哮：用清肺经，加清天河水。

冷哮：用补肺经，加推三关、揉外劳宫。

久病体虚，肾不纳气者，加推三关、补脾经、补肾经、揉二马。

3. 注意事项

推拿每日1次，重者每日2次，6日为1个疗程。一般治疗1～5个疗程后即可减轻或停止发作，每个疗程之间可间隔1～2日，也可连续治疗。

遗　尿

遗尿是指3周岁以上的儿童反复出现不随意的排尿，多在睡眠中发生，醒后方觉，故又称"尿床"。由于3岁以下儿童，脑髓未充，正常的排尿习惯尚未形成，亦可发生遗尿，不属病态。中医认为，本证多因肾气不足，下元虚冷，或病后脾肺两虚，气虚失摄所致。

【主证】

睡眠中不自主排尿，白天疲劳或阴雨天更易发生，轻者数夜1次，重则每夜1～2次，甚或更多。病久可见患儿面色萎黄、

once or twice or more every night for severe patients. If the disease lasts longer the patient may have sallow complexion listlessness, lassitude, dizziness, soreness of loins, spontaneous perspiration, night sweat, cold extremities, pale tongue with thin and whitish fur and deep and thready pulse.

TREATMENT

1. Essential Prescription: Reinforcing Pijing, Feijing and Shenjing, kneading Erma and Wailaogong, pushing Sanguan, pressing-kneading Baihui (Du 20), kneading Dantian (Elixir Field), pressing-kneading Shenshu (UB 23), scrubbing the lumbosacral portion, and pressing-kneading Sanyinjiao (Sp 6).

2. Modification of Prescription according to Syndromes

Pushing Dachang for patients with diarrhea; arc-pushing Neibagua for patients with anorexia and abdominal distention; and kneading Shending for patients with spontaneous perspiration and night sweat. Clinically, The above manipulations can be used in the combination with moxa roll moxibustion on the points of Baihui (Du 20), Dantian (Elixir Field), Shenshu (UB 23) and Sanyinjiao (Sp 6) for better results.

3. Points for Attention

The massase is performed once a day. One course of treatment includes 6 times. Generally, the patient can recover after 1 course of treatment. If there is no effect, another course should be continued 1 or 2 days later.

Uroschesis

Uroschesis refers to difficulty in micturition. Though there is a lot of urine in the bladder, it is difficult to pass out. is named "*long bi*" (uroschesis) in TCM. The cause of the disease is downward flow of damp-heat to the bladder or deficiency of the kidney-*yang* and disturbance in *qi* transformation.

MAIN SYMPTOMS

1. Downward Flow of Damp-heat: The patient feels

智力减退、精神不振、头晕腰酸、自汗盗汗、四肢不温等，舌质淡，苔薄白，脉沉细。

【治疗】

1. 基本处方

补脾经，补肺经，补肾经，揉二马，揉外劳宫，推三关，按揉百会，揉丹田，按揉肾俞，擦腰骶部，按揉三阴交。

2. 随证加减

大便溏泻者，加推大肠；食欲不振、腹胀者，加运内八卦；自汗、盗汗者，加揉肾顶。在临床上，如配用艾条灸百会、丹田、肾俞、三阴交等穴，效果更佳。

3. 注意事项

推拿每日1次，6次为1个疗程。一般治疗1个疗程后即可痊愈。若不愈，可间隔1～2天后进行下一个疗程。

尿潴留

尿潴留，是指排尿障碍，膀胱蓄有大量尿液，而小便不通的病症。中医称为"癃闭"。是因湿热下注，结于膀胱，或肾阳不足，气化不利所致。

【主证】

1. 湿热下注

distention and pain in the lower abdomen and wants to pass urine very much. But it is very difficult to do so. Sometimes it is accompanied with retention of feces and thirst without inclination for drink. The patient has yellow and greasy fur on the tongue and smooth and rapid pulse.

2. Deficiency of the Kidney-*yang*: Manifested as uroschesis, pale face, lassitude in loins and knees, spiritless and lassitude, aversion to cold, pale tongue with whitish and moist fur and deep slow and weak pulse.

TREATMENT

1. Essential Prescription

Pushing Jimen, pressing-kneading Dantian (Elixir Field) and Sanyinjiao (Sp 6).

2. Modification of Prescription according to Different Syndromes

Downward flow of damp-heat: Add Clearing Xiaochang, kneading Xiaotianxin and reducing Liu Fu.

Deficiency of the Kidney-*yang*: Reinforcing Shenjing, Kneading Erma, pushing Sanguan, and kneading Shenshu (UB 23) can be added. Apart from the manipulations mentioned above, clearing Dachang and pushing-down Qijiegu can be added for patients with constipation.

3. Points for Attention

The massage is performed once a day. In severe cases, it is done twice a day or repeatedly until urination happens. If there is no effect, the duration of manipulation can be prolonged or some other therapies may be taken.

Night Crying

The child looks normal during day time, but cries during night intermittently or continously. Some children cry all the night or at regular hours every night. The symptom occurs most often in children under 6 months. TCM holds that it is due to insufficiency and cold of the spleen, retention of

小腹胀满疼痛，有强烈尿意，而小便不得排出，或伴有大便不畅、口渴不欲饮，舌苔黄腻，脉滑数。

2. 肾阳不足

小便不通，面色㿠白，腰膝酸软，神疲乏力，畏寒，舌质淡，苔白润，脉沉迟无力。

【治疗】

1. 基本处方

推箕门，按揉丹田、三阴交。

2. 随证加减

湿热下注：加清小肠、揉小天心、退六腑。

肾阳不足：加补肾经、揉二马、推三关、揉肾俞。

此外，伴有大便秘结者，加清大肠、推下七节骨。

3. 注意事项

推拿每日1次，重者每日2次，或推至排出小便。若不愈，应适当延长推拿时间或采取其他治疗措施。

夜　啼

凡小儿白天如常，入夜啼哭，间歇发作或持续不已，甚则通宵达旦，或每夜定时啼哭者，称为"夜啼"。本症常见于6个月以内的婴儿。中医认为多因脾脏虚寒、心经积热或受惊吓所致。

heat in the heart or fright.

MAIN SYMPTOMS

1. Insufficiency and Cold of the Spleen

The child cries lying prostrate with his back arched. Other symptoms and signs may include curled and cold extremities, pale and blue face, poor appetite with diarrhea, pale tongue with thin and whitish fur and reddish superficial venule of the index finger.

2. Retention of Heat in the Heart

The child cries lying supine, with flushed face, red lip, restlessness, constipation, difficult and dark urine, reddish tip of the tongue with thin and yellowish fur and black purple superficial venule of the index finger.

3. Night Cry due to Fright

It is manifested as paroxysmal crying with restlessness due to fright during sleep, timidness which can be relieved by being carried in arms, changeable face and lip colour and black superficial venule of the index finger.

Besides, abdominal pain and distention due to retention of food and milk in the stomach may also cause night crying, which must be differentiated from the above three types.

TREATMENT

1. Essential Prescription

Pinching-kneading Xiaotianxin, Zongjin and Wuzhijie, rubbing the abdomen and pressing-kneading Zusanli (St 36).

2. Modification of Prescription according to Different Syndromes

Insufficiency and Cold of the Spleen Type: Reinforcing Pijing, pushing Sanguan and kneading Wailaogong can be added.

Retention of Heat in the Heart: Clearing Xinjing and Tianheshui can be added.

Fright Type: Kneading Baihui (Du 20), opening Tianmen and clearing Ganjing can be added. Clearing-reinforcing Pijing, separating abdominal Yin-Yang and kneading Zhong-

【主征】

1．脾脏虚寒型

患儿俯卧屈腰而啼，四肢踡缩不温，面色青白相兼，食少便溏，舌质淡，苔薄白，指纹淡红。

2．心热型

患儿仰身而啼，面赤唇红，烦躁不安，便干或燥结，小便赤涩，舌尖红，苔薄黄，指纹青紫。

3．惊吓型

患儿常于睡中惊惕不安，阵发啼哭，神气虚怯，喜抚抱而卧，唇与面色乍青乍白，指纹青。

此外，乳食积滞所致的腹痛、腹胀亦可引起本症，应注意鉴别。

【治疗】

1．基本处方

掐揉小天心，掐揉总筋，掐揉五指节，摩腹，按揉足三里。

2．随证加减

脾脏虚寒型：加补脾经、推三关、揉外劳宫。

心热型：加清心经、清天河水。

惊吓型：加揉百会、开天门、清肝经。伤食者，加清补脾经、分

wan (Ren 12) can be added for the patient with dyspepsia.

3. Notes

The massage is performed once a day. One course of treatment includes 3 times. Generally, the patient can recover after 1 course of treatment. If there is no effect, 1 or 2 more courses should be continued.

Infantile Myogenic Torticollis

It is a disease characterized by slanting of the head to the affected side, the neck to the front and the face to the healthy side. Clinically, apart from a few children who suffer from bony torticollis due to deformation of spinal column, compensatory postural torticollis due to visual disturbance and neurogenic torticollis due to myoparalysis of the neck, most of them suffer from myogenic torticollis caused by spasm of sternocleidomastoid muscle on one side. Because a fusiform mass can be found on one side of the neck soon after the child was born with slanting of the head to oneside, so it is also called congenital myogenic torticollis (Fig. 3—72).

There are many version about its causes, including birth trauma, abnormal fetal position, abnormal growth during embryonic period and hereditary factors. Most scholars consider that the cause is in relation to birth trauma and abnormal fetal position, because most of the patients have the history of birth trauma and abnormal fetal position. Sternocleidomastoid muscle bleeds due to pressing of the birth canal, and obstetric forceps during delivery make the muscle become a fusiform mass due to clots after birth, causing fibrocyte multiplication of sternocleidomastoid muscle and myofibrosis on the affected region, which may turn to connective tissue, forming cord. If the fetal head is not in normal position during delivery, blood circulation of sternocleidomastoid muscle on one side will be disturbed, causing ischemic changes of the muscles, resulting in torticollis.

MAIN SYMPTOMS

A fusiform mass can be found on one side of the neck

腹阴阳、揉中院。

3．注意事项

推拿为每日 1 次，3 次为 1 个疗程。一般治疗 1 个疗程即可痊愈。如不效，可继续治疗 1～2 个疗程。

小儿肌性斜颈

小儿肌性斜颈是以头向患侧倾斜、颈前倾、颜面旋向健侧为特点。临床上，除少数患儿是由脊柱畸形引起的骨性斜颈、视力障碍引起的代偿姿势性斜颈和颈部肌麻痹导致的神经性斜颈外，一般系由一侧胸锁乳突肌挛缩造成的肌性斜颈。因多数患儿是在生后即发现颈部一侧有梭形肿块，头向一侧倾斜，故又称先天性肌性斜颈(图3-72)。

有关斜颈病因的说法很多，如产伤、胎位不正、胚胎期发育异常、遗传因素等。但多数学者认为与产伤、胎位不正有关，这是因为大多数病儿有产伤和胎位不正史。分娩时一侧胸锁乳突肌因受产道或产钳挤压受伤出血,生后,凝血块使肌肉呈梭状肿块，久之，血肿可使患侧胸锁乳突肌纤维细胞增生和肌纤维变性，进而变为结缔组织而形成条索状。若分娩时胎儿头位不正，阻碍一侧胸锁乳突肌血运供应，引起该肌缺血性改变，亦可导致斜颈。

【证证】

患儿出生后，多在颈部的一侧发现有梭形肿块，大小不一，

after birth, big or small, in the same direction with the sterno-cleidomastoid muscle. The child may feel pain when the mass is pressed and the head moves. A mass may disappear half year later in some cases. The sternocleidomastoid muscle becomes contractive and stiff gradually. A mass is replaced by cord fibre which is hard, thick and tenderness. When the child slants his head to the affected side his face turns to the healthy side. If it is severe and stays longer, the face of the child may become unsymmetric. Verrucoid mass can be seen round the point of attachment of sternocleidomastoid muscle on the affected side in a few children. If the illness lasts longer, it may be complicated by fixed lateral curvature of cervical vertebrae or thoracic vertebrae.

TREATMENT

1. Manipulations

(1) The doctor uses pushing-kneading manipulation on the sternocleidomastoid muscle of the affected side.

(2) The doctor uses his thumb and index finger to pinch the patient's sternocleidomastoid muscle on the affected side with holding-twisting manipulation in opposite direction.

(3) Grasping the sternocleidomastoid muscle on the affected side.

(4) Stroke the tendon on contracture part with the thumbs, the index and middle fingers of the two hands in different directions.

(5) The doctor holds the patient's shoulder with one hand and the top of the child's head by the other, and makes the child's head slant to the shoulder of the healthy side gradually, and lets the sternocleidomastoid muscle of the affected side be widened gradually. Do this for several times repeatedly.

(6) Use pushing-kneading manipulation on the sternocleidomastoid muscle of the affected side.

(7) Grasping Jianjing (GB 21) on the affected side to finish the treatment.

2. Points for Attention

Early finding and treatment must be stressed here. Treat-

其方向与胸锁乳突肌一致，按压肿块或头部运动牵扯时疼痛。有的肿块经半年后可自行消退，以后患侧的胸锁乳突肌逐渐挛缩紧张，肿块为条索状纤维所代替，且质地较硬、变粗，压痛消失。患儿头部向患侧倾斜，颜面部则旋向健侧。如斜颈明显，久之可出现颜面大小不对称。少数患儿仅见患侧胸锁乳突肌锁骨附着点周围有骨疣样改变的硬状物。病久者，还可伴有颈椎或下胸椎有固定性脊柱侧弯。

【治疗】

1. 操作方法

(1) 医者在患侧的胸锁乳突肌部位施用推揉法。

(2) 医者用拇、食二指捏住患侧胸锁乳突肌，相对用力做捻法。

(3) 拿患侧胸锁乳突肌。

(4) 用双手拇、食、中指在挛缩处做分向牵扯筋腱。

(5) 医者一手扶住患侧肩部，另一手扶患儿头顶，使患儿头部渐向健侧肩部倾斜，逐渐拉长患侧胸锁乳突肌，反复进行数次。

(6) 然后在患侧胸锁乳突肌部位施用推揉法。

(7) 最后，拿患侧肩井穴结束治疗。

2. 注意事项

本病应强调早发现、早治疗。在新生儿期开始治疗，这时

ment beginning at neonatal period when the hematoma is not euplastic may yield best result. Generally the patient can recover from his illness after 1 month's treatment. The older the patient is, the less effective it will be with the organization of hematoma and formation of contracture. The children of 6 months have to be treated for about 3 months. The course of the treatment lasts longer for the children above the age of one year. The massage can be done once a day or every other day. One course of treatment includes 1 month. The child can continue his treatment for another course immediately after the first course or several days later.

Child Massage for Health Care

Child massage for health care refers to using certain manipulations to operate on some points to improve children's health. It can invigorate the spleen, regulate the stomach-*qi*, promote appetite, build up the constitution, prevent diseases and promote growth. The manipulations can be done anytime and are convenient and painless, so they are easy to be accepted by children .

1. Manipulation

Reinforcing Pijing 200—500 times, rubbing the abdomen 2—5 minutes, pressing-kneading Zusanli (St 36) 50—100 times and pinching the spine 3—5 times.

2. Points for Attention

(1) Generally it is suitable to be done in the morning or before meal, once a day. One course of treatment includes 7 days. Another course can be done 1 day later. The child will recover from his illness 3—4 courses later. The children's height and weight will increase after 3—6 months of treatment.

(2) Massage must be suspended when the child has acute infectious disease and can be resumed after the child recovers from his illness.

血肿尚未机化，效果最佳，一般经治疗1个月即可痊愈。随着血肿的机化，形成挛缩，月龄越大，效果越差。半岁的患儿一般须治疗3个月左右，1岁以上的患儿疗程更长。推拿每日1次或隔日1次，1个月为1个疗程。两疗程之间可间隔数日，也可连续进行。

小儿推拿保健

小儿推拿保健是指在小儿的某些穴位上运用一定的手法进行操作，以起到保健作用的方法。它具有健脾和胃、增进食欲、强壮身体、预防疾病、促进发育等作用。其操作方法简便易行，朝夕可作，又无痛苦，故易为小儿所接受。

1. 操作方法

补脾经200～500次，摩腹2～5分钟，按揉足三里50～100次，捏脊3～5遍。

2. 注意事项

(1) 一般宜在清晨或饭前进行，每天操作1次，7天为1个疗程。休息1天后，继续进行下一疗程。一般治疗3～4个疗程即可见效，经3～6个月后，小儿的身高、体重都会较前有明显的增长。

(2) 急性传染病期间应暂停推拿，待病愈后再继续进行。

Chapter Four

Self-massage

Massage by using such simple manipulations as pushing, rubbing, pressing, kneading and thumping with one's own hands on certain points or in certain special areas of the body surface for the purpose of health care, health preservation and autotherapy of illnesses, is called "self-massage". Self-massage for health care or preservation is called "self-health-care massage", that for autotherapy of illness is called "self treatment massage" or "self-massage therapy".

As an important component of Chinese massage, self-massage acts as a remedy by means of stimulation through manipulation to activate the channel, qi and blood systems of oneself. Meanwhile the manipulation process itself is actually an active exercise. So long as one can select proper channels, points and areas based on the conditions of the individual and carry out self-massage seriously, presistently, orderly and step by step, he is sure to achieve satisfactory results.

Self-massage can be done in a sitting, standing or lying position depending on the conditions of the individual. The practitioner should carry out manipulations calmly and attentively with a proper posture, get manipulation, strength, mental activities and qi flow well coordinated, viz. mind concentration should follow the manipulating hand to the area being massaged and, coordinated by breathing, direct qi through concentration to the channels and points at the area being massaged. When manipulations such as pressing are conducted, one should exert strength step by step to, so much

第 四 章
自 我 推 拿

通过自己的双手，运用推、摩、按、揉、捶等简单手法在自身体表经穴与特定部位进行推拿，以达到保健、养生及疾病自疗的方法称为"自我推拿"。其中以保健、养生为目的者称"自我保健推拿"；以疾病自疗为目的者叫"自我医疗推拿"或"自 我 推 拿 疗法"。

自我推拿是中国推拿的重要组成部分，它主要是因为自我手法的刺激，激发了自身的经穴、气血系统而发挥治疗作用的；同时，自我手法的动作过程，本身也是一种主动的运动锻练。所以，只要根据自身的具体情况，辨证地选择好治疗经穴与部位，认真操作，循序渐进，持之以恒地进行自我推拿，一定会取得理想的功效。

自我推拿在施术时，可根据自身的具体情况，选取坐位、站位或卧位。操作时要心平气和、精神集中，呼吸自然不要憋气，在正确的体位下做到"手"到、"力"到、"心"到、"气"到，即要求意念也要随着手的动作转移至操作部位，并配合呼吸将"气"在意想中输送到受术部位的经穴。在施行按压类手法时，用力先轻渐重，以

the better, get the feeling of *qi* manifested as soreness and distension at the channels and points. The hand and the skin of the treated area should be kept dry when rubbing or scrubbing manipulations are performed. Toilet powder or a kind of proper media may be applied if there is sweat. The strength exerted should be appropriate; the manipulation should give one a feeling of local warmth. Violent strength and prolonged rubbing or scrubing should be avoided lest the skin be injured. Self-massage is usually performd twice a day, in the morning and evening, 20—30 minutes each time.

At the initial stage of self-massage, general fatigue, especially aching-pain in the manipulating hand, may occur after massage. Those are the normal phenomena occuring only because of inadaptability of one's physical strength to it. The discomforts may disappear naturally so long as one perseveres in doing the self-massage, which is called "self-exercise" in the traditional Chinese doctrine of health preservation and protection, and becomes skillful in manipulation, powerful in strength and fruitful in attainments. On the contrary, one may feel warm all over, light-hearted and cheerful. Further more, one can, after some self exercises, select points at any part of the body for self-massage and will not abstrain from selection of some effective points on hesitancy of "impossibility to reach the points", provided that the motor function of the joints of the upper extremities is basically normal.

In addition, self-massage is often done in combination with *qigong* (breathing exercise) which has synergism with it. This usually brings complementary effect. Details about *qigong* are introduced in **Chinese Qigong** of this Library. Introduced here are some common self-massage methods.

经穴处有酸胀等得气感为宜;在做摩擦类手法时,手与受术处皮肤要保持干燥,如有汗水可搽些爽身粉或使用介质,用力要适中,手法以局部产生温热感为度,不要加力太重,摩擦太久,以免擦破皮肤。自我推拿一般每日早、晚各做1次,每次在20~30分钟即可。

自我推拿在开始时,由于体力不适应,往往在做后觉得全身疲乏,特别是施术的双手会出现酸痛等不适感,这是正常现象。只要坚持进行这种在中国传统养生保健学中被称为"自我行功"的功法锻炼,随着手法的熟练、体力的增长与功夫的长进,不但这些不适感会自行消失,而且还可在行功后感到通体温热,身心轻松、愉快。再者,只要两个上肢的各个环节的运动功能基本正常,通过锻炼便可以在自己身体上的任何部位"自由"地进行自我手法操作,无需顾虑"可能无法触及"而放弃选用分布在该部位的有效经穴。

另外,在中国传统保健学中,自我推拿经常结合其他与之有协同作用的"气功"功法一起锻炼,往往会起到相得益彰的效果。有关其他练功方法的介绍,读者可参阅本文库《中国气功》分册,这里不再赘述。下面向大家推荐几种常用的自我推拿法。

Section 1

Self-health-care Massage

1. Local Massage

Local massage, also called "local exercising" in antient times, is a kind of self-massage carried out on certain parts of the body.

1) Health Care of the Head, Face, Eyes, Nose, and Ears

(1) Head-face Health Care

MANIPULATION

① Pushing the Forehead on Either Side

Bend the two index fingers and push with their radial sides from the midline of the forehead which runs from Yintang (Extra 1) to the anterior hairline separately toward the left and right Taiyang (Extra 2), Sizhukong (SJ 23) and Touwei (St 8) on the two sides of the forehead, respectively for altogether 30—50 times (Fig. 4—1).

② Wiping the Temples

Press the temples with the whorled surfaces of the thumbs and wipe backwards repeatedly with force for about 30 times. The massage should give a sensation of soreness and distention (Fig. 4—2).

③ Pressing-Kneading the Back of the Head

Put the whorled surfaces or the tips of the thumbs tightly on the points of Fengchi (GB 20) and press them intervally for over 10 times followed by rotative kneading. Then knead Naohoukong for about 30 times until the patient has a sensation of soreness and distention (Fig. 4—3).

④ Patting the Vertex

Sit upright with eyes looking straight ahead and teeth

第一节　　自我保健推拿

1. 分部自我保健推拿

分部自我保健推拿在古代又称作推拿的分部行功法，是一种以肢体部位为单元进行的自我推拿法。

1) 头面、五官保健

（1）头面部

【操作】

①分推前额以印堂至前发际正中之连线为中线，两手食指屈成弓状，用第二指节的桡侧面为着力面，由下而上，自中线向前额两侧分别推至丝竹空、太阳、头维穴处，约30～50次左右（图4-1）

②双抹两颞以两手拇指罗纹面，紧按两侧鬓角处，由前向后反复用力推抹，约30次左右，以酸胀为宜（图4-2）。

③按揉脑后　以两拇指罗纹或指端，紧按风池穴，先用力按压10余次，再作旋转按揉，随后再按揉脑后空穴约30次左右，以酸胀为宜（图4-3）。

④拍击头顶　人正坐，眼睛睁开前视，牙齿咬紧，用手掌心

clenched. Pat rhythmically on the fontanel area with the palm for about 10 times (Fig. 4—4).

⑤ "Bathing the Face" with Hands

Rub the hands against each other to get them warm and, with the palms put lightly against the forehead, rub forcefully down to the mandibles, and along the mandible margins sidewise to the points of Jiache (St 6), then upwards via the preauricular area and the temples to the midpoint of the forehead, Repeat the procedure for 20—30 times until the face feels warm (Fig. 4—5).

FUNCTION

The exercise has the functions of invigorating the brain, improving intelligence and tranquilizing the mind. It is effective in the treatment of headache, dizziness, insomnia, amnesia, neurosis and facial paralysis.

(2) Health Care of the Eye

MANIPULATION

① Kneading Zanzhu (UB 2)

Apply the whorled surfaces of the thumbs on the two points of Zanzhu (UB 2) in the depressions proximal to the medial ends of the eyebrows and knead for 20 times respectively. The force of kneading should be increased gradually to get a feeling of soreness and distention (Fig. 4—6).

② Kneading Jingming (UB 1)

Put the thumb and the index finger of the right hand on the point Jingming (UB 1) which is located in the depression 0.1 *cun* above the inner canthus. Press down and pinch alternatively for about 20—30 times (Fig. 4—7).

③ Pressing – Kneading Sibai (St 2)

Put the index fingers on the points of Sibai (St 2) each of which is 1 *cun* under the midpoint of the lower orbit, and press – knead for about 20 times to get the sensation of soreness and distention (Fig. 4—8).

④ Scrapping the Orbits

在囟门穴处做有节律的拍击动作，约10次左右(图4-4)。

⑤搓手浴面 先将两手搓热，随后掌心紧贴前额，用力向下擦到下颌，再沿下颌下缘向外至颊车，再向上经耳前、鬓角转推至前额中间，如此反复旋转推摩面颊，每次约20～30遍左右，以面部有热感为宜(图4-5)。

【作用】

上法有健脑、益智、安神之功，对防治头痛、头晕、失眠、健忘、神经衰弱、面瘫等病症有效。

（2）眼部

【操作】

①揉攒竹 以双手拇指罗纹面，分别按在双眉内侧头凹陷处的攒竹穴处，由轻而重反复轻揉约20次左右，以酸胀为宜（图4-6）。

②揉睛明 以右手拇、食二指罗纹面，揉压在两目内眦角上1分凹陷中之睛明穴，先用力向下按压；然后向上挤捏，如此一按一挤，反复进行，每次约20～30遍左右(图4-7)。

③按揉四白 以双手食指罗纹面，分别按在眼下眶正中下1寸处的四白穴，反复按揉20次左右，以酸胀为宜(图4-8)。

Bend the index fingers, apply their radial sides against the internal aspects of the upper orbits and scrape from the inner canthi to the outer, followed by scraping the lower orbits in the same way, for about 20—30 times (Fig 4—9).

⑤ "Ironing" the Eyes

Close the eyes slightly. Rub the hands against each other until they are hot and cover the eyes with the palm readiculus to "Iron" the eyes for about 30 seconds followed by rubbing them 10 times or more (Fig. 4—10).

⑥ Kneading Tiayang (Extra 2)

Press the points of Taiyang (Extra 2) hard with the whorled surfaces of the thumbs and knead them for about 30 times to get the sensation of soreness and distention (Fig. 4—11).

FUNCTION

These manipulations are effective for prevention and treatment of myopia, blurred vision, glaucoma, optic atrophy and other eye diseases.

(3) Health Care of the Nose

MANIPULATION

① Pressing-Kneading Yingxiang (LI 20)

Rest the whorled surfaces of the index fingers on the points of Yingxiang (LI 20) and press and knead them for about 30 times toget the sensation of soreness and distention (Fig 4—12).

② Rubbing the Sides of the Nose

Rub the index or middle fingers of the two hands against each other to get them hot and rub with them the nasolabial grooves up and down to get them hot too. Do it about 30 times each time (Fig. 4—13).

FUNCTION

These manipulations are effective for prevention and treatment of cold, stuffy and running nose, allergic rhinitis, chronic rhinitis, paranasal sinusitis, etc.

(4) Health Care of the Ear

MANIPULATION

④刮眼轮　双手食指屈曲，以第二指节的桡侧面紧贴上眼眶的内侧端，自内向外推抹至眼眶的外侧端；然后再如此推抹下眼眶，如此先上后下，自内向外反复刮推约 20～30 次（图4-9）。

⑤熨眼双目轻闭，先将两掌搓热，用双手掌根处轻压热熨双目30秒钟，再轻轻揉动10余次（图4-10）。

⑥揉太阳　以两手拇指罗纹面紧贴双侧太阳穴处，反复按揉30次左右，以酸胀为宜（图4-11）。

【作用】

上法可防治近视眼、视物不清、青光眼、视神经萎缩等各种目疾。

（3）鼻部

【操作】

①按揉迎香　以两手中指罗纹面，按压在双侧迎香穴处，用力反复按揉30次左右，以酸胀为宜（图4-12）。

②搓擦鼻旁　先将两手食指或中指掌面相对搓热，趁热在鼻翼两侧的鼻唇沟处，上、下搓擦，以热为宜。每次擦30次左右（图4-13）。

【作用】

上法对防治感冒、鼻塞流涕、过敏性鼻炎、慢性鼻炎、副鼻窦炎等病症有效。

（4）耳部

【操作】

① Pressing-Kneading the Points Around the Ear

Press and knead, with the tips of the thumbs or the middle fingers, the points Ermen (SJ 21), Tinggong (SI 19), Tinghui (GB 2), Yifeng (SJ 17) and others for about 20 times each to get the sensation of soreness or distention (Fig. 4—14).

② Rubbing the Helix

Pinch the helices gently with the thumbs and the radial sides of the index fingers, and rub down and up repeatedly for about 30 times to get the helices hot (Fig. 4—15).

③ Ming Tiangu

Apply the two palms to the ears, with the bases of the palms pointing to the front and the fingers to the back, and use the index and middle fingers, with the former being on top of the latter, to flick-hit the protruded bones behind the ears 20 times to produce a booming sound in the ears (Fig. 4—16).

④ Rubbing and Scrubbing the Part in Front of the Ear

Apply the radial parts of the two thumbs or the palm faces of the index fingers to the areas in front of the ears and do repeated up and down rubbing and scrubbing about 30 times until a proper sensation of heat is achieved.

FUNCTION

These manipulations are effective for prevention and treatment of tinnitus, dysacousis, deafness and otitis media.

2) Health Care of the Extremities

(1) Health Care of the Upper Limbs

MANIPULATION

① Pressing – Keading the Points of the Upper Limbs

With the whorled surface of the thumb or the middle finger, press and knead the points in the order of Jianneishu, Jianyu (LI 15) and Jianjing (GB 21) around the shoulder joints, Quchi (LI 11), Shousanli (LI 10), Chize (Lu 5), Quze (P 3), Shaohai (H 3) and Xiaohai (SI 8) around the elbows, and

①按揉耳周诸穴　以双手拇指端或中指端为着力点，分别按揉耳周围之耳门、听宫、听会与翳风等穴，每穴按揉20次左右，以酸胀为宜（图4-14）。

②摩擦耳轮　以双手拇指罗纹面与屈曲成弓状的食指桡侧面，轻轻捏住两侧耳轮，上下反复摩擦20～30次左右（图4-15）。

③鸣天鼓　以两手掌心掩住两耳孔，掌根在前，手指指向脑后，用食指搭在中指上，向下弹击耳后高骨20次左右，使耳中隆隆作响（图4-16）。

④搓擦耳前　以双手拇指桡侧，或食指掌面，紧贴在耳前，由上而下、由下而上的反复搓擦约30次左右，以热为宜。

【作用】

上法对防治耳鸣、重听、耳聋、中耳炎等病症有效。

2）四肢部保健

（1）上肢部

【操作】

①按揉上肢诸穴　用拇指罗纹面，或中指指面先后按揉肩关节周围的肩内俞、肩髃、肩井穴；肘关节周围的曲池、手三里、尺泽、曲泽、少海、小海穴；前臂与腕关节围周的外关、内关、

Waiguan (SJ 5), Neiguan (P 6), Yangchi (SJ 4), Yangxi (LI 5) and Hegu (LI 4) around the forearms and wrists. Press and knead these points 20 times each and try to get the "feeling of *qi*" manifested as soreness, distention and tingle. Massage the points of the left arm with the right hand and vice versa (Fig. 4—17).

② Pushing-Rubbing the Upper Limbs

Rub with the right palm the points on the left arm (vice versa) in the order of the anterior, posterior, medial and lateral aspects of the shoulder, the elbow and the wrist till they are warm (about 10—20 times for each aspect). Then rub the lateral side of the arm with the palm from the dorsal carpal cross striation up along the channel to the point Jianyu (LI 15) at the exterior aspect of the shoulder, then move the palm to the anterior side of the shoulder and rub the medial side down to the intracarpal cross striation. Repeat the procedures about 30 times to get a warm sensation in the arm (Fig. 4—18).

③ Rubbing the Hand and Twirling the Knuckles

Apply the major thenar eminence of one hand on the back of the other and rub to get the intermetacarpal muscles warm. Then with the thumb and index finger of one hand, twirl the interphalangeal joints of the other hand one by one (Fig. 4—19).

FUNCTION

These manipulations can be used to prevent and treat scapulohumeral periarthritis, subacrominal bursitis, tennis elbow, wrist tenosynovitis and other disorders of the upper limbs. They are also effective for relaxing the muscles of the upper limbs, relieving fatigue and improving the motor function of the upper limbs and for the prevention and treamtnet of occupational injury.

(2) Health Care of the Lower Limbs

MANIPULATION

① Pressing-Kneading the Points on the Legs

阳池、阳溪、合谷等穴，每穴按揉 20 次左右，以有酸、胀、麻等得气感为宜。左上肢诸穴由右手操作，右上肢诸穴由左手操作（图4-17）。

②推擦上肢　先用一手掌心分别将对侧上肢的肩、肘、腕关节的前、后、内、外各面擦热，每面擦 10～20 次左右；再沿经络循行方向，用一手掌心在对侧上肢的外侧，自腕背横纹处向上直擦至肩外侧之肩髃穴，再转向肩前方，沿上肢内侧向下直擦到腕内侧横纹处。如此在上肢的外侧由下而上、在上肢的内侧由上向下地反复推擦 30 遍左右，以擦热为宜（图4-18）。

③擦捻掌指　先用一手之大鱼际，将另手之手背各掌骨间的肌肉分别擦热；再以一手之拇、食二指，分别将另一手的各个指间关节一一揉捻（图4-19）。

【作用】

上法可防治肩周炎、肩峰下滑液囊炎、网球肘、腕部腱鞘炎等上肢各关节疾患；并有放松上肢肌肉、解除疲劳、增强上肢关节运动功能、预防职业性创伤等功效。

（2）下肢部

【操作】

①按揉下肢诸穴　先用拇指指面，或指端，或中指端，自上

Press and knead hard the points, with the whorled surface or the tip of the thumb or the tip of the middle finger, in the order of Juliao (St 3), Huantiao (GB 30), Futu (St 32), Zusanli (St 36), Yanglingquan (GB 34), Chengshan (UB 57) and Sanyinjiao (Sp 6), for about 20 times each. Try to get the feeling of *qi* (Fig. 4—20).

② Pressing-kneading the Thigh

Press and knead hard the muscles of the lateral, medial and anterior sides of the thigh from above to below with the palm roots for 3—5 times to get the sensation of soreness and distention (Fig. 4—21).

③ Pressing-kneading the Knee-cap

Stretch the legs naturally with the muscles relaxed. Carry out grasping-pinching and pressing-kneading with the thumb and the radial surface of the index finger, which is bent like a bow, on the knee-caps (Fig. 4—22).

④ Grasping the Shank

With the thumb and the tip of the index and middle fingers, conduct lifting-up, grasping, pinching and kneading manipulations gently on the gastrocnemius muscle from above to below to the Achilles tendon, for about 10 times. Try to get the sensation of soreness and distention (Fig. 4-23).

⑤ Patting the Lower Limb

Pat the leg with the centres or the roots of palms with forces in the opposite directions from the bend of the upper thigh to the lower part of the shank for about 10-15 times (Fig. 4-24).

⑥ Scrubbing Yongquan (K 1)

Scrub hard and rapidly the point Yongquan (K 1) at the sole with the minor thenar eminence. Use the right hand to rub the left foot and vice versa for about 30 times each to get the point hot (Fig. 4-25).

⑦ Rocking the Ankle Joint

Sit upright. Hold the malleolar part with one hand and the metatarsophalangeal part with the other hand. Rotate

而下分别用力按揉居髎、环跳、伏兔、足三里、阳陵泉、承山、三阴交等穴，每穴按揉 20 次左右，以有得气感为宜(图4-20)。

②按揉大腿　以两手掌根，自上而下，分别用力按揉大腿外侧、内侧与前侧肌肉 3～5 遍，以酸胀为宜(图4-21)。

③按揉髌骨　下肢自然伸直，肢肉放松。以一手拇指指面及屈成弓状的食指桡侧面，拿捏并按揉髌骨(图4-22)。

④拿小腿　以一手拇指与食、中指指端，提拿捏揉腓肠肌，自上而下直至跟腱，用力柔和，每次操作 10 遍左右，以酸胀为宜(图 4-23)。

⑤拍击下肢　以两手掌心或掌根，自大腿根部起，以上而下，相对用力拍击下肢，直至小腿下端，约 10～15 遍左右(图4-24)。

⑥擦涌泉　用一手小鱼际掌侧面，快速用力摩擦对侧足心之涌泉穴 30 次左右，以发热为宜，两足交替进行(图 4-25)。

⑦摇踝关节　正坐搁腿，一手抓踝上，一手握住足跖趾部，

the ankle joint clockwise and counterclockwise for about 20 times each (Fig. 4–26).

FUNCTION

These manipulations are effective for the prevention and treatment of injury of the superior clunial nerves, strain of the gluteal fascia, swelling and pain in the knees, systremma and injury of the ankle joints. It may also help to relax the muscles of the lower limbs, relieve fatigue, improve the motor function of the lower limb joints and prevent various kinds of occupational injuries. Besides, kneading Zusanli (St 36) and Sanyinjiao (Sp 6) and scrubbing Yongquan (K 1) in combination with the manipulations operated on the abdomen and head are salutary to the digestive, urinary, reproductive and central nervous systems.

3) Health Care of the Chest and Abdomen

(1) Health Care of the Chest

MANIPULATION

① Pressing-Kneading the Points at the Chest and Intercostal Spaces

Press and knead the the points at the chest and the intercostal spaces with the cushion of the middle finger. Press and knead Tanzhong (Ren 17), Zhongfu (Lu 1), Rugen (St 18) and Rupang for 20 times each. Then press and knead hard every intercostal space starting from the one on the infraclavicular part, from the midline to the sides and from above to below, to get the sensatin of soreness and distention (Fig. 4–27).

② Grasping Muscles of the Thorax

Apply one thumb tightly against the chest and the index and middle fingers against the side of it below the armpit. Lift up and down the anterior axillary fold at the lateral side of the greater pectoral muscle. The lifting-up-and-down should be cooperated with slow and gentle pinching and kneading movements. Do it 5 times each session (Fig. 4–28).

③ Patting the Chest

作顺时针及逆时针方向的旋转摇动踝关节，约 20 次左右（图 4-26）。

【作用】

上法对防治臀上皮神经损伤、臀筋膜劳损、膝关节肿痛、腓肠肌痉挛、踝关节损伤等病症有效，并有放松下肢肌肉、恢复疲劳、增强下肢各关节运动功能、预防各种职业性损伤等功效。另外，按揉足三里、三阴交，擦涌泉等法配合腹部及头部自我推拿手法，对胃肠消化系统、泌尿生殖系统与中枢神经等有保健作用。

3）胸腹部保健

（1）胸部

【操作】

①按揉胸部诸穴及肋间　以一手中指罗纹面，先分别按揉膻中、中府、乳根、乳旁等穴，每穴 20 次左右；再自锁骨下肋骨间隙开始，从上而下，由内向外，用力按揉每个肋间隙，以酸胀为宜(图 4-27)。

②拿胸肌　一手拇指紧贴胸前，食、中两指紧贴腋下相对用力提拿由胸大肌外侧组成的腋前壁，一提一拿并加以缓慢柔和的捏揉动作，每次操作 5 遍左右(图 4-28)。

③拍胸　以一手握虚拳，沿胸前正中线与两侧乳中线，自上

Make one hand a "hollow" fist and hit the chest with it from above to below along the thoracic median line and the breast median lines for about 10 times each. Holding breath while hitting should be avoided (Fig. 4–29).

④ Scrubbing the Chest

Apply the major thenar eminance or the whole palm of one hand tightly against the chest surface and scrub hard to and fror horizontally for about 20 times. The proper manipulation should produce a feeling of warmth (Fig. 4–30).

FUNCTION

These manipulations may be applied to the prevention and treatment of pain in the chest on breathing and chest pain, stuffiness in the chest, cough, dyspnea, disorder of functional activities of *qi* as well as palpitation.

(2) Abdominal Health Care

MANIPULATION

① Pressing-Kneading the Points on the Abdomen

By means of the tip of the middle finger or the major thenar eminance or the palm root, press and knead Zhongwan (Ren 12), Zhangmen (Liv 13), Tianshu (St 25), Qihai (Ren 6), Guanyuan (Ren 4) and Zhongji (Ren 3) for about 20–30 times each. Try to get the feeling of *qi* during manipulation (Fig. 4–31).

② Rubbing the Abdomen

Move the palm of one hand around Zhongwan (Ren 12), Shenque (Ren 8) and Guanyuan (Ren 4) clockwise and then counterclockwise for about 30–50 times respectively each (Fig. 4–32).

③ Scrubbing the Lower Abdomen

Apply the ulnar sides of the minor thenar eminances against the two points of Tianshu (St 25) about 2 *cun* beside the navel, rub up and down for about 30 times (Fig. 4–33).

④ Pressing the Points Digitally

Carry out digital-pressing with the middle finger of on.

而下，叩击胸部，在每条操作路线上叩击10次左右，叩击时不要屏气(图4-29)。

④擦胸　用一手大鱼际，或全掌紧贴胸部体表，横向用力来回摩擦20次左右，以产生热感为宜(图4-30)。

【作用】

上法对岔气、胸痛、胸闷、咳嗽、气喘、气机不畅、心悸等病症有防治作用。

（2）腹部

【操作】

①按揉腹部诸穴　用中指端、或大鱼际、或掌根为着力面，分别按揉中脘、章门、天枢、气海、关元、中极等穴，每穴20～30次左右，以产生得气感为宜(图4-31)。

②　摩腹　以一手掌心分别在中脘、神阙与关元穴周围，先沿顺时针方向，再沿逆时针方向旋转摩运，每个部位顺、逆各30～50次左右(图4-32)。

③擦少腹　以两手小鱼际掌侧贴紧脐旁2寸处的天枢穴，做上、下往返摩擦30次左右(图4-33)。

④点气海、关元、中极穴　以一手中指端分别点击气海、

hand on Qihai (Ren 6), Guanyuan (Ren 4) and Zhongji (Ren 3) for about 30–50 times respectively. A feeling of distention and tingle which transmits to the external genital organs is desirable.

FUNCTION

These manipulations are effective for prevention and treatment of discomfort in the stomach, indigestion, constipation, pain in the abdomen, irregular menstruation and impotency.

4) Health Care of the Back and Lumbosacral Portion

MANIPULATION

① Pressing-Kneading the Neck and Back

First, use the tips of the index, middle and ring fingers of both hands to press and knead from Fengchi (GB 20) at both sides downward via Tianzhu (UB 10) to the root of the neck for about 5–10 times; then with the tips of the three fingers of one hand push from Fengfu (Du 16) down to Dazhui (Du 14) for 5–10 times. Stop pushing at the points to press and knead for 20–30 times each. Lastly, use the middle finger of one hand to press and knead Dazhui (Du 14), Dazhu (UB 11), Shenzhu (Du 12), Fengmen (UB 12) and Feishu (UB 13) for about 30 times at each session. It is desirable to get a feeling of soreness and distention (Fg. 4–34).

② Patting the Back

Pat the right side of the back with the left palm and vice versa alternatively for about 10 times each(Fig. 4–35).

③ Hitting Jianjing (GB 21)

Sit upright or stand erect with the back straightened. Make a fist and hit with it the point Jianjing (GB 21) at the opposite side for 20–30 times. Hit the other Jianjing (GB 21) with the other fist for the same times.

④ Rubbing Gaohuang

With the upper body upright, abduct the upper limbs to form an angle of 90 degrees and bend the elbows. Rotate

关元、中极穴，每穴 30～50 次左右，以向外生殖器有胀、麻等传导感为宜。

【作用】

上法对防治胃脘不适、消化不良、大便秘结、腹痛、月经不调、阳痿等病症有效。

4）项背腰骶部保健

（1）项背部

【操作】

①按揉项背　先以双手食、中、无名指端,沿双侧风池向下,经天柱至项根按揉5～10 遍左右；再以一手食、中、无名指端,沿风府向下至大椎穴一线按揉5～10 遍, 在穴位处稍停按揉 20～30 次左右。再用一手中指向后伸向对侧背后, 按揉大椎、大杼、身柱、风门、肺俞等穴, 每次按揉 30 次左右, 以酸胀 为宜（图4-34）。

②　拍背　以一手虚掌, 向后伸向对侧背后, 拍打上背部10 次左右。左右交替操作（图4—35）。

③　捶击肩井　正坐或直立, 上身挺直, 一手握成空拳捶击对侧肩井穴 20～30 次；再以另一手用同法捶击另一侧肩井。

④　摩膏肓　上身挺直, 两上肢外展90°, 屈肘。作肩 关节

the shoulder joints with the amplitude of the backward movement being as large as possible to stimulate through the rotative movements of the scapula, the points, such as Gaohuang (GB 43), located the lateral to the interscapular region (Fig. 4-36).

FUNCTION

These manipulations are effective for the prevention and treatment of pain, soreness and distention in the back, cervical spondylopathy, stiffneck, cough, asthma, accumulation of phlegm, consumptive diseases, stiffness and pain in the chest, palpitation and angina pectoris.

(2) Health Care of the Waist

MANIPULATION

① Kneading the Points at the Waist

Clench the fists and knead hard with the knuckles of metacarpophalangeal of the index fingers the paired points of Shenshu (UB 23), Zhishi (UB 52) and Yaoyan (Extra) of for about 30 times each. Try to get the feeling of soreness and distention (Fig. 4-37).

② Thumping and Vibrating the Lumbar Region

Clench the fists and thump with their ulnar side along the three lines: from Shenshu (UB 23) to Pangguangshu (UB 28), from Zhishi (UB 52) via Yaoyan (Extra) to Baohuang (UB 53) and from Mingmen (Du 4) to the lumbosacral joint respectively for 5-10 times each to provide vibrations to the waist (Fig. 4-38).

③ Scrubbing the Waist

Stick the two palms tightly on the skin of the waist and rub-scrub with them up and down from the second lumbar vertebra to the sacro-iliac articulation till the region is hot (Fig. 4-39).

FUNCTION

These manipulations can be used to prevent and treat soreness and pain in the loins caused by various factors, general

的环转动作，并尽量增大向后的伸展幅度，以利用肩胛骨的环转动作来刺激位于两侧肩胛间区的膏肓等穴（图4-36）。

【作用】

上法对防治背痛酸胀、颈椎病、落枕、咳嗽、哮喘、痰结、虚劳、胸闷、胸痛、心悸、心绞痛等病证有效。

（2）腰部

【操作】

①揉腰部诸穴　两手握拳，用食指掌指关节突起处用力，分别按揉肾俞、志室、腰眼诸穴，每穴按揉30次左右，以酸胀为宜（图4-37）。

②捶振腰区　两手握拳，以拳眼处着力，自上而下，分别沿肾俞至膀胱俞一线，志室经腰眼至胞肓一线与命门至腰骶关节一线，叩击捶振腰部5～10遍（图4-38）。

③擦腰　用两手掌紧按腰部皮肤，自第二腰椎水平向下至骶髂关节处，上下往返摩擦，以局部发热为宜（图4-39）。

【作用】

上法可防治各种原因引起的腰部酸痛、无力、失眠、阳痿、

weakness, insomnia, impotency, frequency of micturition, proliferation of the lumbar vertebrae, prolapse of lumbar intervertebral disc, lumbar muscle strain, irregular menstruation and diarrhea. It also functions in soothing the loins, relieving fatigue and strengthening the motor function of the lumbar region.

The local self-massage manipulations introduced above may be carried out in diffecent ways for different purposes. For general health care, one can carry through these procedures once or twice a day in the order of: head and face → neck → upper back → chest and abdomen → lumbosacral portion → lower limbs. For local health care or treatment of diseases in a certain part or a certain organ of the body, one can select some of the above manipulations according to needs. For those engaged in professions which may easily cause regional fatigue or injury that affects their working efficiency, and for those who get occupational diseases easily, self-massage of the related areas can be conducted to raise the working efficiency or prevent occupational diseases. For example, long-distance runner or workers who have to stand long may carry out self-massage of the lower limbs every day before and after training or working, a method otherwise called "professional self-health-care massage". The manipulations can also be made into prescriptions of point massage for self health care or prescriptions of self-treatment massage.

2. Point Self-massage for Self Health Care

"Point self-massage for self health care" means a selection of certain points or areas as a prescription for self-massage.

1) The Manipulations for Easing Mental Stress and Refreshing the Mind

尿频、腰椎增生、腰椎间盘突出症、腰肌劳损、月经不调、腹泻等病证，并有放松腰部肌肉、恢复疲劳、增强腰部运动功能等功效。

以上介绍的分部自我推拿法可用于多方面。如作为全身性保健推拿，可按头部→颈项→上背→胸腹→腰骶→下肢的顺序，每天全部操作1～2遍；也可根据需要选做其中的一部分或某一部位的操作，以作为肢体或五官的局部保健治疗；另外，如因从事某种职业而使身体的某些部位容易疲劳，或发生劳损而影响工作效率与好发职业病的人，则可选择其中相关的部位进行自我推拿，以提高工作效率或预防职业病。如长跑运动员或取站姿工作的人，可在每天训练与工作的前后做下肢部的自我推拿操作，这种方法又可称为"职业性自我保健推拿"。再者，分部自我推拿中的各种单一的操作方法，也可作为处方的成分，组成经穴自我保健推拿与自我医疗推拿时的操作处方。

2. 经穴自我保健推拿

为特定的保健目的，以有效经穴与部位组成推拿处方而进行的自我推拿法谓之经穴自我保健推拿。

1）安神醒脑法

PRESCRIPTION

Pat the vertex 20 times, press and knead Zanzhu (UB 2) 30 times, push the forehead on either side 20 times, press and knead Touwei (St 8) 30 times, knead Fengfu (Du 16) and Fengchi (GB 20) 30 times each, press and knead Shenmen (H 7) and Sanyinjiao (Sp 6) 30 times respectively and rub Yongquan (K 1) 30 times.

FUNCTION

Being able to ease mental stress, refresh the mind and enhance vigour, these manipulatons are effective for the treatment of insomnia, mental fatigue, muddle-headedness, drowsiness and listlessness.

2) The Manipulations for Invigorating the Mind and Improving the Intelligence

PRESCRIPTION

Press and knead Baihui (Du 20) 50 times, push the forehead on either side 30 times, press and knead Taiyang (Extra 2) 30 times, wipe the temples 30 times, press and knead the back of the head 30 times, pat the upper back 20 times, press and knead Xinshu (UB 15), Neiguan (P 6), Shenmen (H 7) and Sanyinjiao (Sp 6) 30 times respectively and rub Yongquan (K 1) 30 times.

FUNCTION

These manipulations have the functions of invigorating the mind to facilitate mentality, improving the intelligence and raising the working efficiency of the mind. It is effective for neurosis, amnesia, incoherence of thinking and distractibility.

3) The Manipulations for Soothing Chest Oppression and Regulating Qi

PRESCRIPTION

Press and knead Tanzhong (Ren 17) 30 times, scrape the chest 20 times respectively for each side, pat the prothorax 30 times, hit Jianjing (GB 21) 20 times and press and knead Neiguan (P 6) 30 times.

【推拿处方】

拍击头顶 20 次，按揉攒竹 30 次，分推前额 20 遍，按揉头维 30 次，揉风府、风池各 30 次，按揉神门、三阴交各 30 次，擦涌泉 30 次。

【作用】

本法有提神、清脑、振奋精神之功效，对失眠、神倦、头脑不清、昏昏欲睡、精神萎靡者有效。

2）健脑益智法

【推拿处方】

按揉百会 50 次，分推前额 30 次，按揉太阳 30 次，分抹两颞 30 次，按揉脑后 30 次，拍上背 20 次，按揉心俞、内关、神门、三阴交各 30 次。擦涌泉 30 次。

【作用】

本法有健脑助神、增长智慧、提高大脑工作效率的功效，对神经衰弱、健忘、思维混乱、注意力不集中等病证有效。

3）宽胸理气法

【推拿处方】

按揉膻中 30 次，擦胸左右各 20 次，拍前胸 30 次，捶击肩

FUNCTION

Capable of making the lung-*qi* descend and clearing up the air passage, it is indicated for chest stuffiness, deficiency of *qi*, pain in the chest and breathing disturbance.

4) The Manipulations for Normalizing the Lung and Replenishing *Qi*

PRESCRIPTION

Press and knead Tanzhong (Ren 17) and Zhongfu (Lu 1) 30 times each, push and scrape the prothorax 30 times, knead Feishu (UB 13) 30 times, rub Gaohuang (UB 43) 20 times and press and knead Neiguan (P 6) and Zusanli (St 36) 30 times each.

FUNCTION

With the functions of replenishing and invigorating the lung-*qi*, these manipulations are effective for insufficiency of the lung-*qi* and failure of superficial-*qi* to protect the body against diseases, and are indicated for patinets liable to lung diseases and for patients suffering from persistent cough.

5) The Manipulations for Nourishing the Heart to Benefit the Mind

PRESCRIPTION

Knead Baihui (Du 20) and Fengfu (Du 16) 30 and 20 times respectively, press and knead Tanzhong (Ren 17), Rugan (St 18) and Rupang 30 times each, scrub the chest 30 times, press and knead Xinshu (UB 15) 30 times, Rub Gaohuang (UB 43) and Dantian 30 times each, press and knead Zusanli (St 36) and Sanyinjiao (Sp 6) 30 times each, and scrub Yongquan (K 1) 30 times.

FUNCTION

These manipulations have the virtues of transquilizing the mind by strengthening the heart, being beneficial to patients suffering from deficiency of heart-*qi* and for the old and middle-aged who suffer from heart failure.

6) The Manipulations for Strengthening the Spleen and

井 20 次，按揉内关 30 次。

【作用】

本法有肃降肺气、清理气道的功效，对胸闷、少气、胸痛、呼吸不畅者有效。

4）利肺益气法

【推拿处方】

按揉膻中、中府各 30 次，推擦前胸 30 次，揉肺俞 30 次，摩膏肓 20 次，按揉内关、足三里各 30 次。

【作用】

常行本法有补益肺气之功，对肺气虚弱、易患肺疾、卫外不固、久咳者有效。

5）养心益神法

【推拿处方】

揉百会 30 次，揉风府 20 次，按揉膻中、乳根、乳旁各 30 次，擦胸 30 次，按揉心俞 30 次，摩膏肓、丹田各 30 次，按揉足三里、三阴交各 30 次，擦涌泉 30 次。

【作用】

久行本法有强心安神之功，对心气怯弱、中老年心衰者有良好的保健作用。

6）健脾益胃法

Reinforcing the Stomach

PRESCRIPTION

Press and knead Zhongwan (Ren 12) and Zhangmen (Liv 13) 30 times each, rub Zhongwan (Ren 12) clockwise and counterclockwise 30 times each, and press and knead Pishu (UB 20), Weishu (UB 21) Neiguan (P 6) and Zusanli (St 36) 30 times each.

FUNCTION

These manipulations are effective for warming the middle-*jiao*, regulating the stomach and improving the functions of the spleen and stomach in transport and digestion, being indicated in syndromes of deficiency of the spleen and stomach manifested as poor appetite, indigestion and coldness in the epigastric region or aversion to cold.

7) The Manipulations for Promoting Digestion and Removing Stagnated Food

PRESCRIPTION

Rub Zhongwan (Ren 12) clockwise and counterclockwise 30 times respectively, knead Zhongwan (Ren 12) 30 times, push and rub from Jiuwei (Ren 15) to the navel 30 times, scrub the lower abdomen 30 times, hit Pishu (UB 20) and Weishu (UB 21) 30 times each, and knead Neiguan (P 6) and Zusanli (St 36) 30 times each.

FUNCTION

These manipulations can improve the digestive function of the stomach and intestine and are effective for fullness and dull pain in tne gastrial cavity, stagnancy of indigested food as well as belching and constipation.

8) The Manipulations for Enhancing the Waist and Building Up the Constitution

PRESCRIPTION

Rub Dantian 30 times, hit and vibrate the waist 30 times, knead Shenshu (UB 23) 30 times, press and knead Mingmen (Du 4) and Yaoyangguan (Du 3) 30 times each, rub Gao-

【推拿处方】

按揉中脘、章门各 30 次，摩中脘顺逆各 30 次，按揉脾俞、胃俞、内关、足三里各 30 次。

【作用】

本法有温中和胃、增强脾胃运化与受纳的功能，对食欲不振、消化不良、腹中清冷、畏寒等脾胃虚弱诸证有效。

7） 消食导滞法

【推拿处方】

摩中脘顺逆各 30 次，揉中脘 30 次，推摩鸠尾至脐中 30 次，擦少腹捶击脾、胃俞 30 次，揉内关、足三里各 30 次。

【作用】

本法能增强肠胃消化功能，对脘腹胀满闷痛、食滞不化、嗳气、便秘者有效。

8）壮腰强身法

【推拿处方】

摩丹田 30 次，捶振腰区 10 遍，揉肾俞 30 次，按揉命门、腰

huang (UB 43) 20 times, and knead Zusanli (St 36) anu Sanyinjiao (Sp 6) 30 times each.

FUNCTION

These manipulations work to build up the constitution and improve the motor function of the waist, being indicated in the treatment of soreness of waist with difficulty in movement, general lassitude and liability to fatigue.

9) The Manipulations for Tonifying the Kidney and Nourishing the Essence

PRESCRIPTION

Rub and scrub the waist 30 times, knead Shenshu (UB 23) and Zhishi (UB 52) 30 times each, thump from Mingmen (Du 4) to Yaoyangguan (Du 3) 10 times, press digitally Guanyuan (Ren 4) and Zhongji (Ren 3) 20 times each, rub Dantian 30 times, and press and knead Zusanli (St 36) and Sanyinjiao (Sp 6) 30 itmes each.

FUNCTION

Having the functions of tonifying the kidney-*yin* and nourishing *yin* and strengthening *yang*, the prescription is effective for soreness and weakness of the loins and kness, coldness of the extremities, night sweat, insomnia, impotency and seminal emission as well as asthenia in the old-aged.

10) The Manipulations for Warming and Recuperating the Kidney

PRESCRIPTION

Knead Qihai (Ren 6) and Guanyuan (Ren 4) 30 times each, rub Shenque (Ren 8) and Dantian clockwise and counterclockwise 30 times each, rub Yaoyan (Extra) 30 times, rub the lumbosacral portion horizontally 30 times, and press and knead Zusanli (St 36) and Sanyinjiao (Sp 6) 30 times each.

FUNCTION

These manipulations function in warming and nourishing the kidney and strengthening *yang* and restoring *qi* (to promote vital function). Persistent practice of it can treat lingering

阳关各30次，摩膏肓20次，按揉足三里、三阴交各30次。

【作用】

久行本法可增强体力与腰部的运动功能，对腰脊酸软、活动不灵、全身乏力、容易疲劳者有效。

9） 补肾益精法

【推拿处方】

摩擦腰区30次，揉肾俞、志室各30次，捶击命门至腰阳关10遍，点击关元、中极各20次，摩丹田30次，按揉足三里、三阴交各30次。

【作用】

久行本法有补益肾水、滋阴壮阳之功，对腰膝酸软、手足不温、盗汗、失眠、阳痿、遗精及老年体虚均有强壮补益作用。

10） 温补下元法

【推拿处方】

揉气海、关元各30次，摩神阙、丹田顺逆各30次，擦腰眼30次，横擦骶部30次，按揉足三里、三阴交各30次。

【作用】

本法有温养下元、壮阳补虚之功，久行此法对下元虚寒所致

diarrhea, impotency, seminal emission, abdominal pain with gurgling of the intestine and constipation of deficiency type and frequency of micturition due to insufficiency and cold of the kidney and women diseases such as dysmenorrhea and amenorrhea.

11) The Manipulations for Nourishing the Liver to Improve Vision

PRESCRIPTION

Press and knead Fengchi (GB 20) 30 times, scrape the eye orbits 30 times, knead Zanzhu, (UB 2), Jingming (UB 1) and Taiyang (Extra 2) 30 times each, "iron" the eyes 30 seconds, nip and knead Hegu (LI 4) 30 times, and knead Taichong (Liv 3) and Ganshu (UB 18) 30 times each.

FUNCTION

These manipulations can nourish the liver to improve the acuity of vision, can help to keep good eyesight and can prevent and treat juvenile myopia, hypopsia in the old-aged and glaucoma as well as optic atrophy.

12) The Manipulations for Reinforcing the Kidney to Improve Hearing

PRESCRIPTION

Knead Baihui (Du 20) 30 times, press and knead Tinggong (SI 19) 30 times, scrub and rub the preauricular region 30 times, knead Yifeng (SJ 17) 30 times, ming Tiangu 30 times, knead Shenshu (UB 23) 30 times, nip and knead Hegu (LI 4) 30 times and knead Taixi (K 3) 30 times.

FUNCTION

The massage functions in nourishing the kidney, inducing resuscitation and protecting audition. Persistent practice of it can prevent and treat tinnitus, deafness, hypoacusis due to aging and invagination of the tympanic membrance.

13) The Manipulations for Facilitating the Flow of Lung-qi to Clear the Nasal Passage

PRESCRIPTION

的久泄、阳痿遗精、腹痛肠鸣、虚秘、尿频、痛经及闭经等妇科病证均有效。

11）益肝明目法

【推拿处方】

按揉风池 30 次，刮眼轮 30 次，揉攒竹、睛明、太阳各 30 次，熨眼 30 秒钟，掐揉合谷 30 次，揉太冲、肝俞各 30 次。

【作用】

本法能养肝明目、保持视力健康，可防治青少年近视、老年人视力减退、青光眼及视神经萎缩等病证。

12）强肾聪耳法

【推拿处方】

揉百会 30 次，按揉听宫 30 次，搓擦耳前 30 次，揉翳风 30 次，鸣天鼓 30 次，揉肾俞 30 次，掐揉合谷 30 次，揉太溪 30 次。

【作用】

本法有补肾开窍、保护听力的作用，久行可防治耳鸣、耳聋、老年人听力下降及耳膜内陷等病证。

13）宣肺通鼻法

【推拿处方】

Knead Yintang (Extra 1) and Yingxiang (LI 20) 30 times each, scrub and rub the sides of the nose 30 times, press-knead Fengchi (GB 20) 30 times, knead Feishu (UB 13) 30 times, pat the upper back 20 times, and nip-grasp Hegu (LI 4) 30 times.

FUNCTION

These manipulations are effective for clearing the nasal passage by facilitating the flow of the lung-qi. Persistent practice of it can prevent and treat hyposmia of the old and middle-aged and stuffy and running nose caused by frequent attack of exopathogen.

14) The Manipulations for Moistening the Lung to Improve the Voice

PRESCRIPTION

Press-knead Fengchi (GB 20) 30 times, press-knead the nape from Fengchi (GB 20) down to the root of the neck 5 times, press-knead Lianquan (Ren 23) 30 times, knead along the sides of the laryngeal protuberance 30 times, knead Tiantu (Ren 22) 30 times, press-knead Dazhui (Du 14) 20 times, press-knead Feishu (UB 13) 30 times, knead Tanzhong (Ren 17) 30 times and Hegu (LI 4) 30 times, and nip Shaoshang (Lu 11) 10 times.

FUNCTION

These manipulations are beneficial to the voice by moistening the lung and regulating qi. Those who have to raise their voice often, such as singers, opera actors or actresses and teachers, may persist in practising to protect the vocal cords and improve its ability against strain.

Section 2

Self-therapy Massage

Self-massage for self-treatment of diseases through diffe-

揉印堂、迎香各 30 次，搓擦鼻旁 30 次，按揉风池 30 次，揉肺俞 30 次，拍上背 20 次，掐拿合谷 30 次。

【作用】

本法能宣肺气、利鼻窍，久行对中老年人嗅觉减退及经常易患外感、鼻塞流涕者有防治保健作用。

14）润肺清音法

【推拿处方】

按揉风池穴 30 次，按揉项后（风池直下至项 根）5 遍，按揉廉泉穴 30 次，揉喉结旁、天突各 30 次，按揉大椎 20 次，按揉肺俞 30 次，揉膻中、合谷各 30 次，掐少商 10 次。

【作用】

本法有润肺理气、清利嗓音的功效。歌唱戏曲演员、教师等经常用嗓音工作的人，久行本法能保护声带，提高其抗疲劳的能力。

第二节　　自我医疗推拿

以疾病自疗为目的，辨证地选取有效经穴与部位组成推拿治

rential selection of certain effective points and portions to make up a prescription of massage treatment is called "self-therapy massage".

Self-therapy massage can be applied not only as an auxiliary procedure for treatment of some diseases, but also as an important means of autorehabilitation from many chronic diseases. Satisfactory results can be achieved in most patients so long as they practise once or twice every day in accordance with the follwing prescriptions.

Cold
PRESCRIPTION
Push the forehead on either side 30 times, knead Taiyang (Extra 2) 30 times, wipe-separately both the temples 30 times, knead Fengchi (GB 20) 30 times, grasp the posterior cervical ligament 10 times, thump Jianjing (GB 21) 20 times, pat the upper back 20 times, and nip-knead Hegu (LI 4) 30 times.

SYMPTOMATIC POINT SELECTION
For patients sith stuffy and running nose, knead Yingxang (LI 20) and scrub the sides of the nose 30 times each in addition.

For patients with swelling and sore throat, knead the submaxillary region and nip Shaoshang (Lu 11) 30 times each in addition.

For patients with severe cough, knead Feishu (UB 13), press-knead Tiantu (Ren 22), knead Tanzhong (Ren 17), and press-knead Fenglong (St 40) 30 times each, in addition.

For patients with fever, knead Feishu (UB 13), press-knead Dazhui (Du 14) and press-knead Quchi (LI 11) 30 times each, in addition.

Headache
PRESCRIPTION
Press-knead Yintang (Extra 1) 30 times, push the forehead on either side 30 times, press-knead Taiyang (Extra 2) 30 times,

疗处方而进行的自我推拿,谓之自我医疗推拿。本法不仅可作为某些疾病的辅助治疗，而且还可作为许多慢性病自我康复的重要手段。患者只要按下面介绍的常用处方，坚持每日认真操作 1～2 遍，多数会取得满意的疗效。

感冒

【推拿处方】

分推前额 30 次，揉太阳 30 次，分抹两颧 30 次，揉风池 30 次，拿项后大筋 10 遍，捶击肩井 20 次，拍上背 20 次，掐揉合谷 30 次。

【随证取穴】

鼻塞流涕者，加揉迎香 30 次，搓擦鼻旁 30 次。

咽喉肿痛者，加揉颏下 30 次，掐少商 30 次。

咳嗽重者，加揉肺俞 30 次，按揉天突 30 次，揉膻中 30 次，按揉丰隆 30 次。

发热者，加揉肺俞 30 次，按揉大椎、曲池各 30 次

头痛

【推拿处方】

按揉印堂 30 次，分推前额 30 次，按揉太阳 30 次，分抹两

wipe the temples 30 times, press-knead Fengchi (GB 20) 30 times, thump Jianjing (GB 21) 30 times and nip-knead Hegu (L 14) 30 times.

SYMPTOMATIC POINT SELECTION

For patients with migraine, the following manipulations should be added: kneading Touwei (St 8) 20 times, wiping again the temple of the affected side 20 times, nip-kneading Waiguan (SJ 5) 30 times, and nip-kneading Zhongzhu (SJ 3) on the hand 30 times.

Patients with pain in the vertex should carry out the following additional manipulations: kneading Baihui (Du 20) 30 times pressing-kneading Neiguan (P 6) and Taichong (Liv 3) 30 times, each, and scrubbing Yongquan (K 1) 30 times.

Patients with occipital headache should, additionally, knead Naohou (the back of the head) 30 times and press-knead Houxi (SI 3) 30 times.

Insomnia

PRESCRIPTION

Press-knead Baihui (Du 20) 30 times, knead Zanzhu (UB 2) 30 times, scrape the eye orbits 20 times, "iron" the eyes 30 seconds, press-knead Fengchi (GB 20) 30 times, rub Zhongwan (Ren 12) clockwise and counterclockwise for 30 rounds respectively, rub Dantian clockwise and counterclockwise 30 rounds respectively, press-knead Neiguan (P 6), Shenmen (H 7), Zusanli (St 36) and Sanyinjiao (Sp 6) 20 times each, and scrub Yongquan (K 1) 30 times.

SYMPTOMATIC POINT SELECTION

Patients with dreaminess, palpitation and mental fatigue should, for supplement, press-knead Xinshu (UB 15), Pishu (UB 20) and Shenshu (UB 23) 30 times each.

Patients with dizziness, tinnitus and soreness of the loins with nocturnal emission should, additionally, Press-knead Shenshu (UB 23), Zhishi (UB 52) and Taixi (K 3) 30 times each.

Patients with irritability, congested eyes and constipation

颞 30 次，按揉风池 30 次，捶击肩井 30 次，掐揉合谷 30 次。

【随证取穴】

偏头痛者，加揉头维，重抹患侧颞部 20 次，掐揉外关、中渚
各 30 次

头顶痛者，加按揉百会、内关、太冲各 30 次，擦涌泉 30 次。

枕后痛者，加按揉脑后、后溪各 30 次。

失眠

【推拿处方】

按揉百会 30 次，揉攒竹 30 次，刮眼轮 20 次，熨眼 30 秒钟，
按揉风池 30 次，摩中脘、丹田顺逆各 30 次，按揉内关、神门、
足三里、三阴交各 20 次，擦涌泉 30 次。

【随证取穴】

多梦、心悸、神疲者，加按揉心俞、脾俞、肾俞各 30 次。

头晕、耳鸣、腰酸梦遗者，加按揉肾俞、志室、太溪各 30 次。

should add the following manipulations: Scrubbing the hypochondria and the lower abdomen 30 times each, kneading
Ganshu (UB 18) 30 times, and press-kneading Taichong (Liv
3) and Hegu (LI 4) 30 times each.

Hypertension
PRESCRIPTION
Press-knead Baihui (Du 20), Yintang (Extra 1), Taiyang
(Extra 2) and Fengchi (GB 20) 30 times each; push Qiaogong
30 times, rub Shenque (Ren 8) 30 times, scrub the hypochondria (both sides) 30 times, thump Jianjing (GB 21) 30 times,
pat the upper back 30 times, and press-knead Neiguan (P 6),
Quchi (LI 11), Zusanli (St 36) and Sanyinjiao (Sp 6) 30 times
each.

SYMPTOMATIC POINT SELECTION
Hypertensive patients with severe headache may conduct
massage by modifying the prescription for headache.

Hypertensive patients with vetigo and tinnitus, vexation
and amnesia and soreness and weakness of the loins and knees
may, additionally, press-knead Fengfu (Du 16), Tinghui (GB
2), Shenshu (UB 23) and Zhishi (UB 52) 30 times each, scrub
Yaoyan (the small of the back) 30 times, and nip-knead Taixi
(K 3) and Taichong (Liv 3) 30 times each.

Hypertensives with headache and severe dizziness, vertigo, nausea, and stuffiness and distension in the chest and
epigastric region accompanied with poor appetite should add
the following manipulations: rubbing Zhongwan (Ren 12)
30 times, kneading Tanzhong (Ren 17) 30 times, and press-
kneading Pishu (UB 20) and Weishu (UB 21) 30 times each.

Hypertensive patients with stuffiness and pain in the chest,
palpitation, insomnia and dreaminess should, additionally,
knead Xinshu (UB 15) 30 times, push-scrub the prothorax
30 times, and press-knead Tanzhong (Ren 17), Rugen
(St 18), Shenshu (UB 23) and Yongquan (K 1) 30 times
each.

心烦易怒、目赤、便秘者，加擦两胁、少腹各 30 次，揉肝俞 30 次，按揉太冲、合谷各 30 次。

高血压

【推拿处方】

按揉百会、印堂、太阳、风池各 30 次，推桥弓 30 次，摩神阙 30 次，擦两胁 30 次，捶击肩井 30 次，拍上背 30 次，按揉内关、曲池、足三里、三阴交各 30 次。

【随证取穴】

头痛重者，按以上头痛节治疗处方辨证加减。

眩晕耳鸣、心烦健忘、腰膝酸软者，加按揉风府、听会、肾俞、志室各 30 次，擦腰眼 30 次，掐揉太溪、太冲各 30 次。

头痛昏重、眩晕恶心、胸脘闷胀、纳差者，加摩中脘 30 次，揉膻中 30 次，按揉脾俞、胃俞各 30 次。

胸闷痛、心悸、失眠、多梦者，加按揉心俞 30 次，推擦前胸 30 次，按揉膻中、乳根、肾俞、涌泉各 30 次。

Chronic Gastritis
PRESCRIPTION
Press-knead Zhongwan (Ren 12) 30 times, rub Zhongwan (Ren 12) clockwise and counterclockwise 30 turns respectively, scrub the hypochondria 30 times, and press-knead Pishu (UB 20), Weishu (UB 21), Neiguan (P 6), Shousanli (LI 10) and Zusanli(St 36) 30 times each.

SYMPTOMATIC POINT SELECTION
Patients with symptoms of distension and pain in the stomach, vexation, belching, gastric discomfort with acid regurgitation should, additionally, press-knead Zhangmen (Liv 13), Ganshu (UB 18), Liangqiu (St 34) and Taichong (Liv 3) 30 times each.

Patients with burning pain in the stomach that often deteriorates in the afternoon, or when the stomach is empty, which may be relieved by taking food, should add kneading of Liangmen (St 21) Jianli (Ren 11), Neiting (St 44) and Taichong (Liv 3) 30 times each.

Patients with vague pain in the stomach which may be aggravated by cold and relieved by pressure accompanied with lassitude should add kneading Shenshu (UB 23) for 30 times and rubbing Dantian clockwise and counterclockwise for 30 times respectively.

Gastroptosis
PRESCRIPTION
Press-knead Baihui (Du 20) 30 times, rub Zhongwan (Ren 12) and Shenque (Ren 8) clockwise and counterclockwise respectively for 30 times each (The essential of massage on the two points is that when rubbing upwards, a litle more strength should be exerted as if to hold the stomach.), scrub Dazhui (Du 14) 30 times, press-knead Pishu (UB 20), Weishu (UB 21) 30 times each and knead Shenshu (UB 23) 30 times rub Gaohuang (UB 43) 20 times, press-knead Shousanli (LI 10), Neiguan (P 6), Zusanli (St 36) and Sanyinjiao (Sp 6) 30

慢性胃炎

【推拿处方】

按揉中脘 30 次，摩中脘顺逆各 30 次，擦两肋 30 次，按揉脾俞、胃俞、内关、手三里、足三里各 30 次。

【随证取穴】

胃脘胀痛、嗳气泛酸、心烦嘈杂者，加按揉章门、肝俞、梁丘、太冲各 30 次。

胃脘灼痛、午后或空腹时加重、得食即减者，加按揉梁门、建里、内庭、太冲各 30 次。

胃脘隐痛、畏寒喜按、神疲乏力者，加揉肾俞 30 次，摩丹田顺逆各 30 次。

胃下垂

【推拿处方】

按揉百会 30 次，摩中脘、神阙顺逆各 30 次（上二穴操作要领：当向上方摩运时要稍用力兜托）。擦大椎 30 次，按揉脾俞、胃俞各 30 次，揉肾俞 30 次，摩膏肓 20 次，按揉手三里、内关、

times each.

SYMPTOMATIC POINT SELECTION

For gastroptosis accompanied with vertigo, listlessness and asthenia, the following should be done for supplement: kneading Yintang (Extra 1), Taiyang (Extra 2) and Fengchi (GB 20) 30 times each, rubbing-scrubbing Yaoyan (Extra) 30 times and patting the shank 10 times.

For gastroptosis accompanied with palpitation and insomnia, add the following: kneading Xinshu (UB 15) and Fengfu (Du 16) 30 times each, scrubbing the prothorax 20 times, kneading Taixi (K 3) 30 times.

For gastroptosis accompanied with constipation, add kneading Tianshu (St 25) 30 times and rubbing the lower abdomen clockwise 30 times.

For that accompanied with diarrhea, add kneading Tianshu (St 25) 30 times, rubbing the lower abdomen Counterclockwise 30 times and kneading Changqiang (Du 1) 30 times.

Chronic Diarrhea
PRESCRIPTION

Knead Zhongwan (Ren 12), Qihai (Ren 6), Guanyuan (Ren 4) and Tianshu (St 25) 30 times each, rub Shenque (Ren 8) and Dantian (counterclockwise) 50 times each, knead Pishu (UB 20) and Shenshu (UB 23) 30 times each, scrub Yaoyan (Extra) 30 times, scrub horizontally the lumbosacral portion 30 times, press-knead Changqiang (Du 1), Hegu (LI 4), Zusanli (St 36) and Sanyinjiao (Sp 6) 30 times each.

SYMPTOMATIC POINT SELECTION

For treatment of diarrhea that may become severe along with emotional change and is often accompanied with abdominal pain and borborygmus, feeling of stuffiness and choking in the chest and hypochondria, add kneading Ganshu (UB 18) 30 times and pressing-kneading Neiguan (P 6) and Taichong (Liv 3) 30 times each.

Patients having repeated attacks of diarrhea with indi-

足三里、三阴交各 30 次。

【随证取穴】

伴眩晕、神倦、乏力者，加按揉印堂、太阳、风池各 30 次，摩擦腰眼 30 次，拍击小腿 10 遍。

伴心悸、失眠者，加揉心俞、风府各 30 次，擦前胸 20 次，揉太溪 30 次。

伴便秘者，加揉天枢 30 次，向左摩少腹 30 次。

伴腹泻者，加揉天枢 30 次，向右摩少腹 30 次，揉长强 30次。

慢性腹泻

【推拿处方】

揉中脘、气海、关元、天枢各 30 次，摩神阙、丹田向右摩各 50 次，揉脾俞、肾俞各 30 次，擦腰眼 30 次，横擦腰骶 30 次，按揉长强、合谷、足三里、三阴交各 30 次。

【随证取穴】

腹痛肠鸣、胸胁痞闷，常于情绪波动而泄泻加甚者，加揉肝俞 30 次，按揉内关、太冲各 30 次。

gestion which tends to become worse after eating greasy food, sallow complexion and listlessness should be treated by adding the following manipulations: rubbing Zhongwan (Ren 12) 30 times, kneading Jianli (Ren 11) 30 times, and pressing-kneading Weishu (UB 21), Dachangshu (UB 25) and Shousanli (LI 10) 30 times each.

Diarrhea accompanied with periumbilical pain before dawn, instant defecation after borborygmus, aversion of the abdomen to cold, and soreness and weakness of the loins and kness should be treated by adding: scrubbing Dazhui (Du 14) 30 times and pressing-kneading Mingmen (Du 4) and Taixi (K 3) 30 times each.

Habitual Constipation

PRESCRIPTION

Knead Tianshu (St 25) and Guanyuan (Ren 4) 30 times each, rub the lower abdomen clockwise 50 times, press-knead Pishu (UB 20), Weishu (UB 21), Zhigou (SJ 6), Hegu (LI 4) and Zusanli (St 36) 30 times each, pat the shank 10 times and grasp Chengshan (UB 57) 10 times.

SYMPTOMATIC POINT SELECTION

Patients with dry stool, flushed face, fever, dry mouth, vexation and scanty, dark urine should be treated, additionally, by pressing-kneading Dachangshu (UB 25), Shousanli (LI 10) and Taichong (Liv 3) 30 times each and nipping-kneading Neiting (St 44) 30 times.

Dryness and retention of feces, fullness in the abdomen and hypochondria and frequent attacks of belching should be treated by additional massages of the following: press-kneading Zhangmen (Liv 13) 30 times, pushing-scrubbing the hypochondria 30 times and kneading Tanzhong (Ren 17) 30 times.

For treatment of habitual constipation manifested as dyschesia, cold extremities, soreness and coldness of the loins and knees with pain, add: kneading Shenque (Ren 8) clockwise

腹泻反复发作、完谷不化、稍食油腻物即加重、面色萎黄、神疲乏力者，加摩中脘 30 次，揉建里 30 次，按揉胃俞、大肠俞、手三里各 30 次。

每于黎明之前脐周作痛、肠鸣即泻、腹部畏寒、腰膝酸软者，加擦大椎 30 次，按揉命门、太溪各 30 次。

习惯性便秘

【推拿处方】

揉天枢、关元各 30 次，向左摩少腹 50 次，按揉脾俞、胃俞、支沟、合谷、足三里各 30 次，拍击小腿 10 次，拿承山 10 次。

【随证取穴】

大便燥结、面红身热、口干心烦、小便短赤者，加按揉大肠俞、手三里、太冲各 30 次，掐揉内庭 30 次。

大便秘结、胁腹痞满、嗳气频作者，加按揉章门 30 次，推擦两胁 30 次，揉膻中 30 次。

大便艰涩、四肢不温、腰膝酸冷痛者，加揉神阙顺逆各 30

and counterclockwise 30 times respectively, rubbing Zhongwan (Ren 12) 30 times, scrubbing horizontally the lumbosacral portion 30 times, scrubbing Dazhui (Du 14) 30 times and kneading Shenshu (UB 23) 30 times.

For that manifested as dyschesia which makes the patient put forth all his strength on defecation accompanied with sweating, shortness of breath and mental fatigue, add: kneading Shenshu (UB 23) and Zhishi (UB 52) 30 times each, scrubbing Yaoyan (Extra) 30 times, and kneading Tanzhong (Ren 17) and Changqiang (Du 1) 30 times each.

Hiccup
PRESCRIPTION

Press and knead Tanzhong (Ren 17), Zhongwan (Ren 12), Zhangmen (Liv 13) and Tiantu (Ren 22) 30 times each, rub Zhongwan (Ren 12) and Qihai (Ren 6) 30 times each, push-scrub from Tiantu (Ren 22) down to Jiuwei (Ren 15) 30 times, and press-knead Pishu (UB 20), Weishu (UB 21), Neiguan (P 6), Hegu (LI 4) and Zusanli (St 36) 30 times each.

SYMPTOMATIC POINT SELECTION

For treating continuous serious hiccup with loud sound accompanied with stuffiness in the chest and hypochondrium, flushed face and excessive thirst, add: patting the vertex 15 times and pressing-kneading Fengchi (GB 20), Sanyinjiao (Sp 6) and Taichong (Liv 3) 30 times each.

For hiccup with attacks of longer intervals and low sound accompanied with anorexia and abdominal distention, mental fatigue and cold extremities, add: scrubbing Dazhui (Du 14) 30 times and pressing-kneading Shenshu (UB 23) and Sanyinjiao (Sp 6) 30 times each.

Diabetes
PRESCRIPTION

Press-knead Zhongwan (Ren 12), Tanzhong (Ren 17) and Guanyuan (Ren 4) 50 times each, rub Zhongwan (Ren 12) and Shenque (Ren 8) clockwise and counterclockwise

次，摩中脘 30 次，横擦腰骶 30 次，擦大椎 30 次，揉肾俞 30 次。

大便不畅、临便努挣、汗出、气短、神疲者，加揉肾俞、志室各 30 次，擦腰眼 30 次，揉膻中、长强各 30 次。

膈肌挛痉

【推拿处方】

按揉膻中、中脘、章门、天突各 30 次，摩中脘、气海各 30 次，推擦天突至鸠尾 30 次，按揉脾俞、胃俞、内关、合谷、足三里各 30 次。

【随证取穴】

呃声洪亮连续有力、胸胁胀闷、面红烦渴者，加拍击头顶 15 次，按揉风池、三阴交、太冲各 30 次。

呃声微弱间隔较长、厌食腹胀、神疲肢冷者，加擦大椎 30 次，按揉肾俞、三阴交各 30 次。

糖尿病

【推拿处方】

按揉中脘、膻中、关元各 50 次，摩中脘、神阙顺逆各 30 遍，

for 30 times each, press-knead Feishu (UB 13), Shenshu (UB 23) and Mingmen (Du 4) 30 times each, thump the renal region 30 times, rub-scrub Yaoyan (Extra) 30 times, and press-knead Shousanli (LI 10), Neiguan (P 6), Zusanli (St 36) and Sanyinjiao (Sp 6) 30 times each.

SYMPTOMATIC POINT SELECTION

For treatment of thirst with polydipsia, dry mouth and tongue and frequent micturition with increased amount of urine, add digital-pressing of Dazhui (Du 14) and pressing-kneading of Chize (Lu 5) 30 times.

For treatment of excessive drinking and susceptability to hunger, emaciation and constipation, add: pressing-kneading Ganshu (UB 18) 30 times, rubbing the lower abdomen clockwise 30 times and pressing-kneading Chengshan (UB 57), Taichong (Liv 3) and Neiting (St 44) 30 times each.

Peripheral Facial Paralysis

PRESCRIPTION

Press-knead Yintang (Extra 1) 30 times, push the forehead on either side 30 times, press-knead Zanzhu (UB 2) 30 times, scrape the eye orbits 30 times, press-knead Taiyang (Extra 2), Jiache (St 6), Xiaguan (St 7), Dicang (St 4) and Fengchi (GB 20) 30 times each, press-grasp Hegu (LI 4) 30 times, press-knead Zusanli (St 36) 30 times.

SYMPTOMATIC POINT SELECTION

At the onset of the disease with the symptom of posterior auricular pain, add the following manipulations: pressing-kneading Fengfu (Du 16), Yifeng (SJ 17) and Fengmen (UB 12) 30 times each, and patting the upper back 30 times.

For treatment of inability to raise the brows or to close the eyes tightly and epiphora induced by wind, add pressing-kneading Yangbai (GB 14), Sibai (St 2), Jingming (UB 1) and Tong ziliao (GB 1) 30 times each.

For patients with difficulty in blowing up the cheeks, ptosis of labial angle and leakage of water when gargling, add press-

按揉肺俞、肾俞、命门各 30 次，捶击肾区 30 次，摩擦腰眼 30 次，按揉手三里、内关、足三里、三阴交各 30 次。

【随证取穴】

烦渴多饮、口干舌燥、尿频而量多者，加点按大椎 30 次，按揉尺泽 30 次。

多饮易饥、形体消瘦、大便秘结者，加按揉肝俞 30 次，向左摩少腹 30 次，按揉承山、太冲、内庭各 30 次。

面神经麻痹（周围性）

【推拿处方】

按揉印堂 30 次，分推前额 30 次，按揉攒竹 30 次，刮眼轮 30 次，按揉太阳、颊车、下关、地仓、风池各 30 次，按拿合谷 30 次，按揉足三里 30 次。

【随证取穴】

面瘫初起，耳后疼痛者，加按揉风府、翳风、风门各 30 次，拍打上背 30 次。

抬眉不能、闭眼不全、迎风流泪者，加按揉阳白、四白、睛明、瞳子髎各 30 次。

鼓腮无力、口角低垂、漱口漏水、流涎不禁者，加按揉人中、

ing-kneading Renzhong (Du 26), Chengjiang (Ren 24) and Lianquan (Ren 23) 30 times each.

For protracted paralysis which recovers slowly and is accompanied with dizziness, tinnitus, burring and tearful eyes, lacrimation and soreness of the loins and knees, add the following manipulations: pressing-kneading Pishu (UB 20), Weishu (UB 21) and Shenshu (UB 23) 30 times each, rubbing Zhongwan (Ren 12) and Dantian clockwise and counterclockwise respectively for 30 times each, and pressing-kneading Sayinjiao (Sp 6) 30 times.

Cervical Spondylopathy
PRESCRIPTION

Press-knead Fengfu (Du 16) 30 times and from Fengfu (Du 16) down to Dazhui (Du 14) 10 times, press-knead Fengchi (GB 20) 30 times and from Fengchi (GB 20) down to the bottom of the nape 10 times. Press-knead Tianzhu (UB 10) and the pressure pain points along the sides of the neck for 30 times each, thump Jianjing (GB 21) 30 times, press-knead Jianyu (LI 15), Quchi (LI 11), Shousanli (LI 10), Waiguan (SJ 5) and Hegu (LI 4) 30 times each, push-scrub the medial and lateral sides of the upper limbs for 20 times respectively, and scrub-twirl the fingers 5 times each.

SYMPTOMATIC POINT SELECTION

Numbness and pain in the medial side of the upper limbs and muscular atrophy should be treated by adding pressing-kneading Xiaohai (SI 8), Neiguan (P 6), Shenmen (H 7) and Zhongzhu (SJ 3) 30 times each.

For cervical spondylopathy of vertebral artery type with cervical vertigo, add: pushing Qiaogong 30 times, pressing-kneading Yintang (Extra 1) and Taiyang (Rxtra 2) 30 times each, pushing the forehead on either side 30 times, rubbing Zhongwan (Ren 12) clockwise and conterclockwise 30 times each and pressing-kneading Zusanli (St 36) and Sanyinjiao (Sp 6) 30 times each, and bending the neck forward and backward and left and right, and turn it round in cooperation with the massage.

承浆、廉泉各 30 次。

久瘫不愈、恢复缓慢并伴头晕耳鸣、目糊流泪、腰膝酸软者，加按揉脾俞、胃俞、肾俞各 30 次，摩中脘、丹田顺逆各 30 次，按揉三阴交 30 次。

颈椎病

【推拿处方】

按揉风府 30 次，按揉风府至大椎一线 10 遍，按揉风池 30 次，按揉风池至项根一线 10 遍，按揉天柱及项侧压痛点各 30 次，捶击肩井 30 次，按揉肩髃、曲池、手三里、外关、合谷各 30 次，推擦上肢内外各 20 遍，擦捻掌指 5 遍。

【随证取穴】

上肢内侧麻、痛、肌肉萎缩者，加按揉小海、内关、神门、中渚等各 30 次。

椎动脉型颈椎病出现颈性眩晕者，加推桥弓 30 次，按揉印堂、太阳各 30 次，分推前额 30 次，摩中脘顺逆 30 次，按揉足三里、三阴交各 30 次，配合颈部的前后、左右伸展及旋转运动。

For cervical spondylopathy of sympathetic type with occipital pain and stuffiness, dizziness, palpitation and other symptoms, add: pressing-kneading the the back of the head, Pishu (UB 20) and Shenshu (UB 23) 30 times each, rubbing Zhongwan (Ren12) clockwise and counterclockwise 30 times respectively, kneading Qihai (Ren 6) 30 times, and pressing-kneading Zusanli (St 36) and Sanyinjiao (Sp 6) 30 times each.

For cervical spondylopathy of spinal cord type with numbness, soreness and weakness of one side or both sides of the upper or lower extremities, or with paralysis of different degrees, add: pressing-kneading Huantiao (GB 30), Yanglingquan (GB 34) and Chengshan (UB 57) 30 times each, pressing-kneading the thighs 5 times each, grasping the shanks 10 times each, patting the lower limbs 10 times each and scrubbing Yongquan (K 1) 30 times.

Scapulohumeral Periarthritis
PRESCRIPTION
Knead and thump Jianjing (GB 21) 30 times respectively, knead Jianyu (LI 15) and Jianneishu 50 times each, grasp the muscles of the thorax 20 times, and press-knead Quchi (LI 11), Shousanli (LI 10), Waiguan (SJ 5) and Hegu (LI 4) 30 times each. Move the shoulder joint upwards, forwards, backwards and sidewise or move it round in cooperation with the massage.

SYMPTOMATIC POINT SELECTION
At the onset of the disease when there is sevre pain which makes the patient unable to lie down for sleeping, add pressing-kneading Fengchi (GB 20) and Fengmen (UB 12) 30 times each and pushing-scrubbing the painful area until it gets hot.

For treatment of patients having a longer course of illness with apparent shoulder dysfunction and muscular atrophy of the shoulder and arm accompanied with sallow complexion, fear of cold, and mental fatigue and asthenia, add the following manipulations: pressing-kneading Pishu (UB 20) and Shenshu (UB 23) 30 times each, rubbing Zhongwan (Ren 12) clockwise and counterclockwise 30 times respectively, pinching the muscles

交感型颈椎病出现枕项痛沉、头晕心慌等症状者，加按揉脑后、脾俞、肾俞各30次，摩中脘顺逆各30次，揉气海、按揉足三里、三阴交各30次。

脊髓型颈椎病出现上肢或下肢一侧或两侧的麻木、酸软无力或不同程度的瘫痪症状者，加按揉环跳、阳陵泉、承山各30次，按揉大腿5遍，拿小腿10遍，拍击下肢10遍，擦涌泉30次。

肩关节周围炎

【推拿处方】

揉、捶肩井各30次，揉肩髃、肩内俞各50次，拿胸肌20次，按揉曲池、手三里、外关、合谷各30次，配合肩关节的上举、前伸、后背、外展及环转运动锻炼。

【随证取穴】

肩疾初起、疼痛剧甚、夜不能卧者，加按揉风池、风门各30次，推擦肩部痛处以热为度。

病程较久，肩关节功能障碍明显、肩臂肌肉萎缩并面色萎黄、形寒怕冷、神倦乏力者，加按揉脾俞、肾俞各30次，摩中脘顺逆

of the shoulder areas for 50 times each, and pressing-kneading Zusanli (St 36) and Sanyinjiao (Sp 6) 30 times each.

External Humeral Epicondylitis

PRESCRIPTION

Perform massage of the affected side with the hand of the healthy arm. Knead Jianjing (GB 21), Jianyu (LI 15), Quchi (LI 11), Shousanli (LI 10), Waiguan (SJ 5) and Hegu (LI 4) 30 times each, pluck-knead Ashi points at the extra-cubital region for 50 times (pluck the hardened tendon where pain exists left and right), and scrub with the plam the extra-cubital region where pain exists and the redial side of the forearm until they get hot. Stretch and bend the elbows and move the forearm round and round to cooperate with the massage.

Chronic Lumbago

PRESCRIPTION

Press-knead Pishu (UB 20), Shenshu (UB 23), Zhishi (UB 52) and Dachangshu (UB 25) 30 times each. Thump-hit the lumbar region 10 times, scrub Yaoyan (Extra) 30 times, and scrub horizontally the lumbosacral portion till it gets hot. Press-grasp Weizhong (UB 40) and Chengshan. (UB 57) 30 times each. Incline yourself forward, backward, left and right, and rotate your waist to cooperate with the massage.

SYMPTOMATIC POINT SELECTION

For severe lumbago with preference to warmth and aversion to cold which becomes worse in cloudy and rainy days, add pressing-kneading Fengchi (GB 20), Fengmen (UB 12) and Waiguan (SJ 5) 30 times each and grasping Yinlingquan (Sp 9) and Yanglingquan (GB 34) 20 times each.

For lumbago with persistent soreness and weakness of the loins, mental fatigue and cold extremities, add digital pressing on Qihai (Ren 6) and Guanyuan (Ren 4) 30 times each, rubbing Dantian clockwise and counterclockwise 30 times respectively and pressing-kneading Sanyinjiao (Sp 6).

For lumbago with rigidity and soreness of the loins that

30 次，揉捏肩部肌肉萎缩处 50 次，按揉足三里、三阴交 各 30 次。

肱骨外上髁炎

【推拿处方】

用健手按揉患侧肩井、肩髃、曲池、手三里、外关、合谷各 30 次，拨揉肘外阿是穴 50 次（将痛处发硬的筋腱向内、外方向拨动），掌擦肘外痛处及前臂桡侧以热为度，配合肘关节伸屈及前臂旋转运动锻练。

慢性腰痛

【推拿处方】

按揉脾俞、肾俞、志室、大肠俞各 30 次，捶击腰区 10 遍，擦腰眼 30 次，横擦腰骶以热为度，按拿委中、承山各 30 次，配合腰椎前俯、后伸、左右侧屈及旋转等运动锻练。

【随证取穴】

腰痛重着、喜热怕冷、阴雨变天时加重者，加按揉风池、风门、外关各 30 次，拿阴、阳陵泉 20 次。

腰痛酸软无力、缠绵不休、神疲肢冷者，加按点气海、关元各 30 次，摩丹田顺逆各 30 次，按揉三阴交。

腰部僵硬酸痛，不能久坐、有腰椎增生者，加按揉命门、腰

may become unbearable on long-time sitting and with proliferation of the lumbar vertebrae, add pressing-kneading Mingmen (Du 4) , Yaoyangguan (Du 3) and Yanglingquan (GB 34) 30 times each and rubbing Shenque (Ren 8) clockwise and counterclockwise 30 times respectively.

Chronic Prostatitis
PRESCRIPTION

Press-knead Shenshu (UB 23), Mingmen (Du 4) and Yaoyangguan (Du 3) 30 times each, scrub Yaoyan (Extra) 30 times, thump the lumbar region 30 times, strike digitally Guanyuan (Ren 4) and Zhongji (Ren 3) 30 times each, rub Dantian clockwise and counterclockwise 30 times respectively, press-knead Zusanli (St 36), Ququan (Liv 8) and Sanyinjiao (Sp 6) 30 times each and grasp Yinlingquan (Sp 9) and Yanglingquan (GB 34) 20 times each.

SYMPTOMATIC POINT SELECTION

For patients with chronic prostatitis accompanied with soreness and distending pain of the loins, and pain, distention and tenesmus in the perineal, anal and suprapubic regions, add: pressing digitally Huiyin (Ren 1) 30 times, grasping-pinching the medial muscle group 10 times and pressing-kneading Taichong (Liv 3) and Taixi (K 3) 30 times each.

For chronic prostatitis characterized by hesitant, frequent and dripping urination, whitish urine and itching discomfort in the urethra, add: pressing-kneading Pishu (UB 20) 30 times, scrubbing the lower abdomen 30 times, scrubbing horizontally the lumbosacral portion 30 times and pressing-kneading Taixi (K 3) and Kunlun (UB 60) 30 times each.

For chronic prostatitis with dizziness, insomnia, amnesia and asthenia, add: pressing-kneading Fengchi (GB 20), Baihui (Du 20), Touwei (St 8), Pishu (UB 20), Weishu (UB 21), Neiguan (P 6), Shenshu (UB 23) and Taixi (K 3) 30 times each.

For that accompanied with impotency, emission and premature ejaculation, add: pressing-kneading Zhishi (UB 52) 30 tim-

阳关、阳陵泉各 30 次，摩神阙顺逆各 30 次。

慢性前列腺炎

【推拿处方】

按揉肾俞、命门、腰阳关各 30 次，擦腰眼 30 次，捶击腰区 30 次，点击关元、中极各 30 次，摩丹田顺逆各30次，按揉足三里、曲泉、三阴交各 30 次，拿阴、阳陵泉各 20次。

【随证取穴】

伴腰胀疼痛，会阴、肛门、耻骨上区等处疼痛、胀坠不适感者，加按点会阴 30 次，拿捏股内侧肌群 10 遍，按揉太冲、太溪各 30 次。

伴排尿踌躇、尿频数、淋沥、尿白、尿道内刺痒不适者，加按揉脾俞 30 次，擦少腹 30 次，横擦腰骶 30 次，按揉太溪、昆仑各 30 次。

伴头晕、失眠、健忘、乏力者，加按揉风池、百会、头维、脾俞、胃俞、内关、神门、太溪各 30 次。

伴阳痿、遗精、早泄者，加按揉志室 30 次，横擦腰骶 30 次，

es, scrubbing horizontally the lumbosacral portion 30 times and pressing-kneading Taichong (Liv 3) and Taixi (K 3) 30 times each.

Enuresis and Urinary Incontinence

PRESCRIPTION

Press-knead Pishu (UB 20) and Shenshu (UB 23) 30 times each, scrub Yaoyan (Extra) 30 times, scrub horizontally the lumbosacral portion till it gets hot, knead Qihai (Ren 6) and Guanyuan (Ren 4) 30 times each, strike digitally Zhongji (Ren 3) 30 times, rub Dantian clockwise and counterclockwise 30 times respectively, and scrub-knead Hegu (LI 4), Zusanli (St 36) and Sanyinjiao (Sp 6) 30 times each.

SYMPTOMATIC POINT SELECTION

Patients with dripping urination accompanied with dizziness, soreness of the loins and cold extremities should be treated by adding: Pressing-kneading Mingmen (Du 4) and Zhishi (UB 52) 30 times each and kneading Baihui (Du 20), Fengchi (GB 20), Quchi (LI 11) and Taixi (K 3) 30 times each.

Patients with sallow complexion, mental fatigue and weakness, poor appetite and loose stool should be treated by adding: Pressing-kneading Weishu (UB 21) 30 times, rubbing Zhongwan (Ren 12) clockwise and counterclockwise 30 times respectively, scrubbing the lowe abdomen 30 times and pressing-kneading Changqiang (Du 1) and Neiguan (P 6) 30 times each.

Seminal Emission

PRESCRIPTION

Press-knead Pishu (UB 20) and Shenshu (UB 23) 30 times each, scrub Yaoyan (Extra) 30 times, knead Qihai (Ren 6) 30 times, strike digitally Guanyuan (Ren 4) 30 times, rub Dantian and Zhongwan (Ren 12) clockwise and counterclockwise respectively for 30 times each, and press-knead Sanyinjiao (Sp 6) and Taixi (K 3) 30 times each.

SYMPTOMATIC POINT SELECTION

Seminal emission characterized by insomnia, oneirogmus and listlessness should be treated by adding the following:

按揉太冲、太溪各 30 次。

遗尿及尿失禁

【推拿处方】

按揉脾俞、肾俞各 30 次，擦腰眼 30 次，横擦腰骶 以 热为度，揉气海、关元各 30 次，点击中极 30 次，摩丹田顺逆各 30 次，按揉合谷、足三里、三阴交各 30 次。

【随证取穴】

小便滴沥不禁，并伴头晕腰疼、四肢清泠者，加按揉 命 门、志室各 30 次，揉百会、风池、曲池、太溪各 30 次。

面色萎黄、神疲无力、食欲不振、便稀溏者，加按揉胃 俞 30 次，摩中脘顺逆各 30 次，擦少腹 30 次，按揉长强、内关各 30 次。

遗精

【推拿处方】

按揉脾俞、肾俞各 30 次，按腰眼 30 次，揉气海 30 次，点击关元 30 次，摩丹田、中脘顺逆各 30 次，按揉三阴 交、太溪各 30 次。

【随证取穴】

失眠、梦遗、精神萎靡者，加揉百会、风池各 30 次，按 揉 神

kneading Baihui (Du 20) and Fengchi (GB 20) 30 times each and pressing-kneading Shenmen (H 7) and Neiguan (P 6) 30 times each.

Frequent seminal emission or even seminal discharge along with urination accompanied by irritability and insomnia should be treated by adding the following: pressing-kneading Weishu (UB 21) and Xinshu (UB 15) 30 times each, rubbing Gaohuang (UB 43) 30 times, and pressing-kneading Zusanli (St 36) and Ququan (Liv 8) 30 times each.

Seminal emission accompanied by dizziness, tinnitus, soreness of the loins, dim complexion, aversion to cold and cold extremities should be treated by adding: thumping the lumbar region 30 times, scrubbing horizontally the lumbosacral portion 30 times, scrubbing Dazhui (Du 14) 30 times, pressing-kneading Fengchi (GB 20) and Feishu (UB 13) 30 times each and grasping Yinlingquan (Sp 9) and Yanglingquan (GB 34) 30 times each.

Impotency

PRESCRIPTION

Press-knead Shenshu (UB 23) and Zhishi (UB 52) 30 times each, scrub Yaoyen (Extra) 30 times, knead Qihai (Ren 6) and Guanyuan (Ren 4) 30 times each, strike digitally Zhongji (Ren 3) and Qugu (Ren 2) 30 times each, rub Dantian clockwise and counterclockwise for 30 times respectively, and press-knead Sanyinjiao (Sp 6) and Taixi (K 3) 30 times each.

SYMPTOMATIC POINT SELECTION

For impotency accompanied with irritability, restlessness in sleep at night, mental fatigue, sallow complexion and poor appetite, add: kneading Pishu (UB 21) and Weishu (UB 21) 30 times each, rubbing Zhongwan (Ren 12) clockwise and counterclockwise for 30 times respectively and pressing-kneading Zusanli (St 36) 30 times.

For impotency accompanied with dizziness, pale complexion, mental fatigue and soreness and weakness of tne lions and kness, add: kneading Mingmen (Du 4) and Feishu (UB 13) 30 times

门、内关各 30 次。

遗精频作甚或随溺外流、心烦失眠者，加按揉胃俞、心俞 30 次，摩膏盲 30 次，按揉足三里、曲泉各 30 次。

伴头晕目眩、耳鸣腰酸、面色少华、畏寒肢冷者，加捶击腰区 30 次，横擦腰骶 30 次，擦大椎 30 次，按揉风池、肺俞各 30 次，拿按阴、阳陵泉各 30 次。

阳痿

【推拿处方】

按揉肾俞、志室各 30 次，擦腰眼 30 次，揉气海、关元各 30 次，点击中极、曲骨各 30 次，摩丹田顺各逆 30 次，按揉三阴交、太溪各 30 次。

【随证取穴】

阳痿伴心烦、夜寐不安、神疲、面色萎黄、纳差者，加按揉脾俞、胃俞各 30 次，摩中脘顺逆各 30 次，按揉足三里 30 次。

阳痿伴头晕目眩、面色㿠白、神疲腰腿酸软者，加揉命门、肺

each, scrubbing horizontally the lumbosacral portion till it turns hot, and pressing-kneading Baihui (Du 20), Taiyang (Extra 2) and Neiguan (P 6) 30 times each.

Dysmenorrhea

PRESCRIPTION

Press-knead Shenshu (UB 23) 30 times, thump the lumbar region 30 times, scrub Yaoyan (Extra) 30 times, press-knead Qihai (Ren 6) and Guanyuan (Ren 4) 30 times each, scrub the lower abdomen 30 times, rub Dantian 30 times and press-grasp Hegu (LI 4), press-knead Zusanli (St 36) and Sanyinjiao (Sp 6) 30 times each.

SYMPTOMATIC POINT SELECTION

For distending pain in the lower abdomen prior to or during menstruation, aversion to pressure, scanty, impeded menstrual blood drak purple in colour and with clots accompanied by distending pain in the breast, add: kneading Tanzhong (Ren 17) 30 times, scrubbing the prothorax 20 times, pressing-kneading Ganshu (UB 18), Zhangmen (Liv 13), Xuehai (Sp 10) and Taichong (Liv 3) 30 times each.

For coldness and pain in the lower abdomen prior to or during menstruation which can be relieved by warming, scanty menstrual blood dark-red in colour and cold extremities, add: scrubbing Dazhui (Du 14) 30 times, rubbing Zhongwan (Ren 12) 30 times, scrubbing horizontally the lumbosacral portion till it turns hot, striking digitally Guanyuan (Ren 4) 30 times and pressing-kneading Xuehai (Sp 10) 30 times.

For continuous vague pain in the lower abdomen during or after menstruation with preference to pressure, scanty menstrual blood which looks clear and light in colour, mental fatigue, weakness and pale complexion, add: pressing-kneading Zhishi (UB 52) and Zhangmen (Liv 13) 30 times each, rubbing Zhongwan (Ren 12) clockwise and counterclockwise 30 times respectively, scrubbing horizontally the lumbosacral portion 30 times and pressing-kneading Taixi (K 3) and Taichong (Liv 3) 30 times ecah.

俞各 30 次，横擦腰骶以热为度，按揉百会、太阳、内关各 30 次。

痛经

【推拿处方】

按揉肾俞 30 次，捶击腰区 30 次，擦腰眼 30 次，按揉气海、关元各 30 次，擦少腹 30 次，摩丹田 30 次，按拿合谷、按揉足三里、三阴交各 30 次。

【随证取穴】

经前或经期小腹胀痛、拒按，经量少而不畅，色紫暗有血块，且乳房胀痛者，加揉膻中 30 次，擦前胸 30 次，按揉肝俞、章门、血海、太冲各 30 次。

经前或经期少腹冷痛，得热则减，经量少，色暗红，手足不温者，加擦大椎 30 次，摩中脘 30 次，横擦腰骶以热为度，点击关元 30 次，按揉血海 30 次。

经期或经后少腹绵绵作痛、喜按，经量少、色淡质清，神倦无力，面色苍白者，加按揉志室、章门各 30 次，摩中脘顺逆各 30 次，横擦腰骶 30 次，按揉太溪、太冲各 30 次。

Optic Atrophy
PRESCRIPTION
Press-knead Zanzhu, (UB 2) Jingming (UB 1), Chengqi (St 1) and Tongziliao (GB 1) 30 times each. Scrape the upper and lower parts of the eye orbits for 30 times respectively, "iron" the eyes for 30 seconds, press-knead Fengchi (GB 20) and Taiyang (Extra 2) 30 times each, press-grasp Hegu (LI 4) 30 times and press-knead Guangming (GB 37) and Taichong (Liv 3) 30 times each.

SYMPTOMATIC POINT SELECTION
Optic atrophy accompanied with dizziness, dryness and discomfort of the eyes, tinnitus, dry throat, dysphoria with feverish sensation in the chest, palms and soles, and soreness and weakness of the loins and knees should be treated by adding: pressing-kneading Shenshu (UB 23), Ganshu (UB 18) and Sanyinjiao (Sp 6) 30 times each, and kneading Taixi (K 3) and Yongquan (K 1) 30 times each.

That accompanied with palpitation and shortness of breath, sallow complexion, dizziness and asthenia should be treated by adding: pressing-kneading Xinshu (UB 15) and Pishu (UB 20) 30 times each, rubbing Zhongwan (Ren 12) clockwise and counterclockwise 30 times respectively, rubbing Dantian 30 times and pressing-kneading Zusanli (St 36) 30 times.

Tinnitus and Deafness
PRESCRIPTION
Press-knead Baihui (Du 20) 30 times, knead Fengchi (GB 20), Yifeng (SJ 17) and Tinggong (SI 19) 30 times each, scrub the preauricular area 30 times, Ming Tiangu 30 times, knead Shenshu (UB 23) 30 times, scrub Yaoyan (Extra) 30 times and press-knead Hegu (LI 4) and Taixi (K 3) 30 times each.

SYMPTOMATIC POINT SELECTION
Tinnitus that worsens due to emotional depression or anger accompanied with headache, vertigo, vexation and irritability,

视神经萎缩

【推拿处方】

按揉攒竹、睛明、承泣、瞳子髎各 30 次，刮眼轮上下各 30 次，熨眼 30 秒钟，按揉风池、太阳各 30 次，按拿合谷 30 次，按揉光明、太冲各 30 次。

【随证取穴】

伴头晕目眩、眼内干涩、耳鸣咽干、五心烦热、腰膝酸软者，加按揉肾俞、肝俞、三阴交各 30 次，揉太溪、涌泉各 30 次。

伴心悸气短、面色萎黄、头昏倦怠者，加按揉心俞、脾俞各 30 次，摩中脘顺逆各 30 次，摩丹田 30 次，按揉足三里 30 次。

耳鸣　耳聋

【推拿处方】

按揉百会 30 次，揉风池、翳风、听宫各 30 次，擦耳前 30 次，擦腰眼 30 次，按揉合谷、太溪各 30 次。

【随证取穴】

耳鸣于郁怒后加重，并伴头痛眩晕、心烦易怒、咽干口苦、

dry throat and bitterness in the mouth and constipation should be treated by adding: pushing the forehead on either side 30 times, scrubbing the lower abdomen 30 times, pressing-kneading Fengfu (Du 16) and Ganshu (UB 18) 30 times each, grasping Neiguan (P 6) and Waiguan (SJ 5) of both sides 20 times each, and pressing-kneading Taichong (Liv 3) and Qiuxu (GB 40) 30 times each.

To treat tinnitus that is as loud as the singing of a cicada and sometimes so serious as if the sufferer became deaf, accompanied with dizziness and carebaria, stuffiness in the chest and abundant sputum, add: thumping Jianjing (GB 21) 30 times, kneading Feishu (UB 13) and Tanzhong (Ren 17) 30 times each, scrubbing the prothorax 30 times and pushing the forehead 30 times on either side.

To treat tinnitus accompanied with vertigo, pain in the loins and seminal emission, add: pushing the forehead on either side 30 times, kneading Zhishi (UB 52) and Mingmen (Du 4) 30 times each and scrubbing horizontally the lumbosacral portion 30 times.

To treat tinnitus with poor appetite, mental fatigue and shortness of breath, add: pushing the forehead on either side 30 times, rubbing Zhongwan (Ren 12) 30 times and pressing-kneading Pishu (UB 20) and Weishu (UB 21) 30 times.

Chronic Rhinitis

PRESCRIPTION

Press-knead Baihui (Du 20), Shangxing (Du 23) and Yintang (Extra 2) 30 times each, press-knead Yingxiang (LI 20) 50 times, scrub along the sides of the nose for 30 times, press-knead Fengchi (GB 20) 30 times, rub the hands to bathe the face 50 times, grasp-knead Hegu (LI 4) 30 times and nip-knead Shaoshang (Lu 11) 20 times.

SYMPTOMATIC POINT SELECTION

For intermittent nasal obstruction, white, mucous nasal discharge, cough with phlegm and cold extemities which may be aggravated by wind-cold pathogen, add: pressing-kneading

大便干燥者,加分推前额 30 次, 擦少腹 30 次,按揉风府、肝俞各 30 次, 对拿内关、外关各 20 次, 按揉太冲、丘墟各 30 次。

耳鸣如蝉声, 有时闭塞如聋, 兼头昏重、胸闷痰多者, 加捶击肩井 30 次, 揉肺俞、膻中各 30 次, 擦前胸 30 次, 分推前额 30 次。

耳鸣兼头晕目眩、腰痛遗精者, 加分推前额30次, 揉志室、命门各30次, 横擦腰骶30次。

耳鸣兼纳少、神倦、气短者, 加分推前额 30 次, 摩中脘 30 次, 按揉脾俞、胃俞各 30 次。

慢性鼻炎

【推拿处方】

按揉百会、上星、印堂各 30 次, 按揉迎香 50 次,擦鼻旁 30 次, 按揉风池 30 次, 搓手浴面 30 遍, 拿揉合谷 30 次, 掐揉少商 20 次。

【随证取穴】

鼻塞时轻时重、流涕白粘、咳嗽有痰、形寒肢冷、遇风寒加重

Feishu (UB 13) 30 times, kneading Tanzhong (Ren 17) 30 times, pressing-kneading Taiyang (Extra 2) 30 times and rubbing Gaohuang and Dantian 30 times each.

For severe nasal obstruction with white, mucous or yellow, thick discharge relatively abundant in amount and hyposmia accompanied by poor appetite, mental fatigue, sallow complexion, asthenia and loose stool, add: pressing-kneading Pishu (UB 20) and Weishu (UB 21) 30 times each, rubbing Zhongwan (Ren 12) 30 times, kneading Qihai (Ren 6) 30 times and pressing-kneading Zusanli (St 36) and Sanyinjiao (Sp 6) 30 times each.

Rhinallergosis (Allergic Rhinitis)
PRESSRIPTION

Press-knead Fengchi (GB 20), Fengmen (UB 12), Taiyang (Extra 2) and Yintang (Extra 1) 30 times each, part-push the forehead 30 times, rub the hands to "bathe" the face 30 times, press-knead Yingxiang (LI 20) 50 times, scrub along the sides of the nose 30 times, pat the upper part of the back 30 times, knead Tanzhong (Ren 17) 30 times, scrub Dazhui (Du 14) 30 times and press-knead Hegu (LI 4) 30 times.

SYMPTOMATIC POINT SELECTION

Rhinallergosis accompanied with sallow complexion, poor appetite and abdominal distention, mental fatigue, weakness of the extremities and loose stool should be treated by adding: pressing-kneading Pishu (UB 20) and Weishu (UB 21) 30 times each, rubbing Zhongwan (Ren 12) and Dantian 30 times each and pressing-kneading Zusanli (St 36), Chengshan (UB 57) and Sanyinjiao (Sp 6) 30 times each.

That accompanied with dizziness, tinnitus, soreness and weakness of the loins and extremities, fear of cold, seminal emission and frequency of micturition should be treated by adding: pressing-kneading Shenshu (UB 23) and Zhishi (UB 52) 30 times each, scrubbing Yaoyan (Extra) 30 times, striking digitally Guanyuan (Ren 4) and Zhongji (Ren 3) 30 times each, rubbing Dantian 30 times and pressing-kneading Sanyinjiao (Sp 6)

者，加按揉肺俞 30 次，揉膻中 30 次，按揉太阳 30 次，摩膏肓、丹田各 30 次。

鼻塞重、涕白粘或黄稠、量较多、嗅觉减退、兼食少神疲、面色萎黄、倦怠便溏者，加按揉脾俞、胃俞各 30 次，摩中脘 30 次，揉气海 30 次，按揉足三里、三阴交各 30 次。

过敏性鼻炎

【推拿处方】

按揉风池、风门、太阳、印堂各 30 次，分推前额 30 次，搓手浴面 30 次，按揉迎香 50 次，擦鼻旁 30 次，揉肺俞 30 次，拍上背 30 次，揉膻中 30 次，擦大椎 30 次，按揉合谷 30 次。

【随证取穴】

兼面色萎黄、食少腹胀、神疲肢软、大便溏薄者，加按揉脾俞、胃俞各 30 次，摩中脘、丹田各 30 次，按揉足三里、承山、三阴交各 30 次。

兼头晕耳鸣、腰肢酸软、形寒怕冷、遗精尿频者，加：按揉肾俞、志室各 30 次，擦腰眼 30 次，点击关元、中极各 30 次，摩丹田 30 次，按揉三阴交、太溪各 30 次。

and Taixi (K 3) 30 times each.

Toothache

PRESCRIPTION

Press-knead Fengchi (GB 20) and Yifeng (SJ 17), Taiyang (Extra 2) 30 times each, press-knead Xiaguan (St 7) and Jiache (St 6) at the affected side 50 times each and nip-grasp Hegu (LI 4) 30 times.

SYMPTOMATIC POINT SELECTION

For toothache accompanied with fever, aversion to cold and thirst, add: pressing-kneading Feishu (UB 13) and Fengmen (UB 12) 30 times each, patting the upper part of the back 30 times, thumping Jianjing (GB 21) 30 times and pressing-kneading Dazhui (Du 14) and Quchi (LI 11) 30 times each.

For toothache accompanied with headache, halitosis and constipation, add: pressing-kneading Weishu (UB 21) and Pishu (UB 20) 30 times each, rubbing Zhongwan (Ren 12) 30 times, pressing-kneading Tianshu (St 25) 30 times, kneading the lower abdomen counterclockwise 30 times and pressing-kneading Zusanli (St 36), Neiting (St 44) and Chengshan (UB 57) 30 times each.

Toothache accompanied with soreness and weakness of the loins and knees, dizziness and tinnitus, add: pressing-kneading Shenshu (UB 23) and Zhishi (UB 52) 30 times each, rubbing Dantian clockwise and counterclockwise 30 times respectively and pressing-kneading Sanyinjiao (Sp 6) 40 times.

牙痛

【推拿处方】

按揉风池、翳风、太阳各 30 次，按揉患侧下关、颊车各 50 次，掐、拿合谷 30 次。

【随证取穴】

兼有发热、恶寒、口渴者，加按揉肺俞、风门各 30 次，拍击上背 30 次，捶击肩井 30 次，按揉大椎、曲池各 30 次。

兼有头痛、口臭、大便秘结者，加按揉胃俞、脾俞各 30 次，摩中脘 30 次，按揉天枢 30 次，向左揉少腹 30 次，按揉足三里、内庭、承山各 30 次。

兼腰酸膝软、头晕耳鸣者，加按揉肾俞、志室各 30 次，丹摩田顺逆 30 次，按揉三阴交各 30 次。

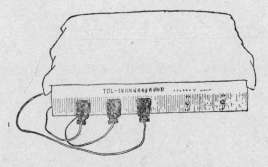

Fig. 1—1 Dynamic Ergograph Model TDL-I for Massage Manipulation

图1-1　　TDL-1型推拿手法动态力测定器

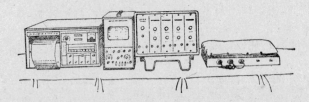

Fig. 1—2 Mechanical Information Test System of Massage Manipulation

图1-2　　推拿手法力学信息测录系统

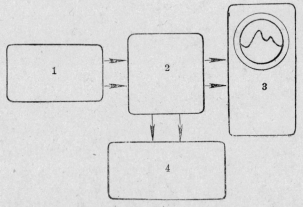

Fig. 1—3 Working Principle Diagram of Manipulation-test System

图1-3　　手法测录系统工作原理框图

1. Dynamic Ergograph Model TDL-I
   TDL-1型手法动态力测定器
2. Dynamic Resistance Responding Strainometer
   动态电阻应变仪
3. Long Afterglow Wave-indicator
   长余辉示波器
4. Light Recording Wave-indicator
   光线记录示波器

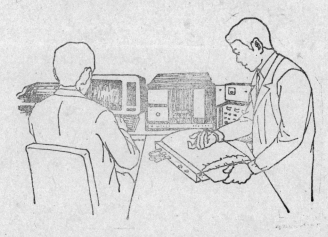

Fig. 1—4 The System of Computer-handled Mechanical Information of
          Massage Manipulation
图1-4   推拿手法力学信息计算机处理系统

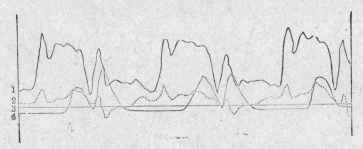

Fig. 1—5 Three-dimensional Co-axial Curve Diagram of Ding Jifeng's Rolling
          Manipulation
图1-5   丁季峰㨰法三维同轴曲线图

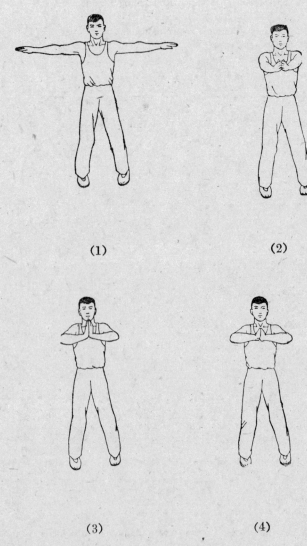

(1)

(2)

(3)

(4)

Fig. 1—6 Wei Tuo's Posture of Presenting the Pestle

图1-6　　韦驮献杵势

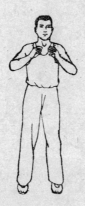

Fig. 1—7 Wei Tuo's Posture of Presenting the Pestle (Ball-holding Posture)

图1-7　　韦驮献杵势(抱球势)

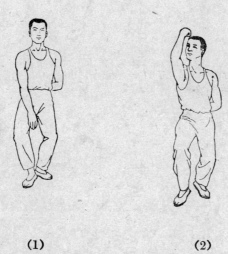

(1)   (2)

Fig. 1—8 The Posture of Plucking and Resetting the Stars

图1-8　　摘星换斗势

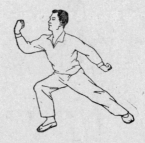

Fig. 1—9 The Posture of Pulling Nine Oxen by the Tails

图1-9　　倒拽九牛尾势

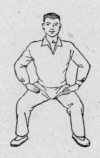

Fig. 1—10 The Posture of Three Dishes Falling to the Ground

图1-10　　三盘落地势

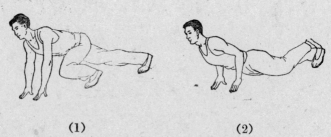

(1)　　　　　　　　　(2)

Fig. 1—11 The Posture of the Prone Tiger Pouncing on Its Prey

图1-11　　卧虎扑食势

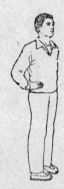

Fig. 1—12 The Posture of the Up-right Standing

图1-12　　站裆势

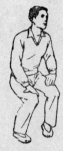

Fig. 1—13 The Horse-riding Stance

图1-13　　马步式

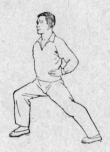

Fig. 1—14 The Posture of the Forward Lunge

图1-14　　弓步势

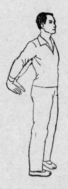

Fig. 1—15 Stretching the Arms and Supporting the Palms
图1-15　　伸臂撑掌

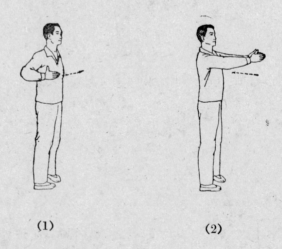

(1)　　　　　　　　　　(2)

Fig. 1—16 Pushing Eight Horses Forward
图1-16　　前推八匹马

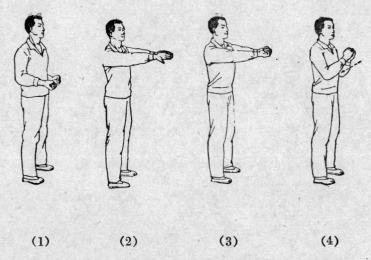

(1)   (2)   (3)   (4)

Fig. 1—17 Pulling Nine Oxen Backward

图1-17   倒拉九头牛

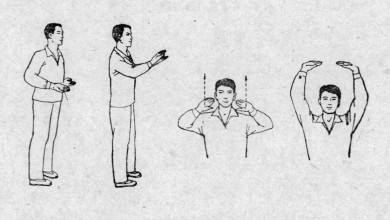

(1)   (2)   (3)   (4)

Fig. 1—18 The Overlord Holding-up the Tripod

图1-18   霸王举鼎

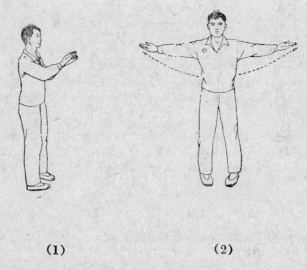

(1)   (2)

Fig. 1—19 The Wind Swaying the Lotus Leaf
图1-19   风摆荷叶

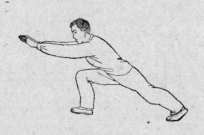

Fig. 1—20 The Entry of the Black Dragon into the Cave
图1-20   乌龙钻洞

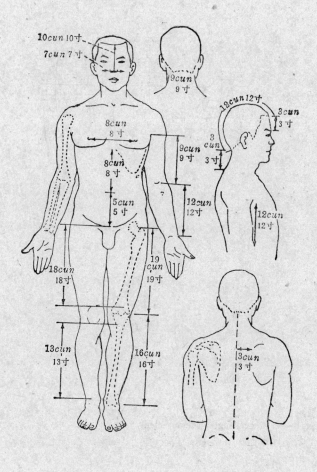

Fig. 1—21 Bone-length Measurement

图1-21　　骨度分寸法

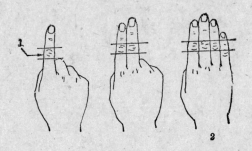

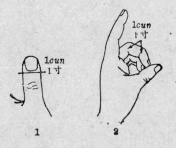

Fig. 1—22 Finger-length Measurement

图1-22 指寸法

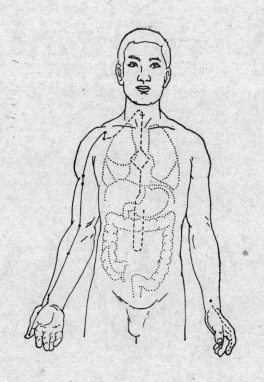

Fig. 1—23 The Lung Channel of Hand-*Taiyin*

图1-23   手太阴肺经

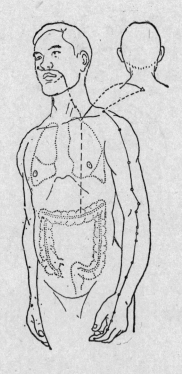

Fig. 1—24 The Large Intestine Channel of Hand-*Yangming*

图1-24　　手阳明大肠经

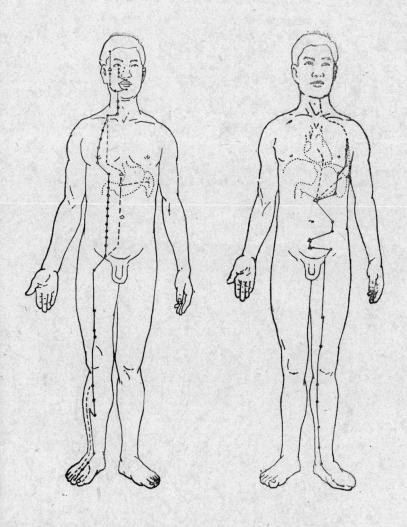

Fig. 1—25 The Stomach Channel of
Foot-*Yangming*

图1-25　足阳明胃经

Fig. 1—26 The Spleen Channel of
Foot-*Taiyin*

图1-26　足太阴脾经

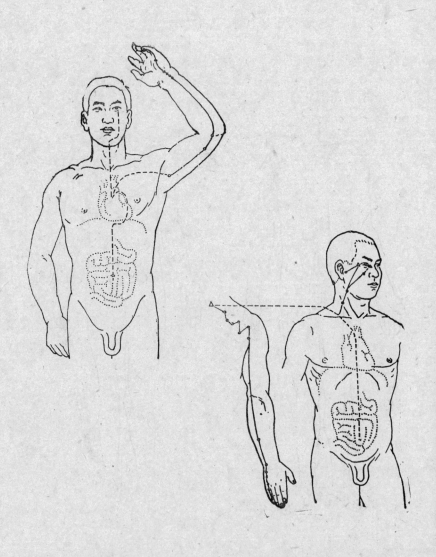

Fig. 1—27 The Heart Channel of
         Hand-*Shaoyin*

图1-27   手少阴心经

Fig. 1—28 The Small Intestine
         Channel of Hand-*Taiyang*

图1-28   手太阳小肠经

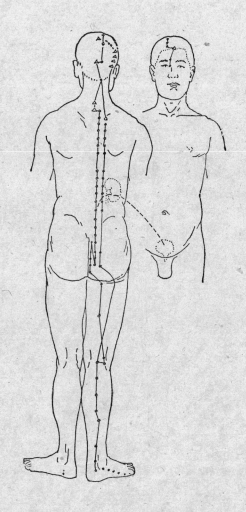

Fig. 1—29 The Urinary Bladder Channel of Foot-*Taiyang*

图1-29　足太阳膀胱经

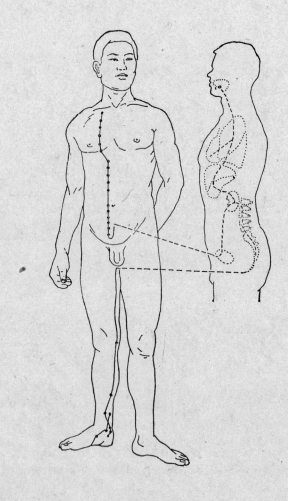

Fig. 1—30 The Kidney Channel of Foot-*Shaoyin*

图1-30　　足少阴肾经

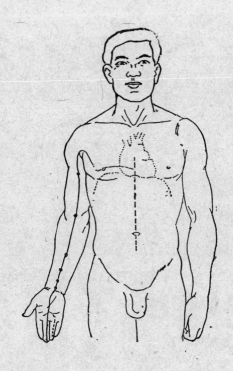

Fig. 1—31 The Pericardium Channel of Hand-*Jueyin*

图1-31　手厥阴心包经

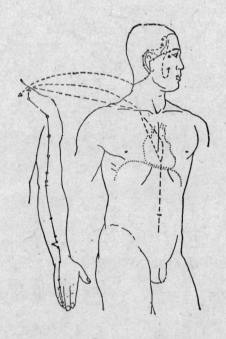

Fig. 1—32 The *Sanjiao* Channel of Hand-*Shaoyang*
图1-32　　手少阳三焦经

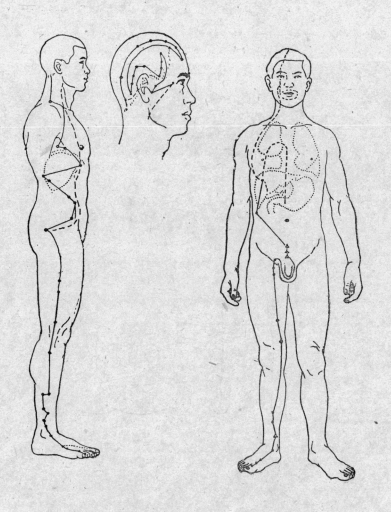

Fig. 1—33 The Gallbladder Channel of Foot-*Shaoyang*

图1-33　足少阳胆经

Fig. 1—34 The Liver Channel of Foot-*Jueyin*

图1-34　足厥阴肝经

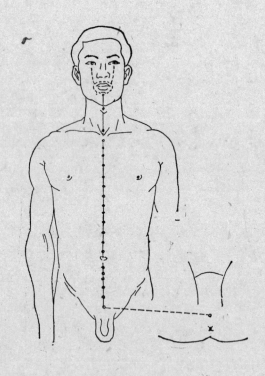

Fig. 1—35 The *Ren* Channel

图1-35 任脉

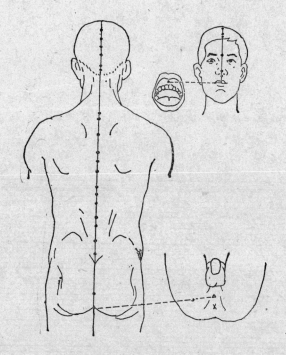

Fig. 1—36 The *Du* Channel
图1-36　　督脉

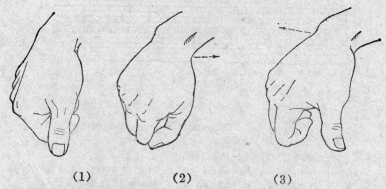

(1)　　　　　　(2)　　　　　　(3)

Fig. 2—1 Pushing Manipulation with One-finger Meditation
图2-1　　一指禅推法

(1) Preparatory Posture 预备姿势
(2) Inside Swinging 内摆
(3) Outside Swinging 外摆

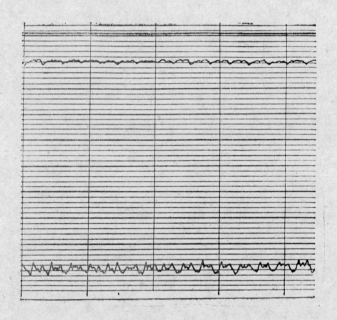

Fig. 2—2 Dynamic Curve Diagram of Pushing Manipulation with One-finger Meditation by Zhu Chunting

图2-2　　朱春霆一指禅推法动态曲线图

period: 0.31 second　　　　　周期：0.31秒
frequency: 193 times/m　　　频率：193次/分
vertical intensity: 1 kg　　　垂直强度：1公斤
upward angle; about 75　　　上升角：75°左右

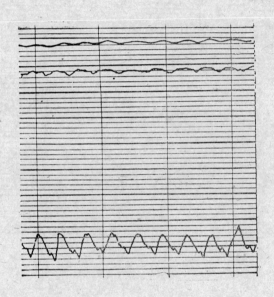

Fig. 2—3 Dynamic Curve Diagram of Pushing Manipulation with
One-finger Meditation by Wang Jisong

图2-3 王纪松一指禅推法动态曲线图

period: 0.37 second   周期：0.37秒

frequency: 160 times/m   频率：160次/分

vertical intensity: 3 kg   垂直强度：3公斤

up ward angle: about 70   上升角：70°左右

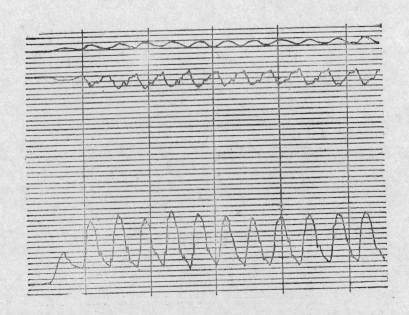

Fig. 2—4 Dynamic Curve Diagram of Whorl-pushing Manipulation by
Wang Baichuan

图2-4　　王百川式罗纹推动态曲线图

period: 0.42 second	周期：0.42秒
frequency: 150 times/m	频率：150次/分
vertical intensity: 4 kg	垂直强度：4公斤
upward angle: 83°	上升角：83°

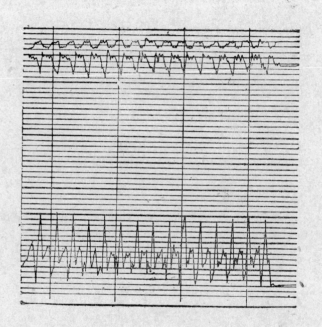

Fig. 2—5 Dynamic Curve Diagram of Vibrating-pushing Manipulation
by Qian Fuqing

图2-5　钱福卿式镟推法动态曲线图

period: 0.24 second　　　　周期：0.24秒
frequency: 255 times/m　　频率：255次/分
vertical intensity: 4 kg　　垂直强度：4公斤
upward angle: 85°　　　　上升角：85°

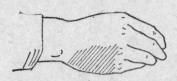

(1) Treating Regions of Rolling
    Manipulation
    滚法的着力部位

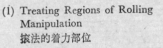

(2) Outward Swinging — Flexing the
    Wrist Joint and Rotating the
    Forearm Backward
    外摆——屈腕和前臂旋后

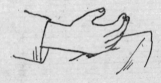

(3) Inward Swinging — Extending the Wrist Joint and Rotating the
    Forearm Forward
    内摆——伸腕和前臂旋前

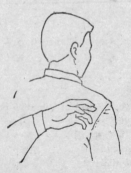

(4) Rolling Manipulation with One Hand at the Shoulders and the Back
    肩背部单手滚法

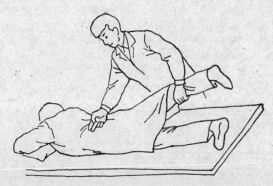

(5) Rolling Manipulation of Lifting the Leg and Extending the Lumbar
Vertebra Backward

抬腿、后伸腰椎之滚法操作

Fig. 2—6 Rolling Manipulations

图2-6　滚法

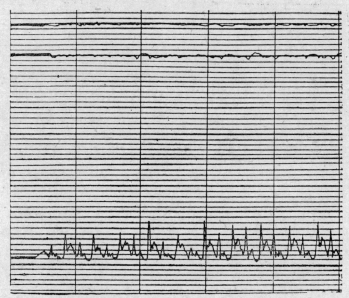

Fig. 2—7 Dynamic Curve Diagram of Light-Type Rolling Manipulation
by Ding Jifeng

图2-7　丁季峰轻型滚法动态曲线图

period: 0.41 second   周期：0.41秒

frequency: 146 times/m   频率：146次/分

vertical intensity: 3 kg   垂直强度： 3公斤

upward angle: 87°   上升角：87°

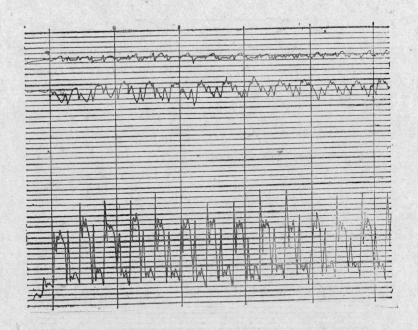

Fig. 2—8 Dynamic Curve Diagram of Medium-Type Rolling Manipulation by Ding Jifeng

图2-8　丁季峰中型㨰法动态曲线图

period: 0.41 second   周期：0.41秒

frequency: 146 times/m   频率：146次/分

vertical intensity: 6 kg   垂直强度： 6公斤

vertical upward angle: 87°   垂向上升角：87°

longitudinal forward

    impulsive force: a little less than 1 kg   纵向前冲力： 1公斤稍弱

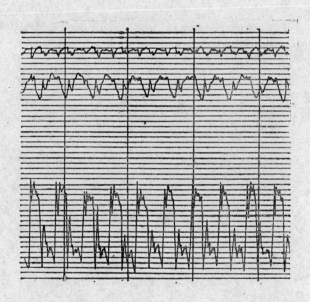

Fig. 2—9 Dynamic Curve Diagram of Heavy-Type Rolling Manipulation
  by Ding Jifeng

图2-9   丁季峰重型𰀀法动态曲线图
  period: 0.41 second
  frequency: 146 times/m
  vertical intensity: 6.6 kg
  vertical upward angle: 87°
  longitudinal forward
    impulsive force: 1 kg

周期：0.41秒
频率：146次/分
垂直强度：6.6公斤
垂向上升角：87°

纵向前冲力：1公斤

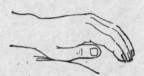 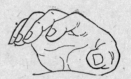

(1) Kneading Manipulation with the Major Thenar
大鱼际揉法

(2) Kneading Manipulation with the Palm Root
掌根揉法

Fig. 2—10 Kneading Manipulations
图2-10　揉法

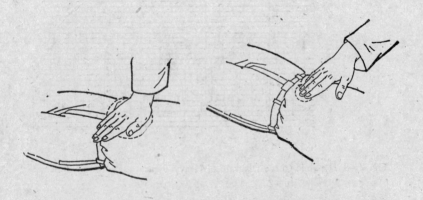

(1) Rubbing Manipulation with the Palm
掌摩法

(2) Rubbing Manipulation with Fingers
指摩法

Fig. 2—11 Rubbing Manipulations
图2-11　摩法

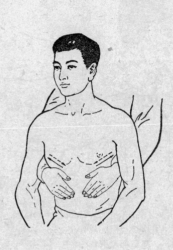

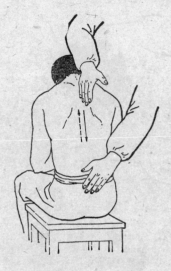

(1) Scrubbing Manipulation with the Palm
掌擦法

(2) Scrubbing Manipulation with the Minor Thenar
小鱼际擦法

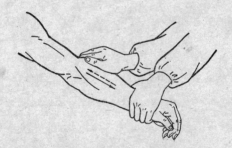

(3) Scrubbing Manipulation with the Major Thenar
大鱼际擦法
Fig. 2—12 Scrubbing Manipulations
图2-12　擦法

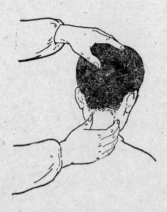 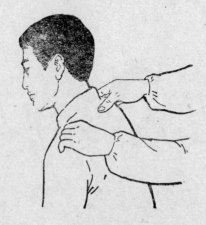

(1) Grasping Neck with One-hand

项部单手拿法

(2) Grasping the Shoulder and Back with Both-hand

肩背部双手拿法

Fig. 2—13 Grasping Manipulations

图2-13 拿法

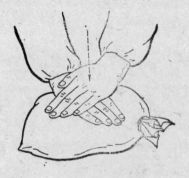 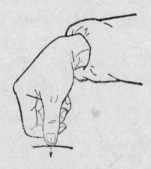

(1) Pressing Manipulation with Both Palms Overlapped

双掌叠按法

(2) Finger-pressing Manipulation

指按法

Fig. 2—14 Pressing Manipulations

图2-14 按法

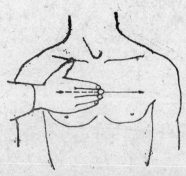

Fig. 2—15 Flat-pushing Manipulation
图2-15   平推法

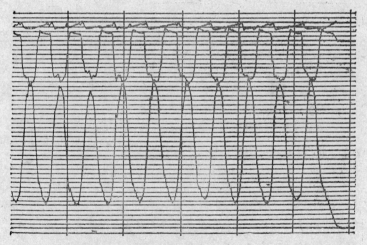

Fig. 2—16 Dynamic Curve Diagram of Flat-pushing (heavy type) by Li Xijiu

图2-16   李锡九平推法动态曲线图(重型)

period: 0.58 second — 周期: 0.58秒

frequency: 104 times/m — 频率: 104次/分

vertical intensity: 10.6 kg — 垂直强度: 10.6 kg

upward angle: 80° — 上升角: 80°

longitudinal forward-pushing force: 3 kg — 向前推力: 3 kg

backward pushing force: 0.66 kg — 纵回推力: 0.66 kg

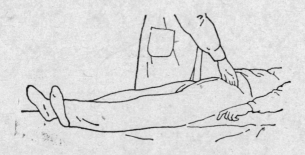

(1) Pressing Manipulation with the Middle Finger
中指点法

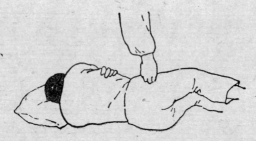

(2) Pressing Manipulation with Interphalangeal Joints of the Middle Finger
中指中节点法

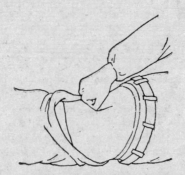

(3) Pressing Manipulation with the Flexed Thumb
屈拇指点法

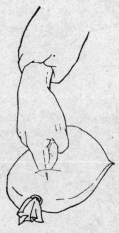

(4) Pressing Manipulation with the Flexed Index Finger
屈食指点法

Fig. 2—17 Digital-pressing Manipulations
图2-17　　按点法

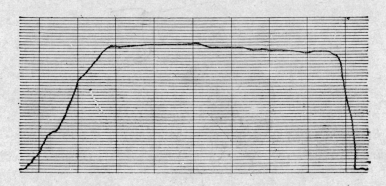

Fig. 2—18 Dynamic Curve Diagram of Digital-pressing Manipulation by Li Xijiu

图2-18　　李锡九按点法动态曲线图

period: 8 seconds　　　　　周期：8 秒

vertical intensity: 12 kg　　垂直强度：12 kg

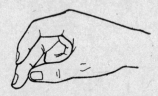

(1) Hand Posture of Striking with the Middle Finger
中指点手式

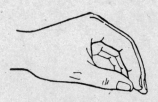

(2) Hand Posture of Striking with the Three Fingers
三指点手式

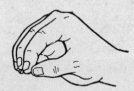

(3) Hand Posture of Striking with the Five Fingers
五指点手式

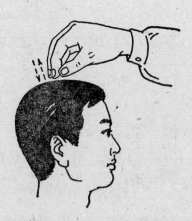

(4) Striking at Point Baihui with the Five Fingers
五指击点百会穴

Fig. 2—19 Digital-striking Manipulations

图2-19　　击点法

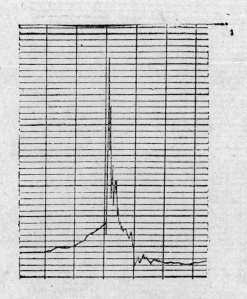

(1) Dynamic Curve Diagram of Single-digital Striking Manipulation
(heavy type)
单点法(重型)动态曲线图
intensity: 60kg (dynamic resistance responding meter reduces 100
paper speed: 100mm/second, 0.1 second for each square)
强度·60kg(动态——电阻应变仪表减100，走纸速度：100mm/秒,每格0.1秒)

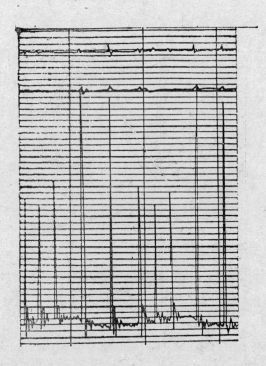

(2) Dynamic Curve Diagram of Rhythem-digital Striking (light type)
　　　节律点法(轻型)动态曲线图
　　　　rhythem: three weak digital strikings
　　　　　and two forceful ones make one rhythem
　　　　intensity of weak striking: 7kg
　　　　intensity of forceful striking: 12.6 kg
　　　　rhythem period: 1.54 seconds

节律：3次虚点，二次实点
　　　为一节律
虚点强度：7 kg
实点强度：12.6 kg
节律周期：1.54秒

Fig. 2—20 Dynamic Curve Diagram of Digital-striking by Jia Lihui
图2-20　　　贾立惠击点法动态曲线图

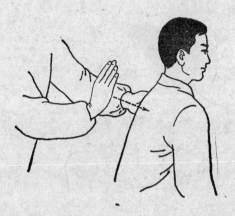

(1) Patting Manipulation with a Single Palm
单掌拍法

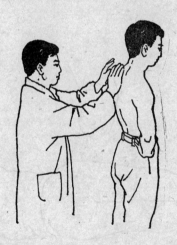

(2) Patting Manipulation with Both Palms
双掌拍法

Fig. 2—21 Patting Manipulations

图2-21   拍法

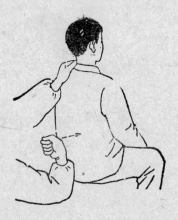

(1) Hitting Manipulation with the Fist Back
拳背击法

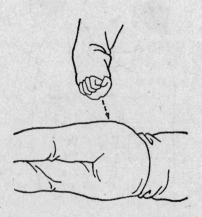

(2) Tapping Manipulation with the Palm Root
掌根击法

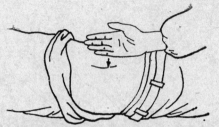

(3) Hitting Manipulation with the Minor Thenar
小鱼际击法

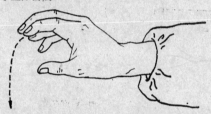

(4) Tapping Manipulation with the Finger Tips
指尖击法

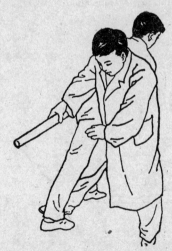

(5) Striking Manipulation with a Stick
棒击法

　　Fig. 2—22 Tapping Manipulations
　　图2-22　　叩击法

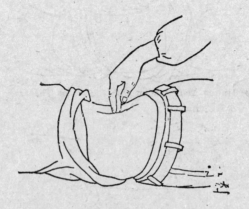

⁽¹⁾ Finger-vibrating Manipulation
指振法

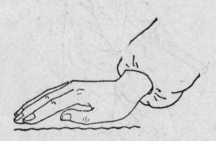

(2) Palm-vibrating Manipulation
掌振法

Fig. 2—23 Vibrating Manipulations
图2-23   振法

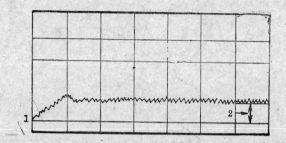

Fig. 2—24 Dynamic Curve Diagram of Calming Vibrating

图2-24　　　平直型振法动态曲线图

　　　　1. vertical curve　　　垂向曲线
　　　　2. base intensity　　　基强度

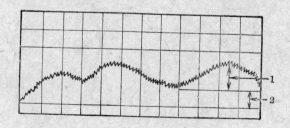

Fig. 2—25 Dynamic Curve Diagram of Undulating Vibrating

图2-25　　　起伏型振法动态曲线图

　　　　1. undulating wave-force value　　起伏波力值
　　　　2. base intensity　　　　　　　　基强度

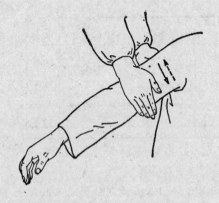

(1) Foulage at the Upper Limb with both Hands
上肢之双手搓法

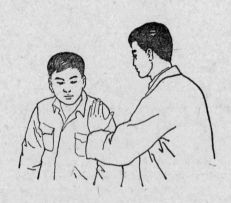

(2) Foulage at the Shoulder with both Hands
肩部之双手搓法

Fig. 2—26 Foulage Manipulations
图2-26　　搓法

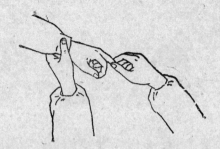

Fig. 2—27 Holding-twisting Manipulation

图2-27　捻法

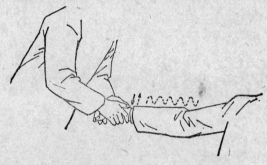

Fig. 2—28 Shaking Manipulation

图2-28　抖法

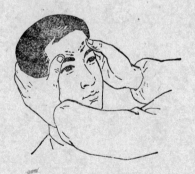

Fig. 2—29 Wiping Manipulation

图2-29　抹法

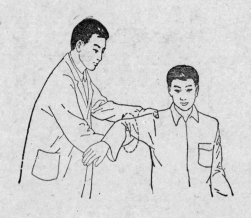

(1) Shoulder Rotating by Holding Elbow
托肘摇肩法

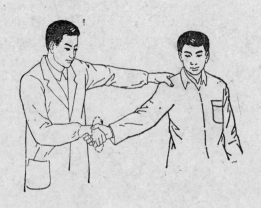

(2) Shoulder Rotating by Holding Hand
握手摇肩法

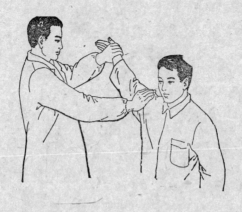

(3) Shoulder Rotating in Big Range (I)
大幅度摇肩法（Ⅰ）

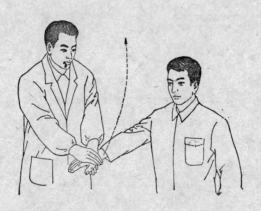

(4) Shoulder Rotating in Big Range (II)
大幅度摇肩法（Ⅱ）

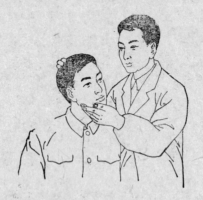

(5) Cervical Vertebrae Rotating Manipulation
颈椎摇法

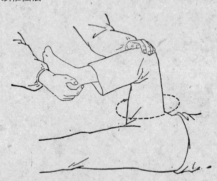

(6) Hip Joint Rotating Manipulation
髋关节摇法

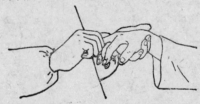

(7) Metacarpophalangeal Joints Rotating Manipulation
掌指关节摇法

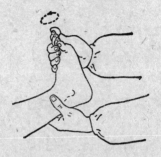

(8) The ankle Joint Rotating Manipulation
踝关节摇法
Fig. 2—30 Rotating Manipulations
图2-30 摇法

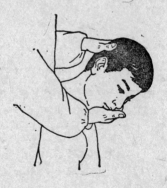

Fig. 2—31 Obliquely-pulling Manipulation of Cervical Vertebrae
图2-31 颈推斜扳法

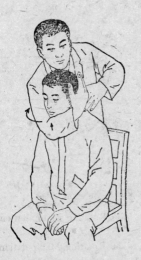

Fig. 2—32 Obliquely-pulling Manipulation after Localizing Cervical
        Vertebrae

图2-32　　颈椎定位斜扳法

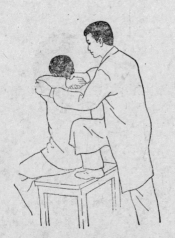

Fig. 2—33 Chest-expansion Pulling Manipulation

图2-33　　扩胸牵伸法

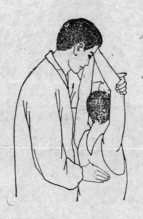

Fig. 2—34 Counter-reduction of Thoracic Vertebrae

图2-34　　　胸椎对抗复位法

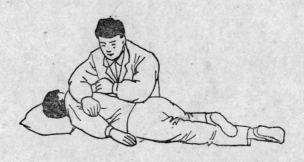

Fig. 2—35 Obliquely-pulling Manipulation of Lumbar Vertebrae with
the Patient in a Lateral Position

图2-35　　　侧卧位腰椎斜扳法

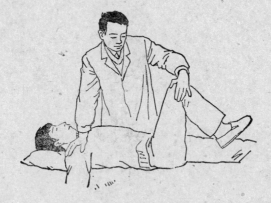

(1)

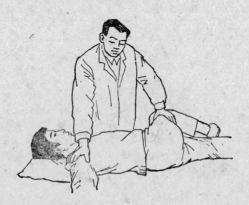

(2)

Fig. 2—36 Long-handle Obliquely-pulling Manipulation of Lumbar
Vertebrae with the Patient in a Supine Position

图2-36　　仰卧位长柄式腰椎斜扳法

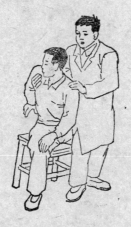

Fig. 2—37 Obliquely-pulling Manipulation of Lumbar Vertebrae with the Patient in a Sitting Position

图2-37　　坐位腰椎斜扳法

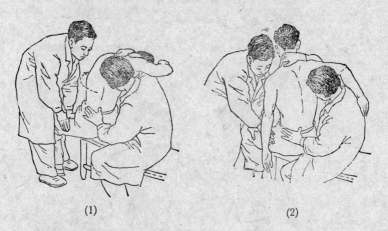

(1)　　　　　　　　　　　　　　(2)

Fig. 2—38 Rotating Reduction of Lumbar Vertebrae

图2-38　　腰椎旋转复位法

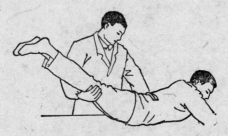

Fig. 2—39 Pulling Manipulation of Lumbar Vertebrae with Backward
Extension of Two Legs

图2-39　　双腿腰椎后伸扳法

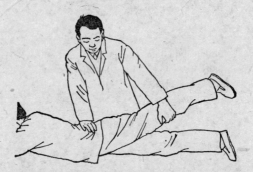

Fig. 2—40 Pulling Manipulation of Lumbar Vertebrae with Backward
Extension of One Leg

图2-40　　单腿腰椎后伸扳法

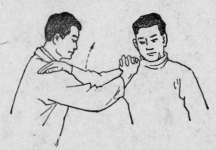

(1) Shoulder-pulling Manipulation in an Abducting Manner
外展扳肩法

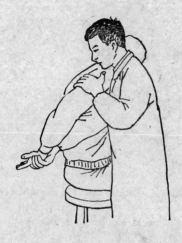

Shoulder-pulling Manipulation with Backward Extension
肩伸扳肩法

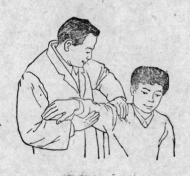

(2) Shoulder-pulling Manipulation with Forward Flexion and Lift
前屈上举扳法

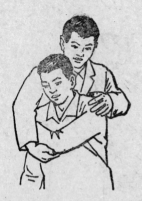

(3) Shouder-pulling Manipulation in an Adducting Manner
内收扳肩法

Fig. 2—41 Pulling Manipulations of Shoulder Joints

图2-41　　肩关节扳法

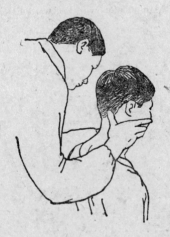

Fig. 2—42 Traction and Counter-traction of Cervical Vertebrae with
the Patient in a Sitting Position

图2-42　　坐位颈椎拔伸法

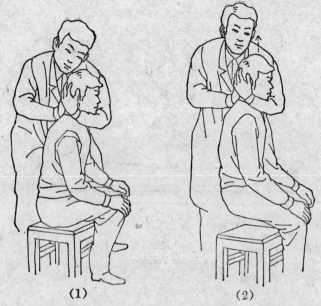

(1)   **(2)**

Fig. 2—43 Traction and Counter-traction of Cervical Vertebrae with
the Patient in a Lower Sitting Position

图2-43　　低坐位颈椎拔伸法

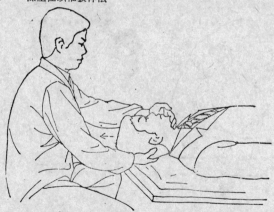

Fig. 2—44 Traction and Counter-traction of Cervical Vertebrae with
the Patient in a Supine Position

图2-44　　仰卧位颈椎拔伸法

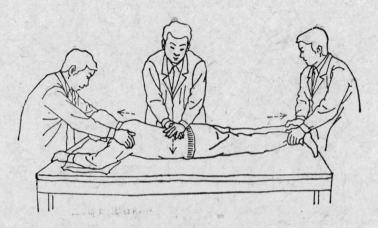

Fig. 2—45 Traction and Counter-traction of the Lumbar Vertebrae with
the Patient in a Prone Position

图2-45　　卧位腰椎拔伸法

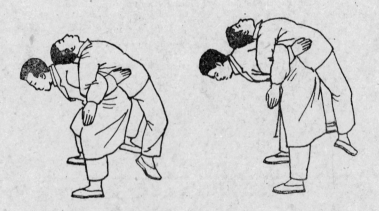

Fig. 2—46 Traction and Counter-traction of the Lumbar Vertebrae with
the Patient in a Back-ward-extension Position

图2-46　　背势腰椎牵引法

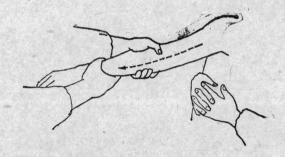

Fig. 2—47 Traction and Counter-traction of Shoulder Joints
图2-47   肩关节拔伸法

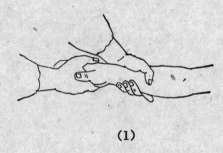

(1)

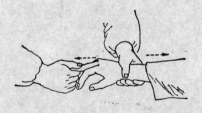

(2)

Fig. 2—48 Traction and Counter-traction of the Wrist and Phalangeal
          Joint of the Hand
图2-48   腕、指关节拔伸法

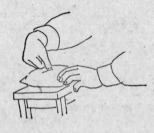

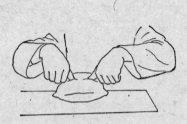

(1) One-hand Practice of the Pushing Manipulation with One-finger Meditation

一指禅推法单手练习

(2) Both-hand Practice of the Pushing Manipulation with One-finger Meditation

一指禅推法双手练习

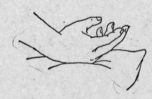

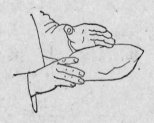

(3) Rolling Manipulation Practice

㨰法练习

(4) One-hand Practice of Rubbing Manipulation

擦法之单手练习

Fig. 2—49 Practice of Basic Skills on Rice Sack

图2-49   在米袋上进行手法基本动作训练

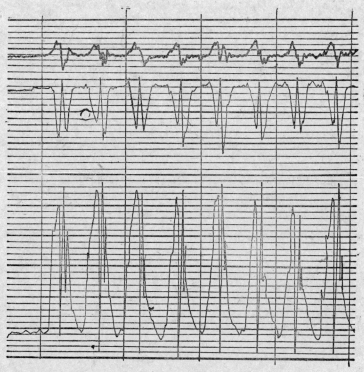

Fig. 2—50 Wave Curve Diagram of Improper Rolling Manipulation with Too Much Forward Force

图2-50　　　前顶力过强的错误𢱟法曲线

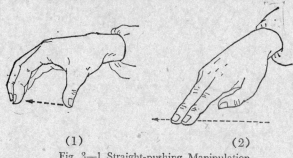

(1)　　　　　　　　　　　(2)

Fig. 3—1 Straight-pushing Manipulation

图3-1　　　直推法

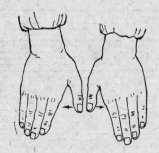
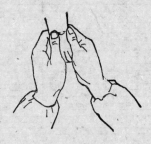

Fig. 3—2 Parting-pushing
      Manipulation

图3-2 　分推法

Fig. 3—3 Meeting-pushing
      Manipulation

图3-3 　合推法

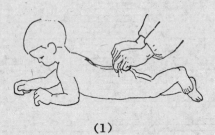

(1)

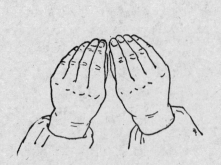
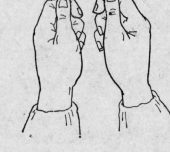

(2)   (3)

Fig. 3—4 Pinching Manipulation

图3-4 　捏法

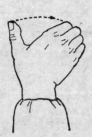
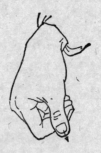

Fig. 3—5 Arc-pushing Manipulation　　Fig. 3—6 Nipping Manipulation
图3-5　运法　　　　　　　　　　　图3-6　掐法

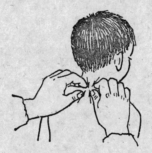

Fig. 3—7 Squeezing Manipulation
图3-7　挤法

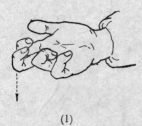
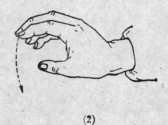

(1)　　　　　　　　　　　　　　(2)

Fig. 3—8 Pounding Manipulation
图3-8　捣法

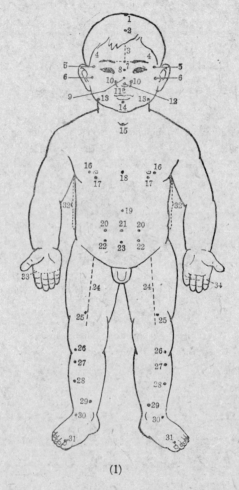

(1)

Fig. 3—9 (1) Points in the Front 正面穴位图

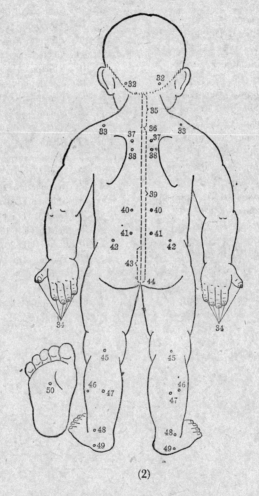

(2)

(2) Points on the Back 背面穴位图

1. Baihui (Du 20) 百会
2. Xinmen 囟门
3. Zanzhu (UB 2) 攒竹
4. Kangong 坎宫
5. Taiyang (Extra 2) 太阳
6. Ermen (SJ 21) 耳门
7. Meixin 眉心
8. Shangen 山根
9. Yannian 延年
10. Yingxiang (LI 20) 迎香
11. Renzhong (Du 26) 人中
12. Zhuntou 准头
13. Yaguan 牙关
14. Chengjiang (Ren 24) 承浆
15. Tiantu (Ren 22) 天突
16. Rupang 乳旁
17. Rugen (St 18) 乳根
18. Tanzhong (Ren 17) 膻中
19. Zhongwan (Ren 12) 中脘
20. Tianshu (St 25) 天枢
21. Qi (Shenque, Ren 8) 脐(神阙)
22. Dujiao 肚角
23. Dantian (Elixir Field) 丹田
24. Jimen 箕门
25. Baichong (Xuehai, Sp 10) 百虫(血海)
26. Xiyan 膝眼
27. Zusanli (St 36) 足三里
28. Qianchengshan 前承山
29. Sanyinjiao (Sp 6) 三阴交
30. Jiexi (St 41) 解溪
31. Dadun (Liv 1) 大敦
32. Erhougaogu 耳后高骨
33. Jianjing (GB 21) 肩井
34. Shixuan (Extra 30) 十宣
35. Tianzhugu 天柱骨
36. Dazhui (Du 14) 大椎
37. Fengmen (UB 12) 风门
38. Feishu (UB 13) 肺俞
39. Ji (Spine) 脊
40. Pishu (UB 20) 脾俞
41. Shenshu (UB 23) 肾俞
42. Yaoshu (Du 2) 腰俞
43. Qijiegu 七节骨
44. Guiwei 龟尾
45. Weizhong (UB 40) 委中
46. Fenglong (St 40) 丰隆
47. Houchengshan 后承山
48. Kunlun (UB 60) 昆仑
49. Pushen (UB 61) 仆参
50. Yongquan (K 1) 涌泉

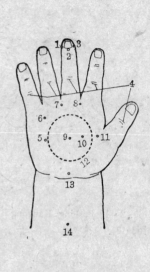
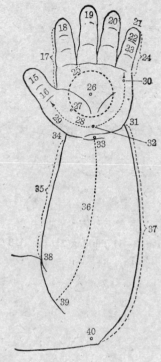

Fig. 3—10 Points on the Upper Limbs

图3-10　　　上肢穴位图

1. Youduanzheng 右端正　2. Laolong 老龙　　3. Zuoduanzheng 左端正
4. Wuzhijie 五指节　　5. Jingning 精宁　　6. Erma 二马
7,8. Ershanmen 二扇门　9. Wailaogong 外劳宫　10. Weiling 威灵
11. Hegu (LI 4) 合谷　12. Waibagua 外八卦　13. Yiwofeng 一窝风
14. Boyangchi 膊阳池　15. Pijing 脾经　　16. Weijing 胃经
17. Dachang 大肠　　18. Ganjing 肝经　　19. Xinjing 心经
20. Feijing 肺经　　21. Shending 肾顶　　22. Shenjing 肾经
23. Shenwen 肾纹　　24. Xiaochang 小肠　25. Neibagua 内八卦
26. Neilaogong (P 8) 内劳宫 27. Banmen 板门　28. Yunshuirutu 运水入土
29. Yunturushui 运土入水 30. Zhangxiaohengwen 掌小横纹
31. Yinchi 阴池　　32. Xiaotianxin 小天心　33. Zongjin 总筋
34. Yangchi 阳池　　35. Sanguan 三关　　36. Tianheshui 天河水
37. Liufu (the Six *Fu*-Organs) 六腑　38. Quchi (LI 11) 曲池
39. Hongchi 洪池　　40. Douzhou 肘肘

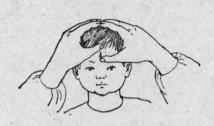

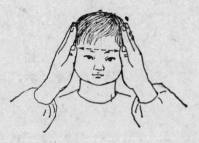

Fig. 3—11 Pushing Zanzhu (UB 2)
图3-11　　推攒竹

Fig. 3—12 Pushing Kangong
图3-12　　推坎宫

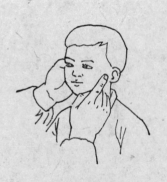

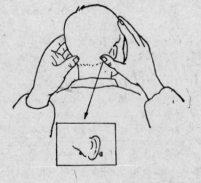

Fig. 3—13 Kneading Taiyang (Extra 2)
图3-13　　揉太阳

Fi7. 3—14 Kneading Erhougaogu
图3-14　　揉耳后高骨

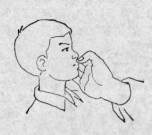
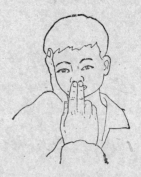

Fig. 3—15 Nipping Renzhong (Du 26)
图3-15　捏人中

Fig. 3—16 Huangfeng Rudong
图3-16　黄蜂入洞

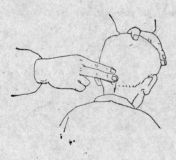
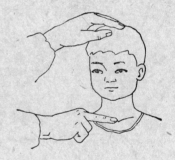

Fig. 3—17 Pushing Tianzhugu
图3-17　推天柱骨

Fig. 3—18 Kneading Tiantu
图3-18　揉天突

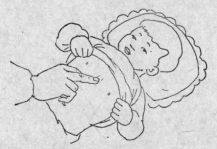

Fig. 3—19 Kneading Tanzhong (Ren 17)
图3-19　揉膻中

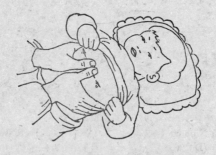

Fig. 3—20 Parting-pushing Tanzhong (Ren 17)

图3-20　　分推膻中

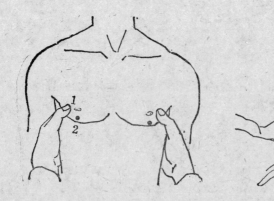

Fig. 3—21 Kneading Rupang and
　　　　Rugen (St 18)

图3-21　　揉乳旁、乳旁

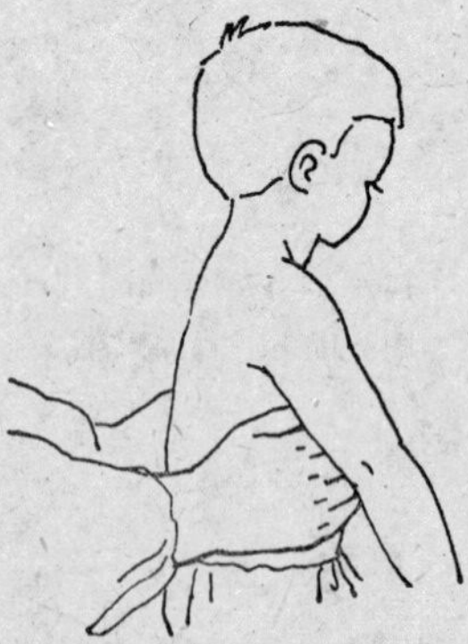

Fig. 3—22 Foulaging-rubbing
　　　　Xielei

图3-22　　搓摩胁肋

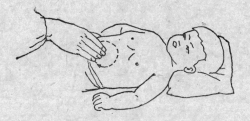

Fig. 3—23 Rubbing Fu (Abdomen)
图3-23　摩腹

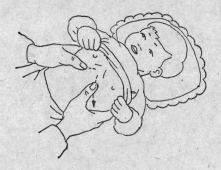

Fig. 3—24 Parting-pushing Fu Yin-Yang
图3-24　分推腹阴阳

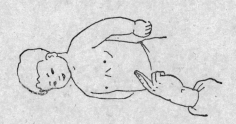

Fig. 3—25 Kneading Qi (Umbilicus)
图3-25　揉脐

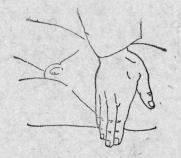

Fig. 3—26 Rubbing Qi (Umbilicus)

图3-26 摩脐

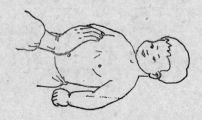

Fig. 3—27 Kneading Dantian (Elixir Field)

图3-27 揉丹田

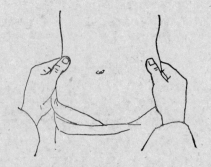

Fig. 3—28 Grasping Dujiao

图3-28 拿肚角.

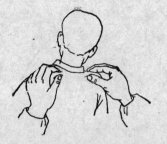 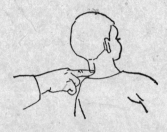

Fig. 3—29 Grasping Jianjing (GB 21) Fig. 3—30 Kneading Dazhui (Du 14)

图3-29　拿肩井　　　　　　　　图3-30　推大椎

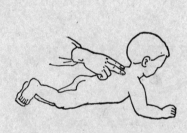 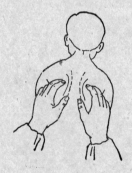

Fig. 3—31 Kneading Feishu (UB 13)　　Fig. 3—32 Parting-pushing Jianjiagu

图3-31　揉肺俞　　　　　　　　图3-32　分推肩胛骨

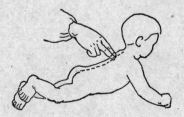

Fig. 3—33 Pushing Ji (Spine)

图3-33　推脊

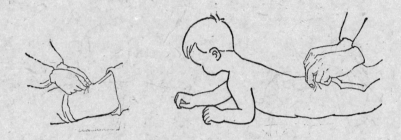

(1)   (2)

Fig. 3—34 Pinching the Spine

图3-34   捏脊

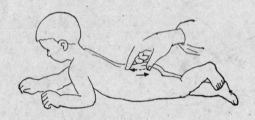

Fig. 3—35 Pushing Qijiegu

图3-35   推七节骨

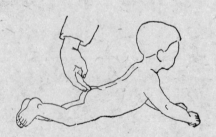

Fig. 3—36 Kneading Guiwei

图3-36   揉龟尾

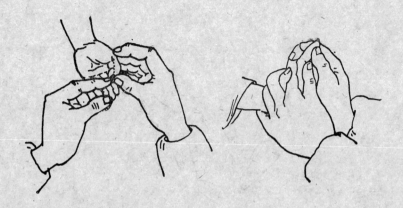

Fig. 3—37 Reinforcing Pijing
图3-37　补脾经

Fig. 3—38 Clearing Ganjing
图3-38　清肝经

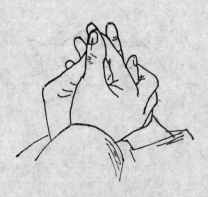

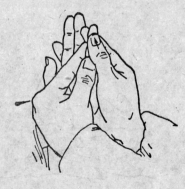

Fig. 3—39 Clearing Xinjing
图3-39　清心经

Fig. 3—40 Clearing Feijing
图3-40　清肺经

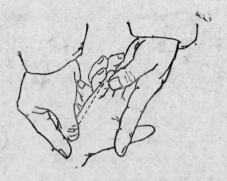

Fig. 3—41 Reinforcing Shenjing

图3-41　补肾经

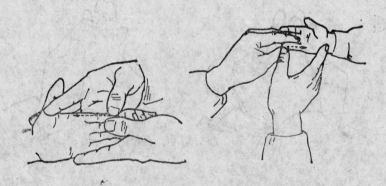

Fig. 3—42 Reinforcing Dachang

图3-42　补大肠

Fig. 3—43 Reinforcing Xiaochang

图3-43　补小肠

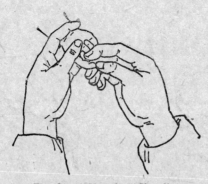

Fig. 3—44 Kneading Shending

图3-44　　揉肾顶

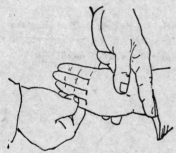

Fig. 3—45 Nipping-kneading
Sihengwen and Xiaohengwen

图3-45　　掐揉四横纹、小横纹

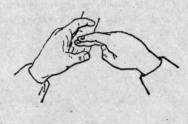

Fig. 3—46 Kneading
Zhangxiaohengwen

图3-46　　揉掌小横纹

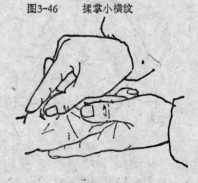

Fig. 3—47 Clearing Weijing

图3-47　　清胃经

Fig. 3—48 Arc-pushing Banmen

图3-48　　运板门

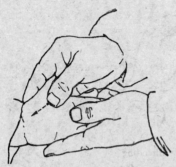 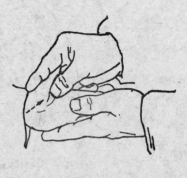

Fig. 3—49 Pushing from Banmen Fig. 3—50 Pushing from Hengwen
to Hengwen   to Banmen

图3-49   板门推向横纹   图3-50   横纹推向板门

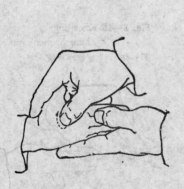 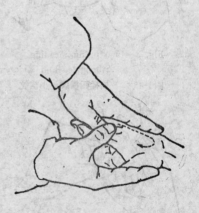

Fig. 3—51 Kneading Neilaogong Fig. 3—52 Shuidilaomingyue (Fishing
(P 8)   for the Moon in the Water)

图3-51   揉内劳官   图3-52   水底捞明月

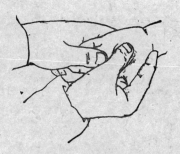

Fig. 3—53 Arc-pushing Neibagua
图3-53　运内八卦

Fig. 3—54 Nipping-kneading Xiaotianxin
图3-54　掐揉小天心

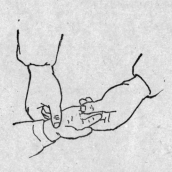

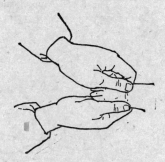

Fig. 3—55 Kneading Zongjin
图3-55　揉总筋

Fig. 3—56 Parting-pushing Dahengwen
图3-56　分推大横纹

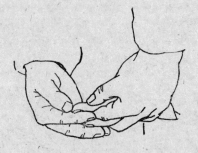

Fig. 3—57 Nipping Shixuan

图3-57　　掐十宣

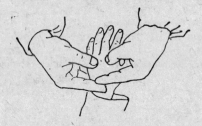

Fig. 3—58 Nipping-kneading Ershanmen

图3-58　　掐揉二扇门

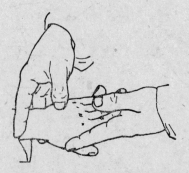

Fig. 3—59 Nipping-kneading Erma

图3-59　　掐揉二马

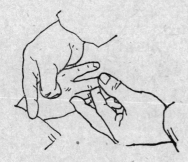 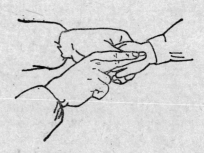

Fig. 3—60 Kneading Wailaogong　　Fig. 3—61 Kneading Yiwofeng
图3-60　　揉外劳官　　　　　　图3-61　　揉一窝风

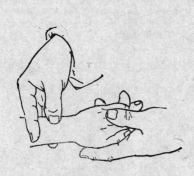 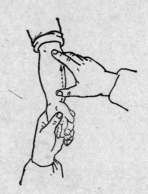

Fig. 3—62 Nipping-kneading Boyangchi　Fig. 3—63 Pushing Sanguan
图3-62　　掐揉膊阳池　　　　　图3-63　　推三关

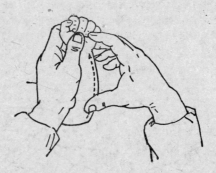

Fig. 3—64 Pushing Liufu
图3-64　　退六腑

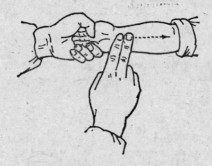

Fig. 3—65 Clearing Tianheshui
图3-65　　清天河水

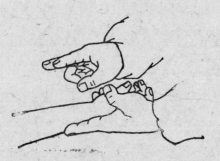

Fig. 3—66 Damaguotianhe (Crossing Tianhe While Beating the Horse)
图3-66　　打马过天河

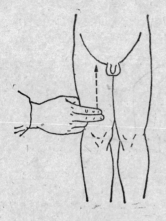

Fig. 3—67 Pushing Jimen
图3-67　推箕门

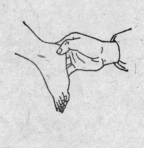

Fig. 3—68 Grasping Baichong
图3-68　拿百虫

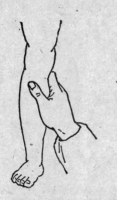

Fig. 3—69 Pressing-kneading
　　　　　Zusanli (St 36)
图3-69　按揉足三里

Fig. 3—70 Grasping Pushen
　　　　　(UB 61)
图3-70　拿仆参

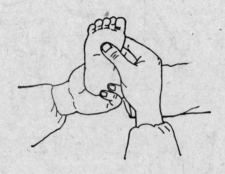

Fig. 3—71 Kneading Yongquan (K 1)
图3-71　　揉涌泉

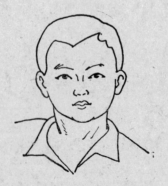

Fig. 3—72 Myogenic Torticollis of Children
图3-72　　小儿肌性斜颈

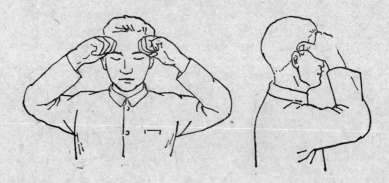

Fig. 4—1 Pushing the Forehead on Either Side

图4-1　分推前额

Fig. 4—2 Wiping the Temples

图4-2　双抹两颞

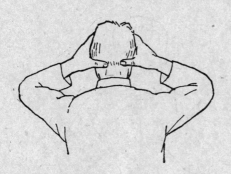
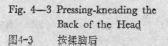
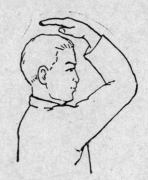

Fig. 4—3 Pressing-kneading the Back of the Head

图4-3　按揉脑后

Fig. 4—4 Patting the Vertex

图4-4　拍击头顶

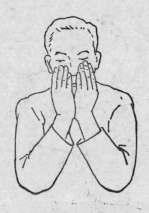

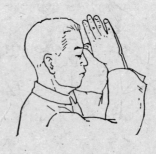

Fig. 4—5 "Bathing the Face" with Hands

图4-5　　搓手浴面

Fig. 4—6 Kneading Zanzhu (UB 2)

图4-6　　揉攒竹

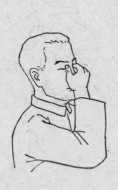

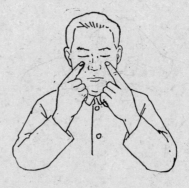

Fig. 4—7 Kneading Jingming (UB 1)

图4-7　　揉睛明

Fig. 4—8 Pressing-kneading Sibai (St 2)

图4-8　　按揉四白

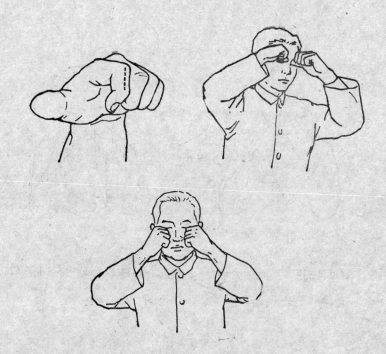

Fig. 4—9 Scraping the Orbits
图4-9   刮眼轮

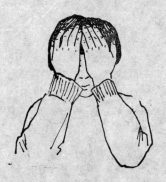

Fig. 4—10 "Ironing" the Eyes
图4-10   熨眼

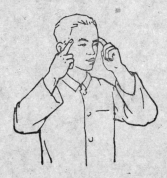

Fig. 4—11 Kneading Taiyang (Extra 2)
图4-11   揉太阳

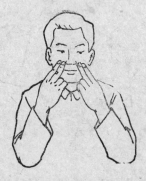

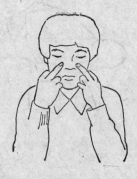

Fig. 4—12 Pressing-kneading
                  Yingxiang (LI 20)

图4-12　按揉迎香

Fig. 4—13 Rubbing the Sides of the
                  Nose

图4-13　　擦鼻旁

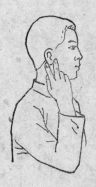

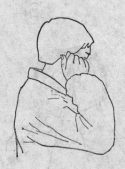

Fig. 4—14 Pressing-kneading the
                  Points around the Ear

图4-14　　按揉耳周诸穴

Fig. 4—15 Rubbing the Helix

图4-15　　摩擦耳轮

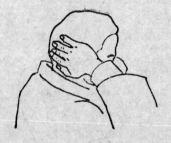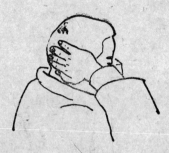

Fig. 4—16 Ming Tiangu
图4-16 鸣天鼓

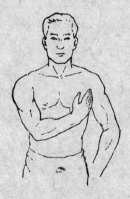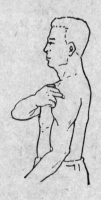

!) Pressing-kneading Jianneishu
按揉肩内俞

(2) Pressing-kneading Jianyu (LI 15)
按揉肩髃

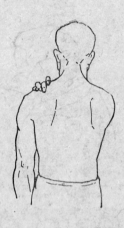

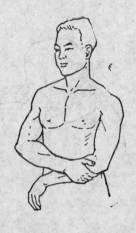

(3) Pressing-kneading Jianjing (GB 21)
按揉肩井

(4) Pressing-kneading Quchi (LI 11)
按揉曲池

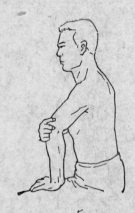

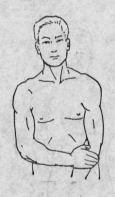

(5) Pressing-kneading Shaohai (H 3) and
Xiaohai (SI 8)
按揉少海、小海

(6) Pressing-kneading Chize (Lu 5)

按揉尺泽

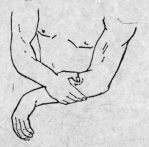

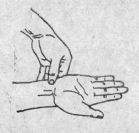

(7) Pressing-kneading Shousanli (LI 10)
　按揉手三里

(8) Pressing-kneading Neiguan (P 6)
　按揉内关

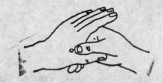

(9) Pressing-kneading Hegu (LI 4)
　按揉合谷

Fig. 4—17 Pressing-kneading the Points of the Upper Limbs
图4-17　　按揉上肢诸穴

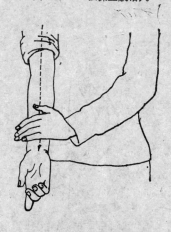

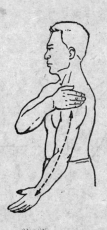

(1)　　　　　　　　　　(2)

Fig. 4—18 Pushing-rubbing the Upper Limbs
图4-18　　推擦上肢

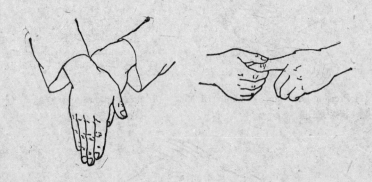

(1) Rubbing the Palms   (2) Twirling the Knuckles

擦掌   捻指

Fig. 4—19 Rubbing the Palms and Twirling the Knuckles

图4-19   擦捻掌指

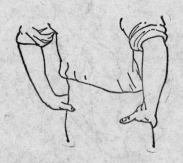

(1) Pressing-kneading Juliao (GB 29)   (2) Pressing-kneading Huantiao (GB 30)

按揉居髎   按揉环跳

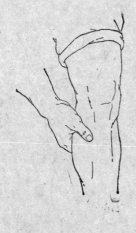

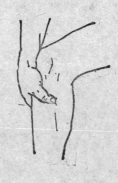

(3) Pressing-kneading Zusanli (St 36)

按揉足三里

(4) Pressing-kneading Yanglingquan (GB 34)

按揉阳陵泉

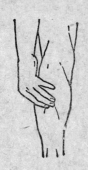

(5) Pressing-kneading Chengshan (UB 57)

按揉承山

(6) Pressing-kneading Sanyinjiao (Sp 6)

按揉三阴交

Fig. 4—20 Pressing-kneading the Points on the Legs

图4-20 按揉下肢请穴

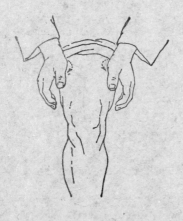

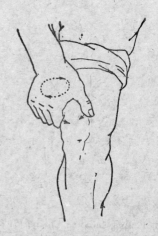

Fig. 4—21 Pressing-kneading the Thigh

图4-21　按揉大腿

Fig. 4—22 Pressing-kneading the Knee-cap

图4-22　按揉髌骨

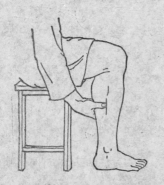

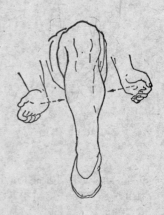

Fig. 4—23 Grasping the Shank

图4-23　拿小腿

Fig. 4—24 Patting the Lower Limb

图4-24　拍击下肢

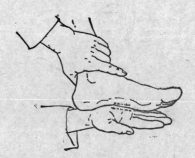

Fig. 4—25 Scrubbing Yongquan (K 1)
图4-25 擦涌泉

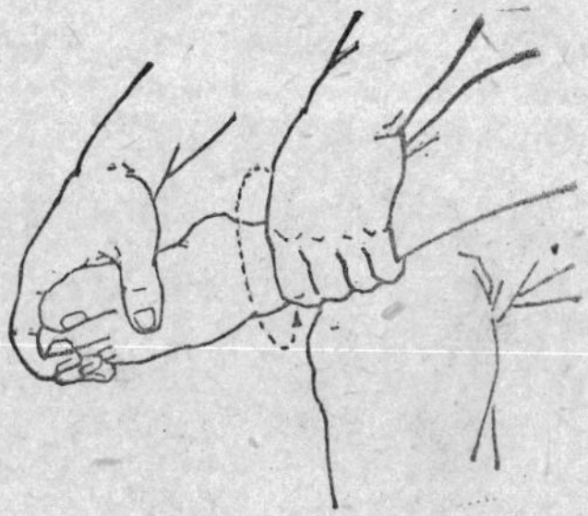

Fig. 4—26 Rocking the Ankle Joint
图4-26 摇踝关节

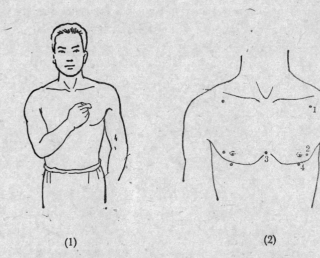

(1)

(2)

1. Zhongfu (Lu 1) 中府   2. Rupang 乳旁
3. Tanzhong (Ren 17) 膻中   4. Rugen (St 18) 乳根

Fig. 4—27 Pressing-kneading the Points at the Chest and Intercostal Spaces
图4-27 按揉胸部诸穴

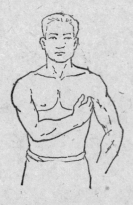
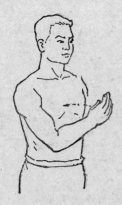

Fig. 4—28 Grasping the Muscles of Thorax
图4-28　拿胸肌

Fig. 4—29 Patting the Chest
图4-29　拍胸

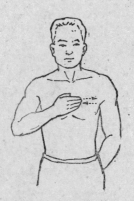

Fig. 4—30 Scrubbing the Chest
图4-30　擦胸

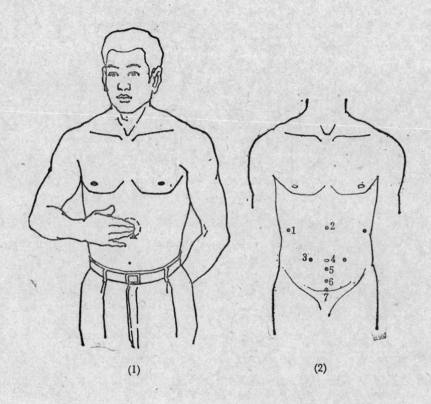

(1)   (2)

1. Zhangmen (Liv 13) 章门
2. Zhongwan (Ren 12) 中脘
3. Tianshu (St 54) 天枢
4. Shenque (Ren 8) 神阙
5. Qihai (Ren 6) 气海
6. Guanyuan (Ren 4) 关元
7. Zhongji (Ren 3) 中极

Fig. 4—31 Pressing-kneading the Points on the Abdomen
图4-31   按揉腹部诸穴

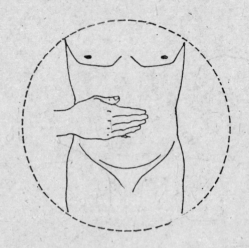

Fig. 4—32 Rubbing the Abdomen
图4-32　　摩腹

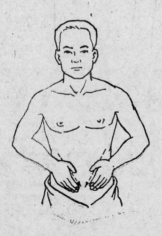

Fig. 4—33 Scrubbing the Lower Abdomen
图4-33　　擦小腹

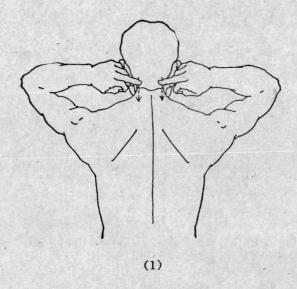

(1)

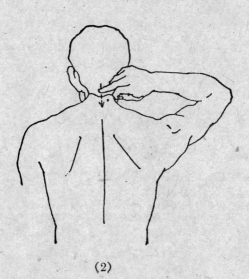

(2)

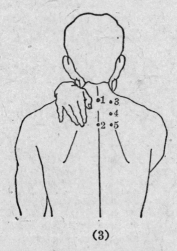

(3)

1. Dazhui (Du 14) 大椎   2. Shenzhu (Du 12) 身柱
3. Dazhu (UB 11) 大杼   4. Fengmen (UB 12) 风门
5. Feishu (UB 13) 肺俞

Fig. 4—34 Pressing-kneading the Neck and Back

图4-34   按揉项背

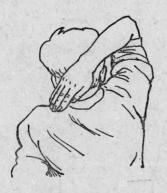

Fig. 4—35 Patting the Back

图4-35   拍背

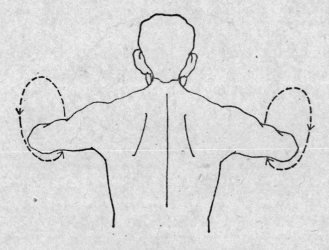

Fig. 4—36 Rubbing Gaohuang (UB 43)
图4-36   摩膏肓

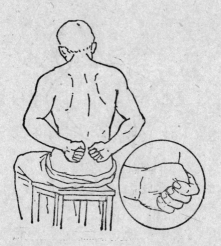

Fig. 4—37 Kneading Shenshu (UB 43), Yaoyan (Extra) and Zhishi (UB 42)
图4-37   揉肾俞、腰眼、志室

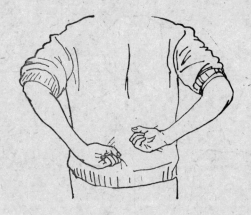

Fig. 4—38 Thumping and Vibrating the Lumbar Region
图4-38　捶振腰区

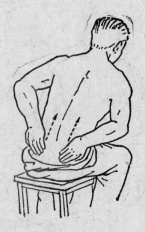

Fig. 4—39 Scrubbing the Waist
图4-39　搽腰